SYSTEM OF OPHTHALMOLOGY

THE proposed scheme for the " System of Ophthalmology " is as follows, but its division into different volumes is liable to alteration.

SYSTEM OF OPHTHALMOLOGY

SIR STEWART DUKE-ELDER

VOL. III

NORMAL AND ABNORMAL DEVELOPMENT

PART 1
EMBRYOLOGY

BY

SIR STEWART DUKE-ELDER
G.C.V.O., F.R.S.

AND

CHARLES COOK
F.R.C.S.

Surgeon, Moorfields Eye Hospital.
Ophthalmic Surgeon, Guy's Hospital, London.

WITH 372 ILLUSTRATIONS AND 4 COLOURED PLATES

THE C. V. MOSBY COMPANY

1963

Reprinted 1970

MADE AND PRINTED IN GREAT BRITAIN

PREFACE

THE combination of normal and abnormal development in one composite volume would seem to be logical since the significance of aberrations cannot be understood without a knowledge of the normal sequence of events, while, on the other hand, the complex story of embryology becomes intensely practical and full of human interest when correlated with the multitude of abnormalities which are so frequently seen in the clinic. So great is the number of these, however, that if they are to be adequately discussed, a single volume would become unmanageable by reason of its bulk; for ease of manipulation and also for ready reference, therefore, I have found it convenient to divide it into two parts. In some ways this is unfortunate, and for a complete understanding both should be read as one.

STEWART DUKE-ELDER.

INSTITUTE OF OPHTHALMOLOGY,
UNIVERSITY OF LONDON,
1963.

ACKNOWLEDGEMENTS

In the provision of illustrations for this book I have incurred a very large debt to many friendly people. The source of each illustration is acknowledged where it appears, but I feel that I must extend my special thanks to those from whom I have borrowed on a large scale:

Dr. Frantisek Vrabec of Prague, who has put at my disposal his quite unusually excellent selection of embryological slides.

The late Dr. Henry Haden, who left his collection of embryological slides to the Department of Pathology at Baylor University, Texas, from which several illustrations were given to me by Dr. Milton Boniuk of that University.

Dr. Aeleta Barber of Louisiana State University, who has provided me with many illustrations most of which have appeared in her *Embryology of the Human Eye*, published by Mosby of St. Louis.

Dr. Dorcas Padget, Dr. Perry Gilbert and Dr. Ronan O'Rahilly, who have allowed me to avail myself on a considerable scale of the unique collection in the Department of Embryology, The Carnegie Institution of Washington, Baltimore.

Dr. Charles Dejean, Dr. François Hervouët and Dr. Georges Leplat, who have given me permission to use many of the illustrations from their *L'Embryologie de l'Œil et sa Tératologie*, published by Masson et Cie, Paris.

Professor W. J. Hamilton of the Charing Cross Hospital Medical School, London, for the use of a number of illustrations from the 2nd Edition of *Human Embryology*, by Hamilton, Boyd and Mossman, published by W. Heffer and Sons of Cambridge.

Dr. Peter Hansell and his staff of the Department of Medical Illustration of the Institute of Ophthalmology, London, who have prepared many of the figures.

I am also greatly indebted to Miss Mina H. T. Yuille and Mr. A. J. B. Goldsmith who have, once again, been kind enough to read the proofs with a due mixture of criticism and care; to Miss Rosamund E. Soley for compiling the index and seeing the book through the press as usual; and finally, to Mr. G. E. Deed of Henry Kimpton for many kindnesses as an unusually forbearant publisher.

STEWART DUKE-ELDER.

CONTENTS OF PART 1
EMBRYOLOGY

SECTION I
INTRODUCTORY

CHAPTER I

HISTORICAL INTRODUCTION

CHAPTER II

THE GENERAL SCHEME OF DEVELOPMENT

CHAPTER III

THE DETERMINATION OF THE EYE

vii

.

SECTION II

EMBRYOLOGY OF THE EYE

Chapter IV

The Differentiation of the Neural Ectoderm

Chapter V

The Development of the Surface Ectoderm

Chapter VI

The Secondary Ectodermal Structures

Chapter VII

The Bulbar Mesoderm

SECTION III

THE DEVELOPMENT OF THE OCULAR ADNEXA AND PIGMENT

CHAPTER VIII

THE OCULAR ADNEXA

CONTENTS

CHAPTER IX

THE OCULAR PIGMENT

SECTION IV

CHRONOLOGY AND POST-NATAL DEVELOPMENT

CHAPTER X

THE CHRONOLOGY OF DEVELOPMENT

CONTENTS OF PART 2
CONGENITAL DEFORMITIES

SECTION V

TERATOGENESIS

CHAPTER XI

HISTORICAL INTRODUCTION

CHAPTER XII

TERATOLOGY

SECTION VI

CONGENITAL DEFORMITIES

CHAPTER XIII

CONGENITAL DEFORMITIES OF THE EYE : I. ANOMALIES IN ORGANOGENESIS

CHAPTER XIV

CONGENITAL DEFORMITIES OF THE EYE : II. ANOMALIES OF DIFFERENTIATION

CHAPTER XV

CONGENITAL ANOMALIES OF THE OCULAR ADNEXA

CHAPTER XVI

ANOMALIES OF OCULAR MOTILITY

CONTENTS xxi

Chapter XVII

Deformities of the Head and Neck

Chapter XVIII

Anomalies of the Central Nervous System

CHAPTER XIX

MULTIPLE SYNDROMES

SECTION I

INTRODUCTORY

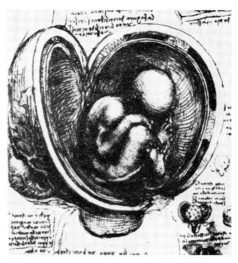

LEONARDO'S DELIGHTFUL DRAWING OF A *FŒTUS IN UTERO*

The fœtus is human, but the uterus is that of a calf—a mixture not unique at the time owing to the difficulty experienced in obtaining human anatomical material.

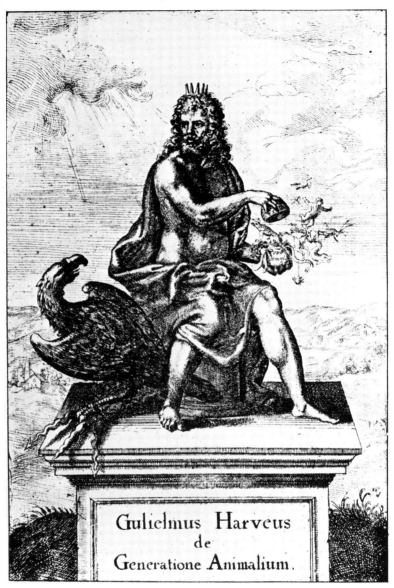

Fig. 1.—Ex Ovo Omnia.

The frontispiece of William Harvey's *De generatione animalium* (1651). The illustration shows Zeus liberating all living creatures from an egg marked with Harvey's dictum (from the copy in the Wellcome Historical Medical Library).

CHAPTER I

HISTORICAL INTRODUCTION

THE development of the embryo and eventually of the adult from the fertilized ovum is an extremely complicated process. Its orderly design in a set pattern so that a new individual is reproduced with the general characteristics of the species and particularly resembling its parents, is essentially genetically determined, although regulated locally by chemical organizers and influenced by environmental factors. It is a process wherein much is still unknown and more is conjectural, but sufficient evidence is available to allow us to outline the main events with considerable certainty and some degree of precision. It is a subject of more than usual importance so far as ophthalmology is concerned, not only on account of its own essential academic interest, but because a clear understanding of the normal ontogeny is necessary for an adequate interpretation of anatomy, much of pathology, and, most particularly, of aberrations in development. These aberrations are more apparent in the eye than in any other organ of the body, and the diagnosis between developmental and diseased conditions is frequently a matter of some difficulty upon which may rest clinical decisions of considerable importance.

It is to be remembered, however, that although ontogeny is usually restricted to the development of the individual between the period of fertilization of the ovum and birth, the latter event is merely an incident in the development of a human being, a process which continues uninterruptedly in the post-natal period. Some organs are not fully developed at birth ; of these, typical examples are the macular area of the retina which is not fully differentiated until 4 months later, the reproductive organs, particularly the prostate and the mammary glands, which are very immature at birth and do not reach full differentiation until puberty, while the lens continues to grow until advanced old age.

THE HISTORY OF EMBRYOLOGY is interesting and can be divided into three distinct epochs : the first, of speculative mysticism or philosophy ; the second, of descriptive morphology ; and the third, of experimental investigation. It is an interesting story, full of nebulous ideas, often tinctured with religious beliefs ; nor is this to be wondered at, for the coming into the world of a new human being is heavily charged with emotional and theological implications. Moreover, the sequence of the events of embryogenesis must be looked at in the perspective that it was not until the year 1677 that van Leeuwenhoek discovered spermatozoa, not until 1827 than von Baer described the mammalian ovum, and not until 1843 that Martin Barry observed the penetration of the former into the latter. Embryology as a science dates back little more than one hundred years.[1]

Although they appear to have learned the art of incubating eggs before 3000 B.C., the ancient Egyptians, to judge from the silence of their early writings, seem to have shown little inquisitiveness about the facts of embryology ; they believed, however, that the child was the product of the two parents, the germ existing in woman and the seed in man, to which the Sun God, Aton, gave life and provided a soul (breath) at birth. Of the two, the father was genetically the important partner and the author of generation, while the mother only provided the nidus and nourishment for the fœtus (see Needham, 1959). This doctrine descended to the pre-classical Greeks ; thus Apollo defended Orestes from the charge of matricide in the *Eumenides* of Æschylus :—

> " She who is called the mother of the child
> Is not its parent, but nurse of seed
> Implanted in begetting. He that sows
> Is author of the shoot, which she, if Heaven
> Prevent not, keeps as in a garden-ground.
> In proof whereof, to show that fatherhood
> May be without the mother, I appeal
> To Pallas, daughter of Olympian Zeus,
> In present witness here. Behold a plant
> Not moulded in the darkness of the womb,
> Yet nobler than all the scions of Heaven's stock."

In early Greece, however, an attempt was made to account for the processes of development. The embryo, according to the Pythagorean philosopher, Empedocles of Agrigentum [*c.* 500–*c.* 430 B.C.] was compounded of earth, air and water animated by the innate heat of the blood, while the Ionian teacher, Anaxagoras of Clazomenæ [500–428 B.C.], held that it was moulded by fire, a view also advanced by HIPPOCRATES of Cos [*c.* 460–375 B.C.],[2] who taught that the embryonic parts were differentiated as they met with water or fire, some parts becoming condensed as the humidity disappeared to become bones and nerves. The embryo was nourished by maternal blood which coagulated to form flesh, the menstrual flow ceasing as it is used up on its way out ; while air was supplied through the umbilical cord. And finally, when the demand for food exceeded the supply, the fœtus was expelled from the womb or the chick from the egg.

It is not to be thought, however, that belief in a dual parenthood was universal ; indeed, the European stork finds its analogy in the folk-lore of many primitive peoples.[3] Certain Australian aborigines, for example, conceive of minute spirit-babies, coming from afar in the East, so small as to be invisible to all but magicians and old women,

---

[1] The word *embryologie* (ἐν, in ; βρύειν, to be full of) was admitted into the French language by the *Académie* in 1762 ; the word did not appear in English until the 19th century.
[2] Vol. II, p. 9.
[3] For a treasury of such folk-lore, see Frazer's *The Golden Bough*, 3rd ed., London, **4** (1), 1927.

which look for kindly females, particularly those with large breasts ; when they find one they enter her body under the fingernail or through the loin or the mouth to find a nidus for development and nourishment in the womb ; the entry of an injured spirit-baby results in the birth of a deformed child, of an animal or a monstrosity.[1] In this scheme the mother has no genetic or biological responsibility for her child for she merely acts first as an incubator and then as a wet nurse ; while the share taken by the father is still less. To some Australian tribes his function is to open up the womb by the act of coitus so that the spirit can enter ; to some East Indian and Polynesian peoples the semen blocks the exit of the uterus so that the menstrual flow is checked and the embryo nourished, an end satisfactorily and happily achieved only after much sexual intercourse.

The science of embryology may be said to commence with ARISTOTLE [c. 384–322 B.C.][2] whose studies covered the whole area of knowledge, for the somewhat scanty writings which had appeared before, even those emanating from the Hippocratic School, were quite unrelated to facts. Dissecting the eggs and embryos of all kinds of animals, cold blooded, avian and mammalian, this great founder of many natural sciences gathered his observations in the five books of his Περὶ ζώων γενέσεως (*On the generation of animals*),[3] wherein he classified the animal kingdom according to embryological characteristics, giving the whole subject coherence. The embryo, he contended, was derived from menstrual blood to which the seminal fluid gave form, a concept which ascribed to the mother a more important role than hitherto. In the determination of form by the male, he considered that the semen played a role comparable to that of rennet in the coagulation of milk, separating the fœtus from the liquid in which it lies, the whole being surrounded by membranes since the surface, like the skin of milk, solidifies on heating and cooling (Fig. 2). In the process of development the tissues are formed by heat and cold to varying degrees as the moisture dries, the nutriment oozes through the blood vessels and the skin develops by the drying of the flesh like the scum upon boiled surfaces. From the morphological point of view, he described embryonic development in remarkable detail considering the technical means at his disposal, and he produced the first textbook of embryology on no other basis than his own tireless observations intermingled, it is true, with many incorrect deductions and much speculative philosophy. For 2,000 years thereafter little or nothing new was added to his clear but rigid teaching, and throughout the Dark and Middle Ages he remained the sole authority ; even the times he postulated at which the various souls entered the embryo were made the basis of legal rulings in Europe concerning abortion.

The Aristotelian view that the menstrual blood constituted the substance of the fœtus has been widespread (see Montague, 1949). In ancient Hindu medicine it was

[1] See Montague. *Coming into Being among the Australian Aborigines*, N.Y. (1938) ; *Ciba Symposia*, **10**, 994, 1009 (1949).
[2] Vol. II, p. 10 ; Fig. 7.
[3] *De generatione animalium*, translated into English by Smith and Ross (1908–31).

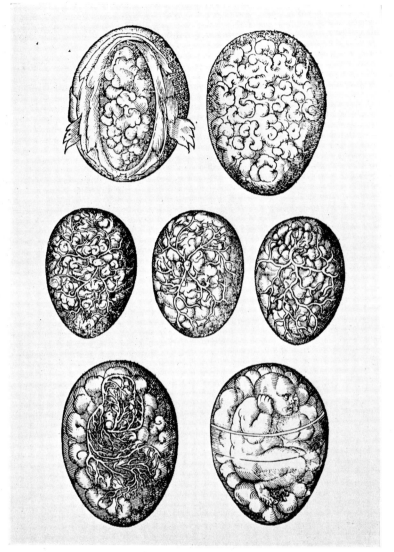

FIG. 2.—DE CONCEPTU ET GENERATIONE HOMINIS.

An illustration from the classical book of Jacob Rueff (1554) showing the Aristotelian conception of the coagulation of blood by seed in the uterus and its development into a fœtus (from the copy in the Wellcome Historical Medical Library).

taught by Charaka and Suśruta,[1] and is said to account for the belief still held in certain parts of India today that a girl should go from her father's house to her husband's before she starts to menstruate. Those early Indian writers also compared the formation of the embryo with the clotting of milk, an analogy which crept into Biblical

[1] For the epoch and the writings of those early Hindu scholars, see Vol. II, p. 17. Possibly they existed about the 5th century B.C.

writings. Thus Job : " Hast thou not poured me out as milk and curdled me like cheese?"[1] ; and again, in the Apocrypha : " And in the womb of a mother was I moulded into flesh, being compacted in blood of the seed of man and pleasure that came with sleep."[2] The Jewish Talmudic commentators believed that the generative process was shared. From the white semen the Talmudists believed that the bones, the brain and the white of the eyes were derived, from the red menstrual flow the flesh, the blood, the hair and the iris. In relatively recent times the learned men who upheld at all costs Aristotle's classical dogma that the fœtus was derived from menstrual blood violently attacked William Harvey when in 1651 he brought forward the theory that all living things were derived from the egg ; and even today the belief survives among the natives of Bechuanaland that in embryogenesis the father's semen clots the menstrual blood from which the child is formed.

The Alexandrian School which carried on the Greek tradition from 330 to 30 B.C. added little to embryological knowledge, accepting without protest the classical teaching embodied in Aristotelian doctrine. The possibility of dissection of the body which the faculty of medicine enjoyed, however, allowed its scholars to contribute some morphological facts ; thus HEROPHILOS of Chalcedon [c. 344–280 B.C.], the greatest of its teachers, described the ovaries and fallopian tubes, while, although his writings are lost, it would seem that ERASISTRATOS of Chios [c. 300–260] studied the growth of the embryo. When with the fall of Alexandria, learning was transferred to Rome, the same authority was ascribed to the teaching of Classical Greece. The most brilliant and authoritative of the Roman writers— CLAUDIUS GALENUS (Galen) of Pergamos [c. A.D. 130–200], however, with his usual acute observation, recorded many new anatomical facts, and in his scholastic way, integrated and systematized the scheme of Aristotle, making it conform with teleological ends. In his voluminous writings, he described the amnion, the allantois and the placenta, and gave an extraordinarily accurate description of the umbilical and fœtal circulations including the ductus arteriosus, the ductus venosus and the foramen ovale. The process of development whereby the embryo evolved from the status of a plant to that of an animal, he divided into four stages : a seminal stage when it remained unformed, a stage wherein the three main organs (*tria principa*— the heart, liver and brain) are generated, a stage wherein all the other organs are mapped out, and a final stage when all parts differentiate.

On the whole, however, from the Alexandrian School or the writings of Galen nothing new of note emerged and for some 14 centuries the teaching of Aristotle as interpreted by Galen was venerated as established doctrine to deny which was sacrilege. Even in the re-awakening of science after the Dark Ages had passed, only a few incidental observations were made without any attempt at the formulation of a comprehensive philosophy by such observers as ALBERTUS MAGNUS [1206–80] of Cologne and Bollstadt,[3] or, with his extraordinary insight, by LEONARDO DA VINCI [1452–1519] in his

[1] Old Testament, *The Book of Job*, x, 10 (475 B.C.).
[2] *The Wisdom of Solomon*, vii, 2, 3 ; (150–50 B.C.).
[3] *De animalibus* and *De secretis muleriorum*.

delightful drawings[1]. Even when biology was becoming rationalized
and even in the School of Padua where successive professors of genius—
ANDREAS VESALIUS [1514–64],[2] GABRIEL FALLOPIO [1523–62],[3] and
HIERONYMUS FABRICIUS AB AQUAPENDENTE [1537–1619][4]—interested
themselves particularly in the subject and made detailed observations on
the anatomy of the uterus, the placenta and the embryo, no revolutionary
concepts appeared. The only real originality was shown by VOLCHER COITER
[1534–?1600], a pupil of Fallopio who gave an excellent account of the reproductive tract of the hen and wrote a minute study of the developing chick[5]
far surpassing in its accuracy that of Aristotle. It was not until the middle
of the 17th century that embryology may be said to have emerged as a
modern science ; its inspiration was derived from the School of Padua and
its commencement dated from William Harvey's classical work, *Exercitationes de generatione* (1651) in which, studying the embryo of the deer and
the developing egg of the chick, he demonstrated the similarity between the
two and concluded that the embryos of mammals were of the same nature
as the eggs of birds ; from this he enunciated the dictum that all animals
were derived from eggs (*ex ovo omnia*) (Fig. 1). He thus abolished the
Aristotelian concept of the female as substance and the male as form and
elevated the role of the egg to its true and proper dignity.

Throughout its evolution as a science, embryology has attracted no outstanding
figure who can compare with Newton and Einstein, Darwin or Freud, each of whom
transformed his science and consolidated it into an integrated philosophy. Minor
luminances have appeared in plenty, most of the pioneers in Germany, but none of all-
embracing genius. For this reason it seems fitting to include in this book the portrait of
WILLIAM HARVEY [1578–1657] (Fig. 3), the great English physician who, above all
others, was responsible for the foundation of the sciences of physiology and medicine
based on experiment and observation by his demonstration of the circulation of the
blood.[6] His interest in embryology, although it occupied his attention mainly in the
later years of his life, was stimulated during his early studies at Padua where his
teacher, Hieronymus Fabricius, as we have seen, conducted a classical research on the
development of the chick in the fertilized egg. It is true that Harvey's generalization
on the origins of life had less effect on the development of embryology than had his
De motu cordis on the progress of medicine, that his book on the former subject lacks
coordination and, although the fruit of patient and extensive observations, is inferior
to its great predecessor which revolutionized ideas on the circulation and laid the
foundations of a rationalized physiology ; nevertheless, had he written only this work
he would have attained immortality. When it is remembered that it dealt with a subject
inaccessible to accurate observation without the aid of a microscope and fixatives—
and of these Harvey had neither—it is astonishing that his account of the development

[1] For drawing see p. 1. *Quaderni d'anatomia.* For Leonardo see Vol. II, p. 32 ; Fig. 23.
[2] Vol. II, p. 33 ; Fig. 35. *De humani corporis fabrica*, 1543, 1565.
[3] Vol. II, p. 37. *Observationes anatomicœ*, Venice, 1561.
[4] Vol. II, p. 37 ; Fig. 36. *De formato fœtu*, Venice, 1600 ; *De formatione ovi et pulli*,
Padua, 1621.
[5] *Externarum et internarum principalium humani corporis partium tabulœ*, Nuremberg,
1572.
[6] For an excellent appreciation of Harvey, see *William Harvey, Englishman*, by K. J.
Franklin, London (1961).

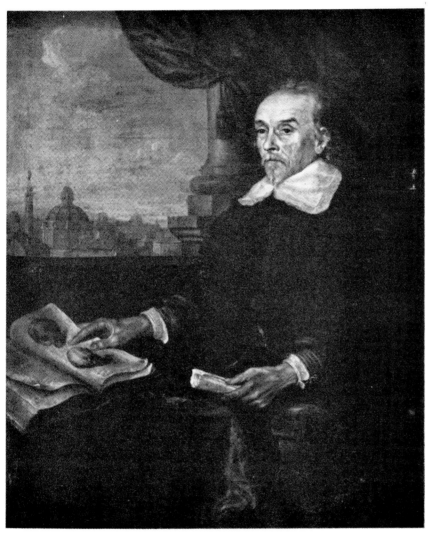

FIG. 3.—WILLIAM HARVEY
[1578–1657].

The founder of scientific embryology.
(Portrait by Wilhelm von Bemmel from the Hunterian Collection of the University of Glasgow.)

of the embryo in the egg remains to this day one of the most accurate ; it constituted
the first systematized factual observations which were exploited to establish embryology
on a scientific basis.

Inaugurated by Volcher Coiter and completed by William Harvey, the
science of gross embryological anatomy may be said to have been established
between 1572 and 1653 and to have escaped from the Aristotelian dogma.
In a short time it was supplemented by the studies of MARCELLO MALPIGHI
[1628–94],[1] who migrated between several Italian universities and, with the
use of the simple microscope which he introduced, studied the development
of the chick embryo during the first few hours after incubation.[2] Thereby
he was able to describe the neural groove, the optic vesicles, the aortic

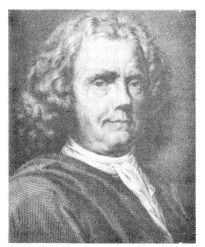

FIG. 4.—HERMANN BOERHAAVE
[1668–1738].
Biochemical embryologist.

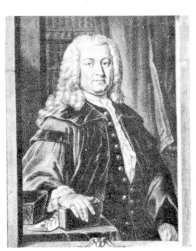

FIG. 5.—ALBRECHT VON HALLER
[1708–1777].
Physiological embryologist.

arch and the somites and can justly be credited with inaugurating the
science of embryological histology. Fifty years later the full potentialities
of this technique were finally realized by the great French surgeon and
ophthalmologist, ANTOINE MAÎTRE-JAN [1650–1730] who introduced fixatives,[3] hardening his embryos in distilled spirits of vinegar so that they could
be accurately dissected and sectioned. Previously to this, embryological
physiology may be said to have had its first disciple in JOHN MAYOW
[1643–79], that remarkable Fellow of Oxford who anticipated Priestley and
Lavoisier by a century and explained respiration and combustion by the
action of oxygen (" spiritus nitro-aereus "), an element distinct from the

[1] Vol. II, p. 39 ; Fig. 39.
[2] *De ovo incubato,* and *De formatione pulli in ovo,* published by the Royal Society of
London, 1672.
[3] *Observations sur la formation du poulet,* Paris (1722).

general mass of air. In 1674 in his work, *De respiratione in utero et ovo*, he showed by ingenious experiments that the umbilical arteries of the placenta aerated the fœtal tissues by " nitro-aerial particles " in the same way as the pulmonary vessels acted in the adult. " I think ", he wrote, " that the placenta should no longer be called a uterine liver but rather a uterine lung." These observations were extended to biochemical embryology by HERMANN BOERHAAVE [1668–1738][1] the Dutch theologian and philosopher, professor of botany, medicine and chemistry in Harderwick (Fig. 4)[2] and to general physiology by J. B. MAZIN of Belgium,[3] JOSEPHUS ONYMOS of Holland,[4] and J. C. HEFFTER[5] and ERHARDIUS HAMBERGER of Germany who first studied such problems as the water content and rate of growth of the embryo.[6] The culmination of early embryological physiology may be said to have been achieved by ALBRECHT VON HALLER [1708–77],[7] the great professor of botany, anatomy and surgery at Göttingen, who contributed elaborate studies on the functional development of the organs and the growth of bones[8] (Fig. 5).

We must, however, return to Harvey's revolutionary dictum which was followed by a period of philosophical theorizing and discussion concerning the emergence of an individual from an egg. Two theories held the field. Harvey accepted Aristotle's classical doctrine of *embryological epigenesis* whereby it was held that the integrated organism developed from amorphous and homogeneous material, the transformation being accomplished by the stimulation of the sperm by virtue of its own innate and specific " vital force ".[9] An alternative theory of *embryological preformation* claimed that the entire organism with all its component parts was already present and represented in the seed so that the whole of development constituted an increase in growth of elements already there. As a corollary, all future generations of a species were postulated to have been preformed in miniature at the Creation within the first two individuals, and subsequent generations could, therefore, be compared to preformed miniatures like a series of ever-diminishing boxes, one inside the other. The theory had its roots in classical times and was upheld by such writers as Leucippus and Democritus in Greece and Lucretius and Seneca in Rome. The Dutch scientist, JAN SWAMMERDAM [1637–80], for example, observed the emergence of the fully formed butterfly at the chrysalis stage and developed this concept in its most extreme form. " In nature ", he wrote, " there is no generation, but only propagation, the growth of parts. Thus original sin is explained, for

[1] Vol. II, p. 150.
[2] *Elementa chemiæ*, Leyden (1732).
[3] *Conjecturæ physico-medico-hydrostaticæ de respiratione fœtus*, Brixen (1737).
[4] *De natura fœtu*, Leyden (1745).
[5] *De causis in crem. fœtu*, Erfurt (1745).
[6] *Physiologia medica*, Jena (1751).
[7] Vol. II, p. 136.
[8] *Elementa physiologiæ corporis humani*, Lusanne (1757–66) ; *Ad generationem*, Lusanne (1767).
[9] Vol. I, p. 28.

all men were contained in the organs of Adam and Eve. When their stock of eggs is finished, the human race will cease to be."

Some insisted that the preformed individual was present in the male sperm, a view held by VAN LEEUWENHOEK [1632–1723] who, looking at unfixed specimens through his imperfect lenses with the aid of a flickering candle, first observed spermatozoa (1678) with the microscope which he evolved,[1] and supported by scientists of the calibre of J. VON LEIBNIZ [1646–1716] and HERMANN BOERHAAVE (1732). The Dutch microscopist, NICOLAS HARTSOEKER [1656–1725], indeed, published pictures of the preformed men (" homunculi ") which he saw with the eye of faith in the spermatozoa (Fig. 6).

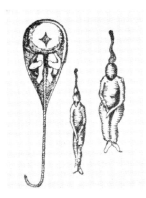

FIG. 6.—EMBRYOLOGICAL PREFORMATION.

Illustrations of spermatozoa of man, containing homunculi, as visualized and drawn by the 17th-century early microscopists. The figure on the left is that of Hartsoeker in 1694 ; the two on the right are those as seen by Plantades (1699), the assumed name of an anonymous author.

Others equally notable, such as MARCELLO MALPIGHI (1672), insisted that the new individual was fully formed in the female egg, and the great ALBRECHT VON HALLER (1766–67) claimed that the vessels and organs of the chick were present in the egg as a fine invisible network surrounding the yolk waiting for the act of fertilization to instigate growth. Indeed, it was not until almost a century had elapsed after Harvey's epoch-making generalization that CASPAR FRIEDRICH WOLFF [1733–94] of Halle (Fig. 7), a member of the Russian Academy under the Empress Catherine the Great, in his *Theoria generationis* (1759), written at the age of 26, established that the theory of epigenesis was true by direct observation of the gradual and complex development of the embryo from the relatively homogeneous matter of the egg.

The imaginative flights of authors of this time are well indicated by the publication of Theodorus Kerkringius of Amsterdam.[2] His observation of a fœtus tethered by the umbilical cord standing nonchalantly in the uterus 15 days after conception is shown in Fig. 8, and the skeleton of a child conceived 3 weeks previously is shown in Fig. 9.

This somewhat speculative period which lasted a hundred years was followed by a long and more fruitful stage wherein the detailed morphology of the development of the embryo was traced with all the resources of the now established science of histology. It was a purely descriptive period which extended throughout the 19th century ; its origin lay in the work of Wolff ; it may be said to have been ushered in by the researches of HEINRICH CHRISTIAN VON PANDER [1794–1865], who was fortunate in being born in Riga of wealthy parents so that he was able to devote his life to his favourite study ; and to have been terminated by the experiments of ERNST HAECKEL [1834–1919], the great disciple of Darwin who occupied the chair of zoology at Jena and excited an immense influence in his time on the progress of

---

[1] Vol. II, p. 39.
[2] *Anthropogeniæ Ichnographia*, Amsterdam (1671).

biology[1] (Fig. 10). This period was dominated by the *germ layer theory*. von Pander (1817) claimed that the development of the various organs of the chick embryo could be traced from three primary tissue-layers (or leaflets), themselves characterized by fixity and specificity : from the outermost there developed the skin and nervous tissue, from the middle layer the muscles, skeleton and excretory system, and from the innermost the alimentary canal. KARL ERNST VON BAER [1792–1876], a native of Esthonia

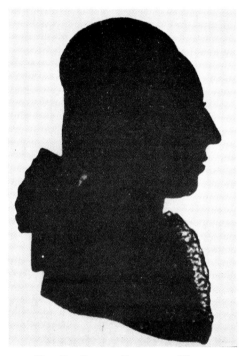

FIG. 7.—CASPAR FRIEDRICH WOLFF
[1733–1794].
A silhouette from the Humboldt University of Berlin (by courtesy of Professor G. Badtke).

and professor of physiology at Königsberg and, like Wolff, an Academician of St. Petersburg, who first saw the mammalian ovum in 1827, elaborated this theory at length, broadening its base by the examination of more varied material and adding a fourth layer which gave rise to the blood vessels (1827–28). Although the original theory of the specificity of the germ layers, implicitly believed in the 19th century, had been considerably modified by later experimental techniques, mechanical and chemical, Baer's philosophy of making metaphysical dogma subservient to practical observation was of

[1] See particularly his *Generelle Morphologie der Organismen* (1866) ; and his extremely popular *Naturliche Schöpfungsgeschichte*, Berlin (1868).

FIGS. 8 and 9.—EARLY CONCEPTIONS OF EMBRYOLOGISTS.

Abstracted from the *Anthropogeniæ Ichnographia* of Theodor Kerkringius (Amstelodami, 1671) by Mr. Oldenburgh : " An account of what has lately been observed by Dr. Kerkringius concerning the eggs to be found in all sorts of females " (*Phil. Trans.*, **7**, 4018, 1672).

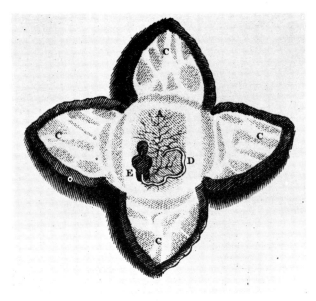

FIG. 8.

FIG. 8.—A fœtus *in utero*, 14 days after conception. " A, the secundine (placenta) ; C, the membrane amnios divided in four places ; D, the navel-string by which the child is fastened to the secundine ; E, the child of 14 days after conception."

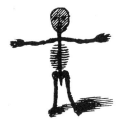

FIG. 9.—The skeleton of a fœtus 21 days after conception. " It is already furnished with all its cartilages though it had been conceived but three weeks."

FIG. 9.

the greatest value in coordinating the observations of a host of subsequent workers who elucidated the morphological changes in the developing embryo. Among these, MARTIN RATHKE [1793–1860] of Dorpat, RUDOLF ALBERT VON KÖLLIKER [1817–1905] of Würzburg[1] and WILHELM HIS [1831–1904] of Leipzig (Fig. 12) were among the most prominent, who, accumulating a wealth of histological detail by looking at embryos instead of looking for hypotheses, succeeded in extricating embryology from theory and establishing it on fact.

The third period in the history of embryological thought in which it

[1] Vol. II, p. 227 ; Fig. 257.

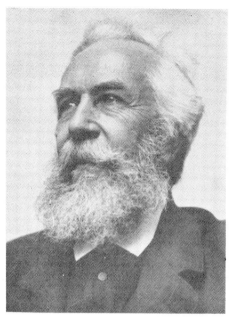

Fig. 10.—Ernst Haeckel
[1834–1919].

The photograph was taken when Haeckel was 71 years of age. (From the University of Jena, through the courtesy of Professor Hollwich.)

broke with the traditions of its purely morphological predecessor, may be said to have been introduced by an experiment of Haeckel (1869) who, working on siphonophore larvæ, demonstrated that half-larvæ were able to form whole organisms. The experimental approach was enthusiastically taken up by his pupil, WILHELM ROUX [1850–1924] (Fig. 11), who occupied chairs at Innsbruck and subsequently at Halle, in a long series of extended and original researches which were destined to lift embryology beyond the stage of anatomical description into that of experiment, and thus to elucidate the mechanics of development (1885–1912). The question "How?" now gave place to that of "Why?". Working on amphibian embryos he came to the conclusion that the development of the egg was determined by mechanical forces within it. A massing of the cytoplasm fixed the point of entry of the sperm, the line of entry of the sperm determined the plane of cleavage and therefore the median plane in an animal with bilateral symmetry, the fates of all parts being determined at the onset of development.

These purely mechanical views were questioned by HANS DRIESCH [1867–1941] who showed that in the sea-urchin all the cells within the egg up to the fourth or fifth division could, if separated, generate complete embryos ; he thus introduced the physiological concept of " prospective potency " to

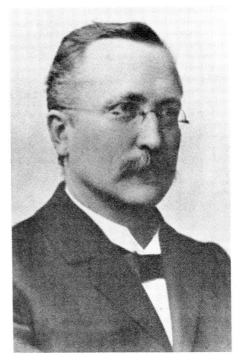

FIG. 11.—WILHELM ROUX
[1850–1924].
From the archives of the University of Halle (by courtesy of Professor G. Badtke).

indicate the several possible fates of the early cells (1894). This work introduced *the organizer concept* largely developed by the German Nobel prizewinner, HANS SPEMANN [1869–1941] of Freiburg and his pupils who, in a long series of experiments showed that chemical substances elaborated within the egg initiated and controlled the later development of the embryo (1912–43) (Fig. 62). Later work, particularly the tissue-culture and microsurgical grafting experiments exploited by R. G. HARRISON (1918–21) in the United States, showed the advisability of supplementing this simple explanation by *the field concept* whereby the developing organism is regarded as a unitary structure wherein the whole and its various constituent parts are dynamically interrelated and are continually reacting to each other and to their environment. This concept of " morphogenetic fields " and its specific application in the idea of the *axial gradient* as elaborated largely by CHARLES MANNING CHILD (1911–46) have undoubtedly provided a basis for research which has proved both stimulating and fruitful. It must be admitted, however, that it is impossible in the present state of our knowledge to decide whether these generalizing concepts of the organizer, the field, and the gradient contain the whole truth or whether they are skirting the periphery rather than penetrating the kernel of a difficult subject ; possibly they are merely aspects of a more all-embracing process the nature of which we do not yet understand.

However that may be, we shall first discuss the morphological aspects of the development of the embryo particularly as it affects the eye, and then take note of the experimental work undertaken to elucidate its determination.

For the history of embryology, see :

Cole. *Early Theories of Sexual Generation*, Oxon. (1930).
Meyer. *The Rise of Embryology*, Stanford (1939).
Needham. *A History of Embryology*, Cantab. (1934, 1959).
Oppenheimer. In *Analysis of Development*, Phila., **1**, 1 (1955).
    Survey of Biological Progress, N.Y., **3**, 1 (1957).
Russell. *The Interpretation of Development and Heredity*, Oxon. (1930).
Seidel. *Naturwissenschaften*, **42**, 275 (1955).

von Baer. *De ovi mammalium et hominis genesi*, Leipzig (1827).
    Ueber Entwickelungsgeschichte der Thiere, Königsberg (1828).
Boerhaave. *Elementa chemiæ*, Leyden (1732).
Child. *J. exp. Zool.*, **10**, 265 (1911).
    Bull. Biol., **23**, 1 (1912).
    Protoplasma, **5**, 447 (1925).
    Anat. Rec., **31**, 369 (1925).
    Patterns and Problems of Development, Chicago (1941).
    Physiol. Zool., **19**, 89 (1946).
Driesch. *Analytische Theorie d. organischen Entwicklung*, Leipzig (1894).
Haeckel. *Zur Entwickelungsgeschichte der Siphonophoren*, Utrecht (1869).
von Haller. *Elementa physiologiæ*, Lusanne, **7–8** (1766).
    Ad generationem, Lusanne (1767).
Harrison. *J. exp. Zool.*, **25**, 413 (1918) ; **32**, 1 (1921).
    Science, **85**, 369 (1937).
    Trans. Conn. Acad. Arts Sci., **36**, 277 (1945).

Harvey. *Exercitationes de generatione animalium*, London (1651).
van Leeuwenhoek. *Phil. Trans.*, **12**, 1040 (1678) ; **15**, 1120 (1685).
Malpighi. *De ovo incubato*, London (1672).
    De formatione pulli in ovo, London (1672).
Montague. *Ciba Symposia*, **10**, 994, 1009 (1949).
Pander. *Diss. sistens historiam metamorphoseos, quam ovum incubatum prioribus quinque diebus subit*, Wirceburgi (1817).
Roux. *Z. Biol.*, **3**, 411 (1885).
    Terminologie d. Entwicklungsmechanik der Tiere u. Pflanzen, Leipzig (1912).
Spemann. *Zool. Jb., Abt. Zool. Physiol.*, **32**, 1 (1912).
    Exp. Beiträge zu einer Theorie der Entwicklung, Berlin (1936).
    Embryonic Development and Induction, Yale (1938).
    Forschung und Leben, Stuttgart (1943).

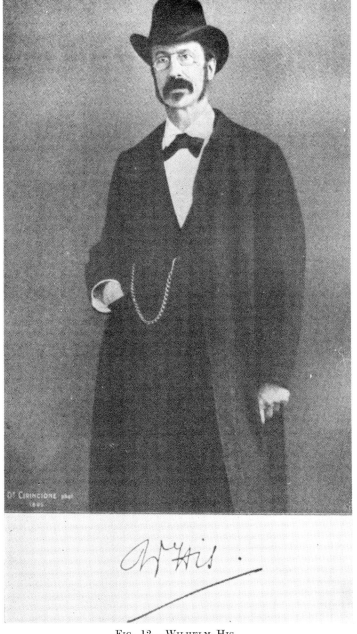

FIG. 12.—WILHELM HIS
[1831–1904].
From the University of Leipzig (through the courtesy of Professor Sachsenweger).

CHAPTER II

THE GENERAL SCHEME OF DEVELOPMENT

THE most suitable introduction to this Chapter on the general scheme of embryo-logical development is the portrait of WILHELM HIS [1831–1904] who was the first to systematize our knowledge of this subject (Fig. 12). A pupil of Johannes Müller, Robert Remak and Rudolf Virchow, to the last of whom his first classical paper (*Beiträge zur normalen und pathologischen Histologie der Cornea*, 1856) was dedicated, he was called to the chair of anatomy and physiology at Basle (1857) where he succeeded Meissner, and subsequently became professor of anatomy at Leipzig (1872). Here for 30 years, together with Carl Ludwig who occupied the chair of physiology, he laboured incessantly, the two masters in their kindred subjects making Leipzig a world-centre of research. His early papers on anatomy, particularly those on the lymphatic system, will always remain classical ; but his great life's work, undertaken from 1865 onwards, was the study of embryological development. For this purpose, instead of laboriously cutting sections by hand, he invented and was the first to use a microtome capable of cutting serial sections (1866). From then onwards not a year passed without the appearance of a paper of fundamental importance, and such were his untiring applica-tion and prodigious energy that, for the first time he traced, both in grand design and considerable detail, with photographs of sections, beautiful drawings and elaborate and accurately scaled models, the entire story of development in all its successive stages from the unfertilized egg through the appearance of the embryonic layers to the evolution of the individual organs in fishes, the chick, and in man. For the first time, early human embryology, particularly that of the central nervous system, was adequately presented to the scientific world in word, section, portrait and model in his immense three-volumed work, *Anatomie menschlicher Embryonen* (1880–85).

The primordium of the eye first appears at a very early stage, developing from that portion of the embryo which forms the anterior part of the central nervous system ; an understanding of the sequence of events at this time therefore necessitates some knowledge of the general development of the embryo as a whole and particularly of this important region. Any attempt to divide this complex process into discrete stages must be artificial since it embraces many diverse activities which proceed simultaneously in an orderly sequence, each accurately coordinated with the others. For the purpose of description, however, it is convenient to divide it into three stages—an initial stage of EMBRYOGENESIS during which the primary layers of the developing embryo are segregated, ORGANOGENESIS during which the segregated material becomes organized into the general pattern of the various organs, and DIFFERENTIATION during which the characteristic structures of each organ are separately elaborated.

EMBRYOGENESIS

The process of EMBRYOGENESIS embraces the early development of the embryo from the stage of the fertilized ovum to the period when the primary germ layers are differentiated and specific masses of cells destined to form the various organs have become segregated. So far as ocular development is concerned, this period may be said to end with the appearance of the optic primordium which occurs prior to the 2·6 mm. stage during the 3rd week after fertilization.

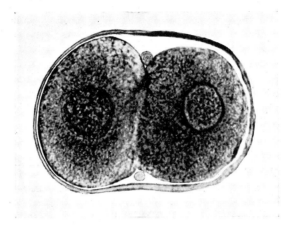

FIG. 13.—THE TWO-CELL STAGE OF THE HUMAN ZYGOTE.

Microphotograph by Hertig and Rock (from Hamilton, Boyd and Mossman's *Human Embryology*, W. Heffer, Cambridge).

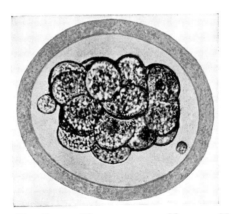

FIG. 14.—THE LIVING MORULA OF THE MACAQUE MONKEY.

(Hamilton, Boyd and Mossman's *Human Embryology*, W. Heffer, Cambridge.)

Immediately after the stimulus of fertilization, while still in the uterine tube, the ovum subdivides by a series of consecutive mitotic divisions to form a solid spherical mass of cells or *blastomeres* called, on account of its mulberry-like appearance, the MORULA (Figs. 13 and 14). In spite of the cellular multiplication occurring during this process of cleavage, there is no increase in protoplasmic volume, the initial disproportion seen in the fertilized ovum between cytoplasm and nucleus being progressively reduced during segmentation until the usual relationship characteristic of the somatic cells of the species is gradually attained. At the same time the individual cells continually alter their relative positions and reorientate themselves to maintain the bilateral symmetry of the ovum.

FIGS. 15 to 17.—THE BLASTULA AND THE GASTRULA.

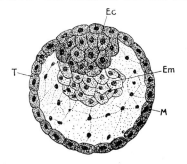

FIG. 15.—Hypothetical stage in development of the ovum.

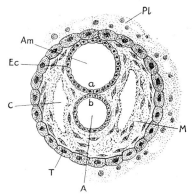

FIG. 16.—The Bryce-Teacher Embryo.

A. Archenteron.
Am. Amniotic cavity.
C. Cœlomic cavity.
E. Primary mesoderm.
Ec. Ectoderm.
Em. Embryonic cell mass.

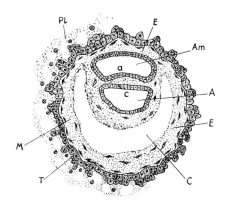

FIG. 17.—Peters's Embryo.

M. Mesoderm.
Pl. Plasmodial trophoblast.
T. Trophoblast.
a. Ectoderm of embryo.
b. Endoderm of embryo.
c. Endoderm separated from
ectoderm by mesoderm.

At about the twelve-cell stage (72 hours after fertilization), the morula reaches the uterus and the first phase of differentiation is thereupon initiated by the segregation of the cells into an outer layer of small slightly flattened cells (the *trophoblast*) and an inner central mass of larger polyhedral cells (Lewis and Hartman, 1933). Fluid from the uterine cavity then passes through the outer layer of cells separating them from the inner cell mass all

around the circumference except at one point, the *upper* or *embryonic pole*.
This introduces the BLASTULA (or BLASTOCYST) stage of development
(Fig. 15). As the fluid accumulates the trophoblastic cells become flattened
and, proliferating rapidly, invade the uterine mucosa to effect the implanting
of the ovum (7½ days after fertilization). This is followed by the stage of

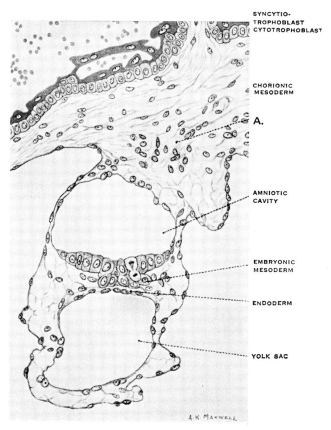

FIG. 18.—TRANSVERSE SECTION THROUGH THE POSTERIOR PART OF A
15-DAY EMBRYO (Edwards–Jones–Brewer).

The section shows the primitive streak, and the early development of the intra-embryonic
mesoderm. A indicates the mesodermal condensation in the body-stalk (Hamilton, Boyd
and Mossman's *Human Embryology*, W. Heffer, Cambridge).

GASTRULATION whereby changes in position of certain cells of the blastula
result in the formation of three germinal layers—ectoderm, endoderm, and
mesoderm—and bring the presumptive organs into the position wherein
they undergo further development. The inner cell-mass is seen to differentiate
into two groups of cells : the *ectoderm* on the outside and the *endoderm*
towards the blastocœle side, each of which rapidly becomes converted into

a hollow vesicle by the accumulation of fluid between the cells. The outer-most vesicle remains in close contact with the trophoblast and constitutes the *ectodermal vesicle* (*amniotic cavity*), whilst the more central and initially smaller vesicle is known as the *endodermal vesicle* or *yolk-sac* (*archenteric cavity*). Except at the embryonic pole, the inner cell-mass is separated from the inner aspect of the trophoblast by a jelly-like tissue (the *primary* or *extra-embryonic* [*chorionic*] *mesoderm*) which in man appears to be derived from the trophoblast. At a later stage, clefts appear in this mesodermal tissue and eventually become confluent to form the *extra-embryonic cœlom* or *cœlomic cavity* which gradually surrounds the developing structures except above where the amnion remains attached to the trophoblast (Fig. 16). At this stage the mesoderm is therefore divided into an outer layer lining

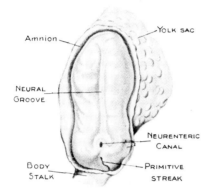

FIG. 19.—HUMAN EMBRYO OF 2 MM. LENGTH.
Dorsal view with the amnion laid open (after Graf Spee).

the trophoblast and an inner layer enveloping the amniotic and archenteric cavities (Fig. 17). The ovum has thus been converted into a large vesicle from the inner wall of which the two embryonic vesicles are suspended. It is in the area where these two vesicles are in apposition that the rudiments of the embryo itself are represented ; this all-important region is called the *embryonic plate* which therefore consists of two apposed layers of cells, one of ectoderm and the other of endoderm (Fig. 18).

The gastrula stage is followed by the NEURULA (or somite) stage wherein the axial embryonic structures and the neural plate are developed. At first nearly circular in shape, the embryonic plate rapidly becomes oval indicating the long axis of the body, and differentiation begins to appear. The first sign of this process is the development of a linear opacity (the *primitive streak*) which runs longitudinally over the caudal part of its dorsal surface (Figs. 19 and 20). This opacity is due to a localized area of ectodermal proliferation at the anterior end of which an ectodermal thickening occurs (*Hensen's node*) with in its centre an invagination of the ectoderm forming the *blastopore*. From this region a proliferation of cells buds forwards from Hensen's node in the axis of the embryonic plate between the ectoderm and the endoderm to form the *notochordal process* into which the invagination of the blastopore extends. Simultaneously, again by proliferation of the cells of Hensen's node, the notochordal process extends caudally, and the invagination of the blastopore burrows throughout its length to form a canal. The process then becomes intercalated in the endoderm and openings appear in the notochordal canal leading into the yolk-sac ; these eventually become

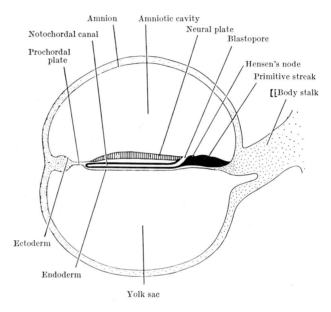

FIG. 20.—DIAGRAMMATIC REPRESENTATION OF THE HUMAN EMBRYO.

In longitudinal section. The mesoderm throughout is dotted. In an early (bilaminar) stage (modified from Harrison).

confluent so that for a time the neural groove is directly connected with the primitive digestive tube, at which stage the blastopore is known as the *neurenteric canal*.

In the meantime, the ectodermal cells on either side of the anterior part of the primitive streak rapidly divide and, migrating laterally and cephalically, infiltrate between the ectoderm and the underlying endoderm of the embryonic plate to form an intervening sheet of cells known as the *intra-embryonic* or *secondary mesoderm* which extends throughout the whole embryonic area with the exception of the median plane (Fig. 18). The ectodermal cells which proliferate to form the notochord on the one hand and the secondary mesoderm on the other, have been termed the *chorda-mesoblast* by Dalcq (1938).

In primitive vertebrates, such as *Amphioxus*, the process of gastrulation is more dramatic (Figs. 21 and 22). The blastula forms a simple hollow sphere, one part of which becomes invaginated to form the endoderm, while the outer layer remains as the ectoderm (the blastocœle). The mouth of the invagination becomes the blastopore, and here the ectoderm and endoderm fuse, just as occurs at the mouth of a hydra. The primitive streak probably represents the fused margins of such an opening, and the blastopore, although it remains patent only a very short time in the higher vertebrates, represents the masked and obscured relic of this important stage. Here the epiblast (of the amniotic cavity) and the hypoblast (of the archenteric cavity) are continuous, and from the line of union the mesoblast is developed and spreads out as a sheet between the two layers (see J. T. Wilson and Hill, 1908 ; Assheton, 1909–10).

FIGS. 21 and 22.—GASTRULATION IN A URODELE.

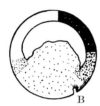

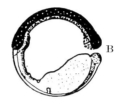

FIG. 21. The blastula stage.

FIG. 22.—The gastrula stage.

White area, epiblast ; black spotted area, ectoblast ; white heavily dotted area, chordomesoblast ; white lightly dotted area, hypoblast ; lined area, the organizing centre. B, blastopore.

The greater part of the central nervous system (which particularly concerns us in this context) is developed from the ectoderm of the embryonic plate anterior to the primitive streak. Here the cells proliferate and thicken to form a curved ridge known as the *neural plate*. This process is initiated by the appearance in the neural plate of a median longitudinal groove (the *neural groove*) on either side of which the ectoderm is elevated to form two parallel curved folds (the *neural folds*) (Figs. 23 and 24). A gradual deepening of the groove and the progressive convergence of the folds ultimately result in the fusion of the dorsal lips of the groove, converting it into a slit-like canal (the *neural tube*) (Fig. 25). These changes begin in the cerebral region and for a long time the anterior and posterior extremities of the canal remain open (the *anterior* and *posterior neuropores*). At the anterior end the two folds expand enormously, their excessive growth causing them to project beyond the margins of the neural plate and to curl round ventrally to form the *head-fold* ; in this way the end of each fold, originally anterior, is now turned to the under surface of the head.

During the conversion of the neural groove into the neural tube, a ridge of ectodermal cells appears along the margin of each of the converging neural folds (the *neural crests*) and, as the folds meet in the middle line, the two neural crests fuse to form a wedge-shaped area along the line of closure of the tube (Fig. 25). Subsequently the cells of the neural crests migrate to the dorso-lateral aspects of the neural tube, thus remaining outside the central nervous system.

The walls of the neural tube become converted into the various parts of the central nervous system—the brain and cord, the retina and optic nerve—

FIGS. 23 to 26.—THE DEVELOPMENT OF THE NEURAL STRUCTURES.

Diagrammatic representation of the development of the neural structures in the human embryo.

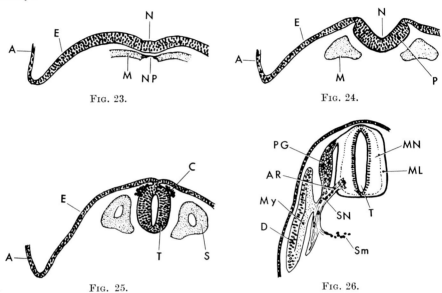

FIG. 23.   FIG. 24.

FIG. 25.   FIG. 26.

Fig. 23 shows the beginning of the development of the neural tube, more fully formed in Fig. 24 and completely formed in Fig. 25. The paraxial mesoderm seen in Fig. 23 becomes segmented in Fig. 24 ; in Fig. 25 the neural crest appears which is responsible for the development of the peripheral nervous system (Fig. 26) and the sympathetic system (modified from Hamilton, Boyd and Mossman).

A, amnion.
AR, anterior spinal root.
C, neural crest.
D, dermatome.
E, embryonic ectoderm.
M, paraxial mesoderm.
ML, marginal layer.
MN, mantle layer.
My, myotome.

N, neural groove.
NP, notochordal plate.
P, neural plate.
PG, posterior root ganglion.
S, somite with cavity.
Sm, sympathetic cells.
SN, spinal nerve.
T, neural tube.

while the neural crest is the rudiment of the ganglia of the cerebro-spinal and sympathetic systems, the neurilemmal sheaths of all the peripheral and sensory nerves (R. G. Harrison, 1937–38), the fundamental basis of the leptomeninges (pia and arachnoid) (Harvey and Burr, 1926 ; Sensenig, 1951), the mesenchyme of the head (mesectoderm) (Stone, 1929 ; Horstadius, 1950), and the chromaffin cells of the chromaffin organs including the medulla of the adrenal gland, the cells of which are therefore postganglionic sympathetic neurons (Hammond and Yntema, 1947 ; Hammond, 1949). There is also much evidence that the melanoblasts of connective tissue are derived from the neural crests (Rawles, 1947–59 ; DuShane, 1948 ; Boyd, 1949 ; Niu, 1954–59) (Fig. 26).[1]

In the meantime the secondary mesoderm throughout the embryonic plate proliferates and becomes subdivided into three zones (Fig. 27) :

(1) A thickened medial portion, the *paraxial mesoderm*, consisting of a mass of cells lying immediately lateral to the neural groove and underlying the neural folds.

(2) A narrower zone, the *intermediate cell-mass*, lying immediately lateral to the paraxial mesoderm.

(3) A flattened lateral sheet, the *lateral plate*, extending from the intermediate cell-mass to the periphery of the embryonic area where it becomes continuous with the primary mesoderm covering the ectodermal and endodermal vesicles.

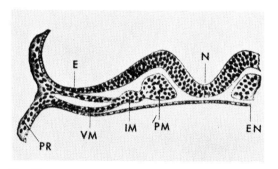

FIG. 27.—THE DEVELOPMENT OF THE MESODERM (after Gray).

E, ectoderm.
EN, endoderm.
IM, intermediate cell mass.
N, neural groove.

PM, paraxial mesoderm.
PR, primary mesoderm.
VM, visceral mesoderm with cœlomic cavity.

At the beginning of the 3rd week after fertilization the paraxial mesoderm shows marked changes. Starting a short distance behind the cephalic tip of the notochord (that is, about the level of the midbrain) it becomes segmented to form symmetrically arranged metameric blocks or *somites* ; the first pair is the occipital and each subsequent successive pair is formed caudally until forty-two eventually appear (cervical, dorsal, lumbar, sacral, coccygeal) (Fig. 28). From these are developed the greater part of the axial skeleton and musculature of the body-wall. In the anterior region, however, this demarcation does not occur and the unsegmented paraxial mesoderm here eventually gives rise to the skeletal and membranous coverings of the brain, the sclera, the greater part of the uveal tract and the extra-ocular muscles. From the lateral mesoderm (called *visceral* in the head region) the structures of the visceral (branchial) arches are formed.

[1] See further, p. 282.

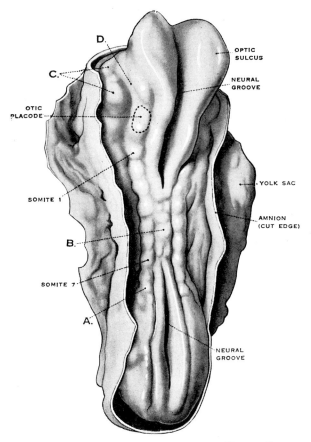

FIG. 28.—RECONSTRUCTION OF A 7-SOMITE HUMAN EMBRYO.

The dorsal aspect at about the 22nd day. The early optic pit (sulcus) is seen in the pros-encephalic region. A, paraxial mesoderm partially segmented into somites. B, roof of the neural tube formed in the central area. C, pericardial area ; D, region of the branchial arches (× *c*. 47) (Hamilton, Boyd and Mossman's *Human Embryology*, W. Heffer, Cambridge).

In the latter part of the 3rd week further changes occur in the development of the central nervous system. Closure of the anterior neuropore is initiated by the fusion of the anterior ends of the neural folds to form an *anterior neural fold* which runs transversely across the lower part of the open neural groove. Meanwhile, as the size of the anterior end of the neural folds increases, the neural groove correspondingly becomes expanded, thus differentiating the dilated rudiment of the brain from the narrower rudiment of the spinal cord. In the former, three secondary dilatations are formed separated by two transverse constrictions, the earliest indication of its division into a hindbrain (rhombencephalon), a midbrain (mesencephalon), and a forebrain (prosencephalon). The latter in its turn develops a constric-

Figs. 29 to 32.—The Evolution of the Brain of Vertebrates.

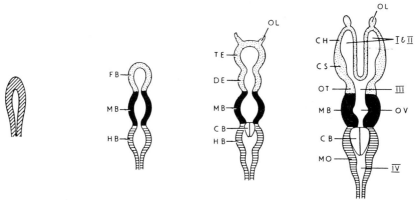

FIG. 29.—The initial archencephalon; a vesicular-shaped swelling at the upper end of the medullary tube.

FIG. 30.—The stage of three primary cerebral vesicles.

FIG. 31.—The stage of five cerebral vesicles.

FIG. 32.—The final division of the telencephalon.

The forebrain and its derivatives are dotted ; the midbrain is in solid black ; the hindbrain is cross-hatched.

CB, cerebellum ; CH, cerebral hemispheres ; CS, corpus striatum ; DE, diencephalon ; FB, forebrain (prosencephalon) ; HB, hindbrain (rhombencephalon), divided into metencephalon and myelencephalon in Figs. 31–32 ; MB, midbrain (mesencephalon) ; MO, medulla oblongata ; OL, olfactory lobe ; OT, optic thalamus ; OV, vesicle which becomes the iter or aqueduct of Sylvius ; TE, telencephalon ; I, II, III and IV, ventricles.

tion dividing itself into a terminal telencephalon and a proximal diencephalon ; from the last of these, growing out from its lateral wall, the anlage of the eye develops (Figs. 29 to 32).

ORGANOGENESIS

THE OPTIC PRIMORDIUM

The process of ORGANOGENESIS may be said to date from the assemblage and segregation of the cells destined to form the eyes near the anterior extremities of the neural plate, when the optic pits appear in the anterior neural folds ; it may be taken to include the period during which the specialized tissues are differentiated and arranged to form the general pattern of the future organ. In this process three different embryonic layers participate : the neural ectoderm which forms the essential visual apparatus, the surface ectoderm which contributes the main elements of the dioptric apparatus, and the mesoderm which is responsible for the stromal and vascular elements. All of these show a complex and interesting evolution. The neural ectoderm of the optic pit develops into the primary optic vesicle which invaginates to form the optic cup and the embryonic fissure, the

FIGS. 33 to 38.—THE ONTOGENETIC DEVELOPMENT OF THE
LATERAL EYE OF VERTEBRATES.

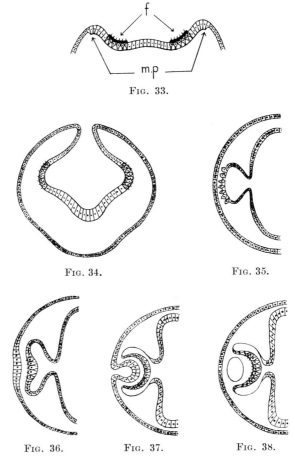

FIG. 33.

FIG. 34.   FIG. 35.

FIG. 36.   FIG. 37.   FIG. 38.

FIG. 33.—The appearance of the optic pits (foveolæ opticæ, f) on the dorsal ectoderm of the cephalic (medullary) plate (m.p.).

FIG. 34.—Invagination of the surface ectoderm with the optical area to form the primitive neural tube.

FIG. 35.—Evagination of the primary optic vesicle.

FIG. 36.—The commencement of secondary invagination of the neural epithelium with thickening of the surface epithelium.

FIG. 37.—Invagination of the surface epithelium.

FIG. 38.—Detachment of the lens from the surface epithelium.

eventual closure of which completes the fundamental process in the development of the organ and prepares the way for the final differentiation of the retina, a process which occurs mainly during the 5th and 6th weeks after fertilization. It is thus evident that the retina is an island of the central nervous system and the optic nerve a tract of this system connecting the outlying part with the main body. The surface ectoderm similarly invaginates to form the lens vesicle over which it closes to form a continuous epithelial covering on the surface ; while the mesoderm supplies the nutritive and most of the supporting elements and the surrounding protective structures as well as a motor apparatus. The development of the two ectodermal vesicles is seen diagrammatically in Figs. 33 to 38.

As the two anterior ends of the neural ridges increase in size and approximate and the termination of the open groove is enclosed in the transverse anterior neural fold, a small recess is formed on either side of the midline terminating in a slight depression on the surface in the region of the cephalic end of the rudimentary forebrain. These are the OPTIC PITS, the first evidences of the rudiments of the eyes ; they appear at the 2·6 mm. stage during the 3rd week (Bartelmez, 1954) (Fig. 28). Viewed externally,

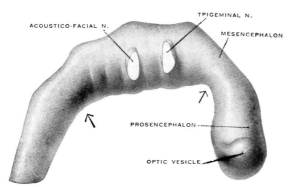

FIG. 39.—THE CENTRAL NERVOUS SYSTEM IN AN EARLY HUMAN EMBRYO

Reconstruction of the external form of the right half of the cranial portion of the central nervous system of a 3·5 mm. length embryo. The arrows indicate the positions of the cervical and mesencephalic flexures ($\times$ c. 50) (Hamilton, Boyd and Mossman's *Human Embryology*, W. Heffer, Cambridge).

they form two lateral outpouchings of the anterior end of the neural tube and, since the cephalic extremity of the tube is still open at the time of their formation, they actually form ectodermal depressions on the surface of the body. When the roof of the neural tube closes, these evaginations enlarge to form two globular projections on the ventro-lateral aspect of the brain (about the 3·2 mm. stage), the PRIMARY OPTIC VESICLES (Fig. 39).

There is still some doubt as to the original position of the optic anlage. The early writers stated that it was single and median (Huschke, 1832), a view supported by Lankester (1880) and Jelgersma (1906) who traced the vertebrate eye phylogenetically from an ascidian ancestor. It was shown, however, by Froriep (1906) that the apparently unpaired eye of this sea-squirt in the tadpole stage[1] was one of a pair of which its fellow had degenerated[2] ; moreover, the facts of embryology seemed to contradict this unitary view so that it was abandoned in favour of the concept of the simultaneous appearance of two optic primordia. A reversion to the original view was advocated by Stockard (1909). As a result of his experimental production of cyclopic deformities

[1] Vol. I, p. 228.   [2] Vol. I, p. 245.

by exposing developing eggs to magnesium, he concluded that cyclopia was not a fusion of two eyes but a failure in the division of a single original optic anlage. Later (1913) he attempted to confirm this theory by operative manipulations. He cut out portions of the neural plate in salamanders and found that when the antero-median region was excised the eyes as a rule failed to develop, but, when the lateral parts were excised, both eyes were usually formed. Spemann (1912–23), however, showed that the optic plate cannot be looked upon as a precisely limited area since a considerable displacement of cells takes place during the closure of the neural tube. Petersen (1923–4) claimed that these experiments merely showed that the optic plates tend to form two eyes however much they are cut about. Fischel (1916), moreover, on repeating Stockard's operative experiments, was unable to confirm the view of a single optic primordium. He showed that the action of magnesium ions is only evident at a stage of development before the neural tube appears, some 15 hours after fertilization ; if they are exhibited later than this, two separate optic pits always develop. At the earlier stage Spemann (1923) showed that no optic primordium was present. He transplanted a piece of presumptive abdominal skin and exchanged it for a portion of the neural tube, and subsequent development showed that the presumptive abdominal skin became the optic vesicle. It follows that the action of magnesium salts is not to inhibit the division of a primary single optic anlage ; they act before the optic plate is laid down in the neural tube, and the influence they exert must therefore be upon the initial process of determination or upon the distribution and organization of material. On the other hand, Leplat (1914–58) contended that the original anlage is an area, initially single but diffuse, in the midline which progressively differentiates into the optic pits and vesicles laterally and the chiasma centrally, a view supported by others (Woerdeman, 1929 ; Manchot, 1929 ; Adelmann, 1937). Finally, such authorities as Jolly (1950) and Wolff (1950) say that the optic anlage cannot be ascribed to a specific area but is initially represented diffusely in the most anterior portion of the neural plate. Obviously the matter has not yet reached finality and it will be discussed further in the section dealing with cyclopia and other related deformities.[1]

THE OPTIC VESICLES

During its initial stages the PRIMARY OPTIC VESICLE gradually forms as a spherical outpouching from the optic pit, the columnar ectodermal cells comprising its wall being directly continuous with those of the forebrain (Figs. 34, 35 and 39). As it increases in size its most distal part comes into close apposition to the surface ectoderm clothing the embryo (by the 4 mm. stage), but elsewhere it is surrounded by mesoderm. For the most part this is of the paraxial type, but in its postero-inferior aspect the marked flexure of the head-fold brings the forebrain and the optic vesicle into close relationship with the bar of visceral mesoderm from which the lower and outer walls of the orbit are eventually formed (the maxillary process). At first the two vesicles are directed almost laterally, being widely separated by a broad fronto-nasal process from which the inner walls of the orbits and the nasal capsule are ultimately derived (Fig. 40). As growth proceeds it involves predominantly the more distal portion of the vesicle, a process which, supplemented by the progressive development of the surrounding mesoderm, results in the formation of a localized constriction of the vesicle at its proximal end where it remains connected with the developing forebrain ; this narrowed

[1] Part 2, p. 429.

region becomes the OPTIC STALK and through its open lumen the cavity of the expanded distal portion remains directly continuous with that of the fore-brain (Figs. 41 and 42).

During the 4th week (4 to 5 mm. stage), an important change occurs in the development of the primary optic vesicle whereby it becomes converted into a cup-shaped form. As it increases progressively in size, a process which affects mainly its upper part, the distal and under surface of the vesicle becomes flattened and here an indentation appears which is gradually converted into a deepening depression so that an invagination is eventually formed involving the distal end of the vesicle and its lower medial quadrant

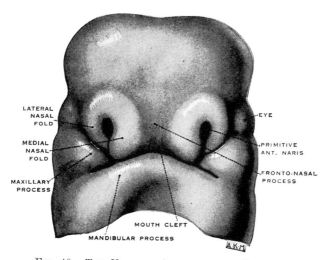

FIG. 40.—THE VENTRAL ASPECT OF THE FACE OF A
10 MM. LENGTH HUMAN EMBRYO.
A drawing from Hamilton, Boyd and Mossman's *Human Embryology*, W. Heffer Cambridge.

(Fig. 45). It is interesting that the invaginated portion concerns the part of the vesicle in intimate association with the surface ectoderm (now forming the lens plate) and the region immediately below this. Even at this early stage the cells constituting this part of the wall of the vesicle are seen to be proliferating to form several rows while the remainder of the wall remains as a single layer of cells. Eventually the invaginating portion (the original outer and lower walls of the vesicle) becomes approximated to the upper and proximal walls and a two-layered cup, widely open distally and below, is formed—the SECONDARY OPTIC VESICLE or OPTIC CUP (Figs. 43 to 45). As the two layers approximate the original lumen of the primary optic vesicle is eventually obliterated to leave a potential cavity only, and the closed space which might be construed as the cavity of a globe is replaced by the open convexity of the optic cup ; its wall is thus formed by two strata of cells continuous with each other at its margins, the outer layer composed of a single stratum of columnar cells[1] formed by the proximal portion of the wall of the primary vesicle, the inner layer showing active cellular proliferation formed by the distal portion (Figs. 47, 49–51).

During this conversion (which is not fully completed until the 6th or

FIGS. 41 and 42.—THE EVOLUTION OF THE OPTIC VESICLE (after Bach and Seefelder).

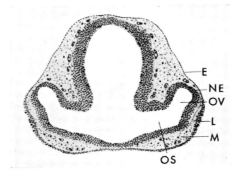

FIG. 41.—Frontal section through the eye of a 4·9 mm. embryo.

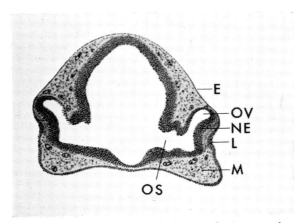

FIG. 42.—Frontal section through the eye of a 5 mm. embryo.

E, Surface ectoderm.   NE, Neural ectoderm.
L, Lens plate.   OS, Optic stalk.
M, Mesoderm.   OV, Primary optic vesicle.

7th week : the 15 to 18 mm. stage) the most proximal portion of the primary vesicle which formed the optic stalk, initially short and relatively wide, elongates and becomes more constricted while its lumen is progressively reduced in size. This structure is also involved in the invaginating process and on its under surface a deep groove appears continuous with the groove on

[1] It is to be noted that in sections the nuclei of the columnar cells of the outer layer are seen to lie at different levels giving the impression of the existence of several layers of cells.

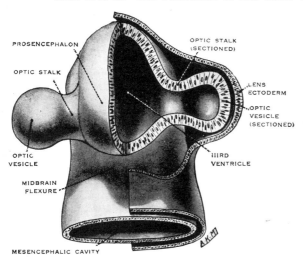

FIG. 43.—In a 4 mm. human embryo.

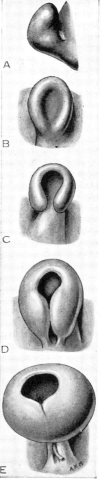

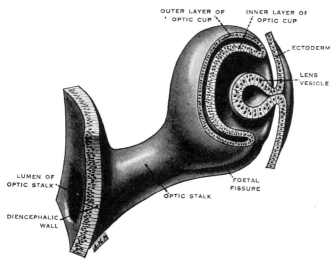

FIG. 44.—In a 7·5 mm. human embryo.

Figs. 43 to 45 from Hamilton, Boyd and Mossman, *Human Embryology*, W. Heffer, Cambridge.

FIG. 45.—The invagination of the optic vesicle (A) through the formation of the embryonic fissure (B, C, D) to form the optic cup (E). In the last the hyaloid artery is seen entering the proximal extremity of the fissure.

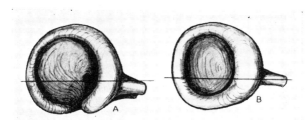

FIG. 46.—A model of the optic cup, showing the embryonic fissure and its continuity up the optic stalk in A. An imaginary model is shown in B demonstrating the condition which would have resulted in the absence of an embryonic fissure if invagination had taken place merely from the external aspect. No communication between the future retina and the optic stalk would have been possible (after Ida Mann).

the under surface of the optic cup ; the two together form the EMBRYONIC FISSURE or CLEFT which thus extends from the peripheral rim of the optic cup almost to reach the lateral wall of the forebrain (Fig. 45). At this stage the fissure is occupied by the immediately adjacent mesoderm which surrounds the optic cup and from this tissue invaginating into the optic cup

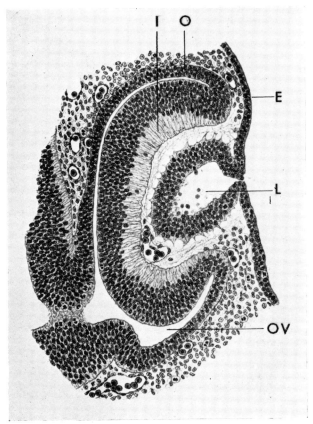

FIG. 47.—SECTION THROUGH THE OPTIC CUP OF A 6·5 MM. EMBRYO
(after Bach and Seefelder) (× 133).

E. Surface ectoderm.	O. Outer layer of optic cup.
I. Inner layer of optic cup.	OV. Cavity of optic vesicle.
L. Lens vesicle.	

the hyaloid system of vessels and the central retinal artery are ultimately formed.

In view of the (correct) belief that a typical coloboma indicated a failure in closure of the embryonic cleft but was interpreted as a failure in the choroid of which the pigmentary epithelium was assumed to be a part, the cleft was initially called the *choroidal fissure*—an obvious misnomer. The subsequent popular change to *fœtal fissure* was unfortunate since the structure forms and closes during embryonic life long before the fœtal stage commences : *embryonic fissure* is the more correct term. In view of the fact that fissures occur in other organs, a still better term would be *optic fissure* (or *cleft*) ; but this is not commonly employed.

Small accessory notches have been noted to occur by Lindahl (1912) on the rim of the optic cup which are clearly marked at the 7·7 mm. stage, are deepest at 10 mm., and are still present at 17·1 mm. This author found four of these notches with great constancy in the eyes of man and the lower vertebrates and considered that they formed part of the normal development. Similar appearances had previously been described by van Duyse (1901), von Szily (1907), Wolfrum (1908), and Bach and Seefelder (1914), but these authors looked upon them as exceptional occurrences[1] (Fig. 48).

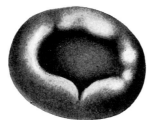

Fig. 48.—The Optic Cup.

From a human embryo of 10 mm., showing the completion of invagination of the optic cup. The embryonic fissure is below and there are accessory notches elsewhere on the rim (after von Szily).

The invagination of the primary optic vesicle is a characteristic of all vertebrates (with the exception of primitive types : *Amphioxus*), and is a necessary consequence of the development of a cerebral eye. We have seen in a previous Volume[2] that the epithelial eye of invertebrates develops from the surface ectoderm, and with few exceptions the sensory end of the sensory cell lies towards the surface of the body and therefore facing the light, while the conducting elements lie deeply to it (the *verted retina*). Initially, in vertebrates when the optic pits formed lateral outpouchings of the neural plate, they were open externally and the cells constituting their floor, which finally differentiate into percipient elements, are exposed directly to the light. The arrangement here, therefore, corresponds to that of the invertebrate eye (Fig. 33). When, however, the sensory layer is enfolded within the neural tube, the percipient end of the sensory cell now lies deeply and the pole from which the nerve fibres issue becomes superficial[3]—the *inverted retina* (Fig. 34). In the vesicular form this type of eye is convex towards the light, and for optical purposes must secondarily assume the more convenient concave form (Fig. 38). This being so, the formation of an embryonic fissure is necessary since it is the only method available which allows the direct conduction of nerve fibres from the inner layer into the optic stalk and up to the brain. If this did not occur and the invagination had involved the distal portion of the vesicle only to form a simple cup, a comparison between A and B in Fig. 46 shows that no direct communication could exist between the inner layer and the stalk. It follows that in the cerebral eye of the vertebrate, light must traverse the whole thickness of the retina in order to reach the sentient layer. The inverted retina may seem an anomalous arrangement from an optical point of view, but it carries the advantage that the visual receptors are brought into immediate contact with the pigment while the part of the

[1] See atypical colobomata, Part 2, pp. 577, 612.
[2] Vol. I, p. 146.　　　　　　　　　　　　　[3] Vol. I, p. 241.

retina in which the greatest activity occurs lies nearest the nutrient capillaries of the choroid ; both of these—pigment and a dense layer of blood vessels—for optical reasons could only be situated deeply to the visual elements. Moreover, an inverted arrangement permits an increase of the resolving power of the central region by the formation of a fovea.

THE CLOSURE OF THE EMBRYONIC FISSURE

Normally the embryonic fissure is a temporary expedient ; its formation dates from the 4·5–5 mm. stage ; during the period from the 5th to the 7th weeks (10–18 mm. stage) it closes except for a small crescent at the posterior pole of the eye, and this also becomes sealed at the 20 mm. stage. The mechanism of its closure has attracted a great deal of study.[1] It is generally true in the process of development that undifferentiated tissues remain plastic so that different layers can be readily moulded into new formations without trace of the changes they have undergone. In the region of the fissure retinal differentiation lags behind the remainder of the retina, but the cells of the inner wall proliferate rapidly throwing up a fold along each margin thus progressively reducing the width of the cleft until, at the 10–11 mm. stage, closure begins to occur. The process commences at the centre of the fissure and proceeds anteriorly towards the rim of the optic cup and posteriorly into the optic stalk ; the margins come together accurately, the two inner layers and the two outer layers fusing rapidly and becoming structurally continuous, thus leaving no trace of the situation of the cleft, while the walls of the optic cup—the outer epithelial and the inner retinal— become two uninterrupted layers forming a complete hemispherical cup (Figs. 49–51).

At the distal end of the fissure fusion is delayed until the 15 mm. stage when a small notch remains at the margin of the optic cup which at this period has reached the equator of the lens ; but this eventually disappears completely and closure is perfected long before the development of the iris. At the proximal end of the fissure this simple mode of fusion is to some extent complicated by the fact that the inner layer of the optic cup in this region grows at first more rapidly than the outer. It is consequently thrown into a number of folds and, in addition, the excessive growth leads to a slight eversion of the inner layer (Fig. 52) ; this prevents the fusion of the outer pigmented layer, thus leaving a small pale area immediately below the optic stalk (Figs. 53 and 54). In some lower animals, particularly in birds, this unpigmented region is more extensive and undergoes further differentiation,[2] but in man it rapidly becomes pigmented and, apart from a small notch at its proximal end, the fissure becomes closed at the 18 mm. stage. This notch marks the site of the enclosure of the hyaloid artery where the inner wall of the cup forms everted folds around the invaginating vessel so

[1] Wolfrum (1908), Nussbaum (1908), Seefelder (1913–23), v. Szily (1921–24), Mann (1922), Leplat (1922), Lindahl and Jokl (1922) and others.
[2] Vol. L p. 410.

FIGS. 49 to 51.—CLOSURE OF THE EMBRYONIC FISSURE OF AN 11·3 MM. EMBRYO
(after Bach and Seefelder) (×50).

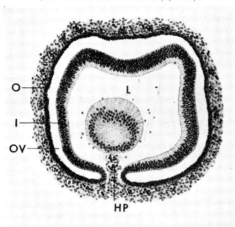

FIG. 49.—Equatorial section anteriorly through the middle of the lens. The lips of the
embryonic fissure have not fused and the hyaloid vessels invaginate between them.

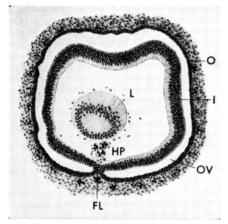

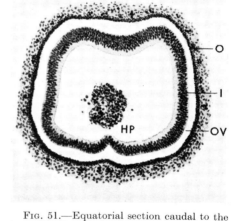

FIG. 50.—Equatorial section more caudally.
The lips of the embryonic fissure are beginning
to fuse.

FIG. 51.—Equatorial section caudal to the
lens. The lips of the fissure have fused and
the hyaloid vessels are within the vesicle.

FL. Fusion of the lips of the
    embryonic fissure.
HP. Invaginating hyaloid
    vessels.

I. Inner layer of optic cup.
L. Lens.
O. Outer layer of optic cup.
OV. Cavity of optic vesicle.

that for a time a crescentic unpigmented portion is left on the lower aspect
of the optic stalk (an inferior crescent) ; but pigment is rapidly acquired
and at the 20 mm. stage fusion is complete around the artery. In a sense,
however, it may be said that the extreme proximal end of the fissure never
closes but remains as the site of entry of the hyaloid vessels and eventually

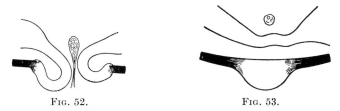

Fig. 52.   Fig. 53.

Figs. 52 and 53.—The Closure of the Embryonic Fissure at the Posterior Pole.

Showing diagrammatically the eversion of the non-pigmented inner wall of the cup (Fig. 52) which results in the formation of a large mass of non-pigmented cells in the outer wall (Fig. 53).

of the central retinal vessels. Subsequently, some time after the fissure has closed, the anterior border of the optic cup grows forwards to form the ectodermal portion of the ciliary region (50 mm. stage) and that of the iris (65 mm. stage).

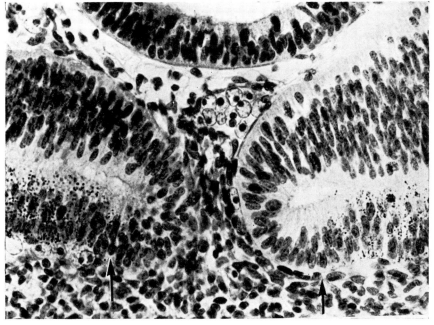

Fig. 54.—The Embryonic Fissure

In a human embryo of 14 mm., showing the slight eversion of the inner (retinal) layer with the result that the pigment of the outer layer does not reach the margin of the cleft (arrowed). Through the cleft mesodermal tissues and vessels penetrate into the cavity of the optic cup (× 373) (F. Vrabec).

The mechanism of the production of the embryonic fissure and the processes associated with its closure in various species of animals have been the subject of much research (v. Hippel, 1903 ; Mann, 1922–28 ; v. Szily, 1922 ; Leplat, 1922 ; Lindahl and Jokl, 1922). This region is characterized by a large number of variations, the structures concerned including the processus falciformis and retractor lentis muscle of bony fishes[1], the cone of reptiles[2] and marsupials[3], the pecten of birds,[4] and the glial tissue on the disc of mammals. Attempts have been made to homologize these structures, but although they all develop in association with the closing fissure, they are in no sense homologous, nor, indeed, are they all developed from the same germ layer. Thus the processus falciformis is entirely mesodermal, and is merely invaginated into the eye through the open fissure ; the retractor lentis, on the other hand, is entirely ectodermal, being developed from the cells of the fold projecting into the eye from the wall of the optic cup in the lower part of the cleft (v. Szily, 1922).[5] The pecten of birds, although considered by some to be mesodermal (Slonaker, 1921 ; Bacsich and Gellért, 1935), appears to be ectodermal at its inception and to be derived from the primitive epithelial papilla ; this becomes secondarily invaded by mesoderm, and finally consists of vascular elements encased in pigmented tissue derived from the retinal surface of the margin of the cleft (Bernd, 1905 ; Franz, 1908 ; v. Szily, 1922 ; Mann, 1922–28 ; Lindahl and Jokl, 1922). The cone of reptiles, although said by von Szily to be mesodermal, is based in its early stages upon the primitive epithelial (ectodermal) papilla and is secondarily invaded by mesoderm, being thus strictly comparable to the cognate structure in the avian eye (Leplat, 1922 ; Mann, 1922) ; this is to be expected in view of the close relationship between all the Sauropsidæ.

It is thus seen that the lower part of the retina is subject to a large number of variations, while the upper part, which subserves the lower field of vision, remains comparatively stable. Not only is the lower part ontogenetically the younger ; it is also phylogenetically the more recently developed and, incidentally, the more prone to congenital deformities. Thus in fish embryos at the stage when the optic nerve fibres first appear, the lower part of the retina is very small and slopes upwards from the optic disc so that the nerve is inserted into the lowest part of the cup ; in amphibians at this stage it is still small and runs horizontally ; in reptiles and birds it is larger and shows a tendency to a downward slope ; and it is not until mammals are reached that the lower part of the retina at this stage of development becomes equal to the upper and curves downwards in the segment of the sphere (Mann, 1928–29).

The arrangement of the optic fibres of the retina diverging from a clear-cut horizontal raphe on the temporal side of the disc,[6] as well as the occurrence of colobomata in the region of the macula,[7] suggested to some early authors that the eye rotated through 80° or 90° from its original position, and that this raphe, which ran through the macula, marked the final position of the embryonic fissure (v. Kölliker, 1861 ; Manz, 1876 ; Vossius, 1888). There was little evidence for this assumption. and the work of Chievitz (1890) definitely showed its falsity.

THE LENS PLATE AND VESICLE

We have seen that during its development the distal end of the primary optic vesicle comes into direct contact with the surface ectoderm. During the first stages of the invagination of the vesicle, early in the 4th week after fertilization (3·2 mm. stage), the cells of this region of the surface layer proliferate actively and assume a columnar shape to form a circumscribed thickened area, the LENS PLATE (Figs. 43 and 171) ; the cells involved are those of the deeper layer of epithelium, not those of the superficial epitrichial layer which may appear contemporaneously or subsequently. Cellular

[1] Vol. I, p. 299.   [2] Vol. I, pp. 362, 372, 378.   [3] Vol. I, p. 440.
[4] Vol. I, p. 410.   [5] Vol. I, p. 298, Figs. 330, 331.   [6] Vol. II, p. 236.
[7] Part 2, p. 614.

proliferation proceeds apace and shortly (5 mm. stage) the ectoderm invaginates inwards to form a depression just below the centre of the plate— the LENS PIT (*fovea lentis*). The depression gradually enlarges, and by a process comparable to the formation of the optic vesicle, its outer part becomes constricted so that during the 4th week a vesicle is formed attached to the surface layer by a short stalk the lumen of which opens onto the outside (Figs. 44 and 47). Before the week is ended or early in the subsequent week (7–9 mm. stage) the stalk atrophies, releasing the lens vesicle from the surface and isolating it as a hollow spherical body composed of a single row of cubical (ectodermal) cells. In this form it sinks inwards within the rim of the optic cup, largely filling its convexity (Fig. 55).

The connection between the optic and lens vesicles is always close. Before the primary optic vesicle commenced to invaginate, its distal wall was in contact with the surface ectoderm ; the invagination of both vesicles is synchronized and as in this process the neural ectoderm retreats from the surface, the two structures are separated by a protein-rich fluid. In histological preparations this becomes coagulated to form fine delicate fibrils which appear to connect the cells of the optic cup with those of the lens vesicle (Fig. 194). From these fibrillæ, derived partly from the surface ectoderm and partly from the neural ectoderm in association with similar elements from the mesoderm which surrounds the lens vesicle, the primary vitreous is developed to fill the remaining cavity of the optic cup (5 to 15 mm. stage).

THE ASSOCIATED MESODERM

While these two epithelial systems are developing the surrounding mesoderm makes its contribution to the ocular structures, a contribution derived mainly from the paraxial mesoderm immediately surrounding the optic cup (Fig. 55). Initially this is highly vaso-formative ; during the 5–6 mm. stage vessels in the form of simple endothelial tubes without differentiation into arteries and veins, grow from the internal carotid artery towards the lower aspect of the optic vesicle where they rapidly separate into three systems, one surrounding the optic cup and two entering the embryonic fissure. Around the external surface of the cup a dense choroidal capillary net develops beginning at the 6 to 7 mm. stage and being well established by the time the embryonic fissure has closed ; proximally, at the 7 to 8 mm. stage, the hyaloid system enters the posterior part of the embryonic fissure to supply the interior of the developing eye, ramifying through the primary vitreous and reaching the lens vesicle ; distally a second system extends anteriorly along the margins of the fissure to reach the rim of the optic cup where its branches anastomose to form an annular vessel (8–9 mm. stage) which makes connection with the hyaloid system. Meantime, the paraxial mesoderm that has been carried into the cavity of the optic cup by the lens vesicle forms the stromal components of the globe, that surrounding the cup forms its tunics as well as the upper and inner walls and contents of the orbit, while the neighbouring visceral mesoderm is responsible for the formation of the maxillary process and contributes the lower and outer walls of the orbit and the structures behind as well as the connective tissue of the lower lids.

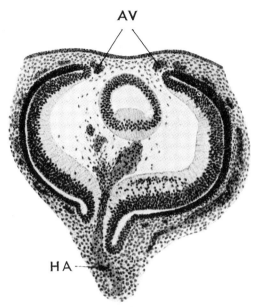

FIG. 55.—THE MESODERMAL INVASION OF THE OPTIC CUP.

By the hyaloid artery posteriorly (HA) and the annular vessel anteriorly (AV). In an embryo of 11·3 mm. (after Bach and Seefelder).

The following summary gives the derivation of the various parts of the fully formed eye from the three types of embryonic tissue (Figs. 56 to 61).

SURFACE ECTODERM gives rise to :

    The lens.
    The epithelium of the cornea.
    The epithelium of the conjunctiva and (hence) the lacrimal gland.
    The epithelium of the lids and its derivatives, the cilia, the meibomian glands, and the glands of Moll and Zeis.
    The epithelial lining of the lacrimal passages.

NEURAL ECTODERM gives rise to :

    The retina (with its pigment epithelium).
    The epithelium covering the ciliary processes.
    The pigment epithelium covering the posterior surface of the iris.
    The sphincter and dilatator pupillæ muscles.
    The optic nerve (neuroglial, nervous elements and leptomeninges).
    Part of the vitreous body.

FIGS. 56 to 61.—THE DEVELOPMENT OF THE EYE.

In each case the solid black is the neural ectoderm, the hatched layer the surface ectoderm and its derivatives, the dotted area is mesoderm ; *a*, cavity of the forebrain ; *b*, cavity of the optic vesicle ; *c*, cavity of the optic cup (or secondary optic vesicle) formed by invagination.

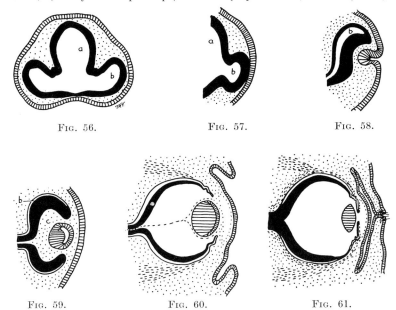

FIG. 56.   FIG. 57.   FIG. 58.

FIG. 59.   FIG. 60.   FIG. 61.

FIG. 56.—Transverse section through the anterior part of the forebrain and optic vesicles of a 4 mm. human embryo.

FIG. 57.—The primary optic vesicle.

FIG. 58.—The formation of the optic cup by invagination at the embryonic fissure ; invagination of the surface epithelium.

FIG. 59.—The optic cup and lens vesicle.

FIG. 60.—The formation of the ciliary region and iris, the anterior chamber, the hyaloid artery and the lid-folds. The lens is formed from the posterior cells of the lens vesicle.

FIG. 61.—The completed eye.

SURFACE AND NEURAL ECTODERM give rise to :

Part of the vitreous body and the suspensory ligament of the lens.

ASSOCIATED PARAXIAL MESODERM gives rise to :

The blood vessels which persist (*i.e.*, the choroidal, the central artery of the retina, the ciliary vessels and other vessels of the orbit), as well as the hyaloid artery, the vasa hyaloidea propria, and the vessels of the vascular tunic of the lens which disappear before birth.

The sclera.

The dural sheath of the optic nerve.

The ciliary muscle.

The substantia propria of the cornea and the endothelium of its posterior surface.

The stroma of the iris.

The extrinsic muscles of the eye.

The fat, ligaments and other connective tissue structures in the orbit.

The upper and inner walls of the orbit.

The connective tissue of the upper lid.

VISCERAL MESODERM (maxillary process) below the eye gives rise to :

The lower and outer walls of the orbit. The structures lying behind and below the
eye (*i.e.*, the ali-sphenoid and malar bones, and the orbital plate of the superior
maxilla).

The connective tissue of the lower lid.

The time-relationships of these developments will be found summarized on p. 291.

In describing the developing embryo or fœtus it is customary to refer a specific
phase either to the reputed time after fertilization or to its length. The latter is the
more accurate method since the time of fertilization is rarely known with certainty
and the rate of development varies with different embryos. On the other hand, the
stage of development is more constantly related to size. The length should be measured
in the fresh state before fixation ; in the embryo it is taken from end to end making
no allowance for curvature, and in the fœtus it should correctly refer to the *crown-rump*
(C.R.) *length* without taking account of the legs. Until the 5th week measurements
are very variable owing to the flexures. At the 32nd day the C.R. length is about
5·0 mm. ; thereafter, from the 32nd to the 55th day, the C.R. length of the embryo
increases approximately by 1·0 mm. per day ; after the 55th day the daily rate of growth
is approximately 1·5 mm. Although better than estimates of time, even this convention
lacks accuracy, particularly in the early stages of development ; from the 1·5 to the
5 mm. stage the most accurate assessment of the degree of development is obtained by
enumerating the number of paired somites.

Table I may be useful in giving very approximate age-length relationships at
representative stages, but the estimates of different embryologists are tantalizingly
variable, particularly up to the 5th week.

TABLE I

Very approximate figures showing the relation between age and (C.R.) length of the embryo and
fœtus

	EMBRYO		11th week	.	.	.	50–60 mm.
4th week	. . .	1 to 25 somites	12th week	.	.	.	60–70 mm.
5th week	. . .	3·4–8 mm.	4th lunar month	.	.		70–110 mm.
6th week	. . .	8–15 mm.	5th lunar month	.	.		110–150 mm.
7th week	. . .	15–22 mm.	6th lunar month	.	.		150–200 mm.
8th week	. . .	22–30 mm.	7th lunar month	.	.		200–230 mm.
	FŒTUS		8th lunar month	.	.		230–265 mm.
9th week	. . .	30–40 mm.	9th lunar month	.	.		265–300 mm.
10th week	. . .	40–50 mm.	10th lunar month	.	.		300–335 mm.

In a book devoted to the development of the eye it is unnecessary to go into
elaborate detail in the description of the stages at which all developmental changes
occur. Such an analysis was compiled by Streeter at the Carnegie Institute (1942–51)
who described 23 stages from the fertilized egg to embryos measuring 30 mm. ; these
(borrowing a term from geology) he called " developmental horizons " (see McKay
et al., 1955 ; Heuser and Corner, 1957).

Descriptions of early human embryos are available in the literature in considerable numbers. Hertig, Rock and Adams (1956), for example, have described 34 human
ova within the first 17 days of development. The following are interesting descriptions
in the literature up to the stage of the formation of the neural plate and folds :

1½ to 2½ days after fertilization (2-cell stage), Hertig and Rock (1951).

3 days (12-cell morula), Hertig *et al.* (1954).

4 to $4\frac{1}{2}$ days (blastocyst), Hertig, Rock and Adams (1956).

$7\frac{1}{2}$ and $9\frac{1}{2}$ days old, Hertig and Rock (1941–45).

$7\frac{1}{2}$ and up to 9 days old, Rock and Hertig (1942–48).

9 to 10 days old, Davies (1944), Davies and Harding (1944).

$10\frac{1}{2}$ to 11 days old, Hamilton *et al.* (1943).

11 days old, Bryce and Teacher (1908), Bryce (1924), Teacher (1924), Dible and West (1941).

13 days old, Peters (1899–1925), Linzenmeier (1914), Krafka (1941), Marchetti (1945).

$13\frac{1}{2}$ days old, Heuser, Rock and Hertig (1945), Morton (1949).

15 days old, Schlagenhaufer and Verocay (1916), von Möllendorff (1921), Brewer (1937).

16 days old, Florian (1927–30), K. M. Wilson (1945), R. G. Harrison and Jeffcoate (1953).

17 days old, Streeter (1920), Stieve (1926), Florian and Hill (1935).

18 days old, Meyer (1924), Grosser (1931), Heuser (1932), Gladstone and Hamilton, (1941).

18 to 19 days old, George (1942).

19 days old, Grosser (1913), Rossenbeck (1923), Thompson and Brash (1923).

20 days old, Spee (1889).

21 days old, Ingalls (1918).

Tissue-culture of mammalian embryos has now become established (see Dalcq, 1954). Thus Brachet (1913), Jolly and Lieure (1938) and Washburn (1951) have successfully cultivated the eggs of rodents *in vitro*, while Runner (1947) has observed the segmentation of the eggs of mice in the anterior chamber. The culture of the human ovum has presented greater difficulties, but Shettles (1954) studied its division into the 32-cell morula stage for 72 hours after fertilization. The tissue-culture of individual organs has also been achieved entirely removed from any embryonic body ; thus Strangeways and Fell (1926) cultured optic vesicles in a mixture of serum and embryonic extract through the various stages of invagination, pigmentation and retinal differentiation. Again, Tansley (1933) and Lucas and Trowell (1958) cultivated the whole eyes and retinæ of the embryos of rats 8 to 17 days old ; cytological differentiation proceeded at the normal rate but the formation of rosettes in the retina was found by the first worker.

Embryonic chick eyes have also been successfully cultivated on plasma clots (Strangeways and Fell, 1926 ; Dorris, 1938) and on an agar-tyrode medium containing embryonic extract (J. R. Harrison, 1951 ; Reinbold, 1954).

Authorities on the general embryology of the eye :

L. Bach and R. Seefelder. *Atlas zur Entwicklungsgeschichte des menschlichen Auges*, Leipzig (1914).

M. Nussbaum. *Entwicklungsgeschichte des menschlichen Auges. Graefe-Saemisch Hb. ges. Augenheilk.*, 2nd ed., Leipzig, **2** (1) (1908).

R. Seefelder. *Kurzes Hb. d. Ophthal.*, Berlin, **1**, 476 (1930).

I. C. Mann. *The Development of the Human Eye*, Cambridge (1928) ; 2nd ed., London (1949).

J. Pérez Llorca. *Arch. Soc. oftal. hisp.-amer.*, **14**, 985 (1954).

A. N. Barber. *Embryology of the Human Eye*, London (1955).

C. Dejean, F. Hervouët and G. Leplat. *L'embryologie de l'œil et sa tératologie*, Paris (1958).

Adelmann. *J. exp. Zool.*, **75**, 199 (1937).

Assheton. *Quart. J. micr. Sci.*, **54**, 221, 631 (1909–10).

Bach and Seefelder. *Atlas z. Entwicklungsges. d. mensch. Auges*, Leipzig (1914).

Bacsich and Gellért. *v. Graefes Arch. Ophthal.*, **133**, 448 (1935).

Bartelmez. *Contr. Embryol. Carneg. Instn.*, **35**, 55 (1954).

Bernd. *Die Entwicklung d. Pekten im Auge d. Hühnchens a. d. Blättern d. Augenblase* (*Diss.*), Bonn (1905).

Boyd. *J. Anat.*, **83**, 74 (1949).

Brachet. *Arch. Biol.* (Liège), **28**, 447 (1913).

Brewer. *Amer. J. Anat.*, **61**, 429 (1937).

Bryce. *Trans. roy. Soc. Edin.*, **53**, 535 (1924).

Bryce and Teacher. *Contrib. to the Study of the Early Development and Imbedding of the Human Ovum. I. An early ovum imbedding in the decidua*, Glasgow (1908).

Chievitz. *Arch. Anat.* (*Physiol.*), 332 (1890).

Dalcq. *Form and Causality in Early Development*, Camb. (1938).
  Ann. Soc. Zool. Belg., **84**, 283 (1954).
  Gaz. Med. Port., **7**, 177 (1954).

Davies. *Nature* (Lond.), **153**, 463, 684 (1944).

Davies and Harding. *J. Obstet. Gynœc. Brit. Emp.*, **51**, 225 (1944).

Dible and West. *J. Anat.*, **75**, 269 (1941).

Dorris. *J. exp. Zool.*, **78**, 385 (1938).

DuShane. *Spec. Pubs. N.Y. Acad. Sci.*, **4**, 1, (1948).

van Duyse. *Arch. Ophtal.* (Paris), **21**, 94 (1901).

Fischel. *Arch. Entwickl.-Mech. Org.*, **42**, 1 (1916).

Florian. *Anat. Anz.*, **63**, Erg., 184 (1927) ; **71**, Erg., 54 (1930).

Florian and Hill. *J. Anat.*, **69**, 399 (1935).

Franz. *Biol. Zbl.*, **28**, 467 (1908).

Froriep. *Anat. Anz.*, **29**, 145 (1906).
  Hertig's *Hb. d. vergl. u. exper. Entwicklungslehre d. Wirbeltiere*, Jena, **2** (1906).

George. *Contr. Embryol. Carneg. Instn.*, **30**, 1 (1942).

Gladstone and Hamilton. *J. Anat.*, **76**, 9 (1941).

Grosser. *Anat. Hefte*, **47**, 649 (1913).
  Z. Anat. Entwickl. Gesch., **94**, 275 (1931).

Hamilton, Barnes and Dodds. *J. Obstet. Gynœc. Brit. Emp.*, **50**, 241 (1943).

Hammond. *J. comp. Neurol.*, **91**, 67 (1949).

Hammond and Yntema. *J. comp. Neurol.*, **86**, 237 (1947).

Harrison, J. R. *J. exp. Zool.*, **118**, 209 (1951).

Harrison, R. G. *Anat. Anz.*, **85**, Erg., 4 (1937–8).

Harrison, R. G., and Jeffcoate. *J. Anat.*, **87**, 124 (1953).

Harvey and Burr. *Arch. Neurol. Psychiat.* (Chicago), **15**, 545 (1926).

Hertig and Rock. *Contr. Embryol. Carneg. Instn.*, **29**, 127 (1941) ; **31**, 65 (1945).
  Amer. J. Obstet. Gynec., *Suppl.*, **61A**, 8 (1951).

Hertig, Rock and Adams. *Amer. J. Anat.*, **98**, 435 (1956).

Hertig, Rock, Adams and Mulligan. *Contr. Embryol. Carneg. Instn.*, **35**, 199 (1954).

Heuser. *Contr. Embryol. Carneg. Instn.*, **23**, 251 (1932).

Heuser and Corner. *Contr. Embryol. Carneg. Instn.*, **36**, 29 (1957).

Heuser, Rock and Hertig. *Contr. Embryol. Carneg. Instn.*, **31**, 85 (1945).

Heuser and Streeter. *Contr. Embryol. Carneg. Instn.*, **29**, 15 (1941).

von Hippel. *v. Graefes Arch. Ophthal.*, **55**, 507, (1903).

Horstadius. *The Neural Crest*, Oxon. (1950).

Huschke. *Arch. Anat. Physiol.*, 1 (1832).

Ingalls. *Contr. Embryol. Carneg. Instn.*, **7**, 111 (1918).

Jelgersma. *Morph. Jb.*, **35**, 377 (1906).

Jolly. *Arch. Anat. micr.*, **39**, 63 (1950).

Jolly and Lieure. *Arch. Anat. micr.*, **34**, 307 (1938).

von Kölliker. *Entwicklungsgeschichte d. Menschen*, Leipzig (1861).

Krafka. *Contr. Embryol. Carneg. Instn.*, **29**, 167 (1941).

Lankester. *Darwinism and Parthenogenesis*, London (1880).

Leplat. *Anat. Anz.*, **46**, 281 (1914).
  Arch. Biol. (Liège), **30**, 231 (1919).
  C.R. Ass. Anat., **17**, 194 (1922).
  L'embryologie de l'œil (Dejean, Hervouët and Leplat), Paris, 32 (1958).

Lewis and Hartman. *Contr. Embryol. Carneg. Instn.*, **24**, 187 (1933).

Lindahl. *Arch. Augenheilk.*, **72**, 213 (1912).

Lindahl and Jokl. *Z. Anat. Entwickl. Gesch.*, **63**, 227 (1922).

Linzenmeier. *Arch. Gynäk.*, **102**, 1 (1914).

Lucas and Trowell. *J. Embryol. exp. Morph.*, **6**, 178 (1958).

McKay, Adams, Hertig and Danziger. *Anat. Rec.*, **122**, 125 (1955).

Manchot. *Arch. Entwickl.-Mech. Org.*, **116**, 689 (1929).

Mann. *J. Anat.*, **55**, 113 (1921).
  Brit. J. Ophthal., **6**, 145 (1922) ; **8**, 208 (1924).
  Development of the Human Eye, Camb. (1928 ; 1949).
  Trans. ophthal. Soc. U.K., **49**, 202 (1929).

Manz. *Klin. Mbl. Augenheilk.*, **14**, 1 (1876).

Marchetti. *Contr. Embryol. Carneg. Instn.*, **31**, 107 (1945).

Meyer. *Arch. Gynäk.*, **122**, 38 (1924).

von Möllendorff. *Z. Anat. Entwickl. Gesch.*, **62**, 352 (1921).

Morton. *J. Anat.*, **83**, 308 (1949).

Niu. *J. exp. Zool.*, **125**, 199 (1954).
  Gordon's *Pigment Cell Growth*, N.Y., 37 (1959).

Nussbaum. *Graefe-Saemisch Hb. d. ges. Augenheilk.*, 2nd ed., Leipzig, **2** (1), 1 (1908).

Peters. *Ueber die Einbettung d. mensch. Eies u. d. früheste bisher bekannte mensch. Placentationsstadium*, Leipzig (1899). *Arch. Gynäk.*, **124**, 625 (1925).

Petersen. *Ergebn. Anat. Entwickl.*, **24**, 327 (1923) ; **25**, 623 (1924).

Rawles. *Physiol. Zool.*, **20**, 248 (1947). *Physiol. Rev.*, **28**, 383 (1948).

Gordon's *Pigment Cell Growth*, N.Y. (1959).

Reinbold. *C.R. Soc. Biol.* (Paris), **148**, 1493 (1954).

Rock and Hertig. *Amer. J. Obstet. Gynec.*, **44**, 973 (1942) ; **45**, 356 (1943) ; **55**, 6 (1948).

Rossenbeck. *Z. Anat. Entwickl. Gesch.*, **68**, 325 (1923).

Runner. *Anat. Rec.*, **98**, 1 (1947).

Schlagenhaufer and Verocay. *Arch. Gynäk.*, **105**, 151 (1916).

Seefelder. *v. Graefes Arch. Ophthal.*, **73**, 419 (1910) ; **111**, 82 (1923). *Anat. Hefte*, **48**, 453 (1913).

Sensenig. *Contr. Embryol. Carneg. Instn.*, **34**, 147 (1951).

Shettles. *Trans. N.Y. Acad. Sci.*, **17**, 99 (1954).

Slonaker. *J. Morph.*, **35**, 263 (1921).

Spee. *Arch. Anat. Entwickl. Gesch.*, 159 (1889).

Spemann. *Zool. Jb., Abt. Zool. Physiol.*, **32**, 1 (1912). *Arch. mikr. Anat.*, **100**, 599 (1923).

Stieve. *Verhdl. anat. Ges. Jena*, **35**, 138 (1926).

Stockard. *J. exp. Zool.*, **6**, 285 (1909). *Amer. J. Anat.*, **10**, 369, 393 (1910) ; **15**, 253 (1913).

Stone. *Z. wiss. Biol., Abt. D.*, **118**, 40 (1929).

Strangeways and Fell. *Proc. roy. Soc. B*, **99**, 340 ; **100**, 273 (1926).

Streeter. *Contr. Embryol. Carneg. Instn.*, **9**, 389 (1920) ; **30**, 211 (1942) ; **31**, 27 (1945) ; **32**, 133 (1948) ; **34**, 165 (1951).

von Szily. *Klin. Mbl. Augenheilk.*, **45**, Beil., 201 (1907). *v. Graefes Arch. Ophthal.*, **106**, 195 (1921) ; **107**, 317 ; **109**, 3 (1922). *Z. Anat. Entwickl. Gesch.*, **74**, 1 (1924).

Tansley. *Brit. J. Ophthal.*, **17**, 321 (1933).

Teacher. *J. Obstet. Gynæc. Brit. Emp.*, **31**, 166 (1924).

Thompson and Brash. *J. Anat.*, **58**, 1 (1923).

Vossius. *Grundriss d. Augenheilkunde*, Leipzig (1888).

Washburn. *Arch. Biol.* (Liège), **62**, 439 (1951).

Wilson, J. T., and Hill. *Phil. Trans. B*, **199**, 31 (1908).

Wilson, K. M. *Contr. Embryol. Carneg. Instn.*, **31**, 101 (1945).

Woerdeman. *Arch. Entwickl.-Mech. Org.*, **116**, 220 (1929).

Wolff. *Ann. biol.* (Paris), **54**, 709 (1950).

Wolfrum. *Klin. Mbl. Augenheilk.*, **46** (2) 27 (1908).

CHAPTER III

THE DETERMINATION OF THE EYE

HANS SPEMANN [1869–1941] (Fig. 62) spent his life in a long series of brilliant researches which threw a new and revealing light on the most fundamental problem of embryology. After studying medicine at Heidelberg, Munich and Würzburg, he became a lecturer in the last university and subsequently occupied chairs in zoology in Rostock (1908–14), the Kaiser Wilhelm Institute in Berlin (1914–18) and Freiburg-im-Breisgau (1919–35). His whole working life was spent with intense concentration in a relatively narrow field of research on the development of amphibians, a subject which proved favourable for an attack on the basic determining factors in embryology which before his time was without an integrated philosophy. Starting with experiments on the mechanical constriction of the embryos of *Triton* and the grafting of their optic rudiments, he evolved the concept of " organizers " whereby he showed that organogenesis in its main outlines and in its details is the result of the interaction between different regions of tissue (1918). From this he and his school elaborated the theory of " embryonic induction ", summarized in his Croonian Lecture to the Royal Society of London (1927) ; thereafter he participated in the physico-chemical investigation of the process until his retirement in 1935, in which year he was awarded a Nobel Prize for Medicine. More than any other he laid the foundations on which a science of experimental morphogenesis has been based.

Embryological Determination

We have seen that at one time embryologists believed that the prospective fates of all parts of the ovum were already fixed or determined at the earliest stage of its development.[1] To some extent this is true since the fertilized ovum carries the full complement of genes from both parents with the potential capacity to produce a new individual reflecting the characteristics of the species. Within this general genetic control, however, three stages can be recognized in the development of any organ. Experimental embryology has shown that the cells formed in the early divisions of the egg are originally *pluripotent* (that is, capable of forming any tissue) ; at this stage the fate of the cells may be said to be " undetermined ". Driesch (1891), for example, demonstrated in the sea-urchin at the 2- and 4-cell stage that whole embryos can develop from single isolated blastomeres, while Spemann (1912), on grafting small portions of an embryo to a different region of the same or even onto another embryo, found that up to a certain stage of gastrulation the grafted tissues differentiated in conformity with the expected developmental fate of the receptor region. At some period during gastrulation, however, this plasticity becomes restricted and the future development of the different parts of the embryo becomes irrevocably fixed so that on subsequent transplantation they retain their own specific identity in the sense that they are able to form only one definite tissue. Thereafter

[1] p. 11.

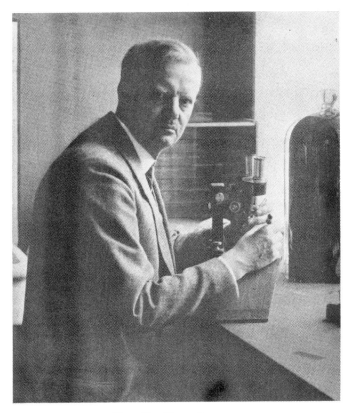

FIG. 62.—HANS SPEMANN
[1869–1941].

the primordial rudiment of the organ assumes the power of working out its own development by itself by a process continued as a result of factors residing within the cells themselves. Once " determined " the organ becomes " self-determining ".

In the earlier stages of development the embryonic tissues may thus be regarded as in a plastic state, but as development proceeds the ability of undifferentiated cells to form a diversity of structures becomes progressively restricted in a process wherein instability is gradually replaced by stability and the original plasticity of the individual parts of the embryo or an organ is replaced by " fixed fates ". The development of neural tissue from ectoderm, for example, occurs normally in the gastrula stage but this faculty is lost after this phase of development has been passed. Indeed, at this early stage the ectoderm can be induced to form any kind of neural or epidermal structure and, if exposed to the appropriate stimulus, can also be transformed into any kind of mesodermal tissue (Mangold, 1923 ; Spemann and Geinitz, 1927 ; Raven, 1935–38 ; Holtfreter, 1936 ; Spofforth, 1948).[1]

Morphogenetic Degeneration. The processes of development are not by any means confined to cellular multiplication and differentiation ; these positive events are associated with the converse change of cellular degeneration whereby structures no longer required are made to disappear. In normal development this is a regularized and tidy process, the importance of which was first stressed by A. Glücksmann (1951) ; it occurs at known times and in typical localities and is more widespread than is often realized. Scaffolding tissues are erected and when their need has passed they are cleared away and structures, usually blurred and temporary, representing the telescoped vestiges of phylogenetic history are rapidly discarded. Thus a considerable degree of cytolysis occurs during the development of the central nervous system, particularly during the transformation of the neural plate into the neural groove and tube, during the subsequent detachment of the neural tube from the overlying ectoderm, and along the dorsal root ganglia (Hamburger and Levi-Montalcini, 1949 ; Källén, 1955 ; Hamburger, 1958 ; Hughes, 1959). The process is seen dramatically in the eye when the hyaloid vascular system disappears, and to a massive degree when the tail region is being resorbed.

THE INDUCTION OF TISSUES

THE CHEMICAL CONTROL. It can well be imagined that a process which involves a series of changes so complicated and necessarily so interrelated can only proceed if subjected to constant and rigorous control both in its temporal and spatial aspects, a control which includes at one time the stimu-

---

[1] Some embryologists make a distinction between embryonic tissues still capable of further segregation and those which have reached their final destination by using the suffix -*blast* for the former and -*derm* for the latter.

lation, at another the inhibition of the genetic potentialities contained within each cell. It is shown in another volume in this series[1] that genetic transmission is chemical in nature, the code being handed down in the nucleic acids of the chromosomes and transferred into structural and metabolic terms by enzymic activity. It is not surprising therefore that, as was first conclusively demonstrated by Spemann (1901–21), the essential control which organizes the development of the embryo and determines how and when this or that genetic potentiality is realized or damped down, is chemical in nature. Such substances, elaborated in the cytoplasm of the cell and apparently unconnected with the nucleus, were first discovered in the dorsal lip of the amphibian blastopore and called ORGANIZERS by Spemann (1912) ; the process by which they influence development has become known as INDUCTION. The first stage of embryogenesis wherein the fundamental tissues are differentiated is controlled by *primary* organizers ; the process of organogenesis (the development of an organ such as the optic cup from the primordial neuroblastic tissue) by *secondary* organizers ; while the differentiation of tissues within the developing organ (the induction of the cornea and lens by the optic cup) forms a process of *tertiary* organization. To achieve the regulated sequence necessary, the action of each of these is related in time to the phase of development, appearing when required and disappearing when the task is done ; indeed, individual organizers do not usually retain their inductive ability for more than a limited period during which the cells or tissues undergoing induction remain competent to react to the organizing influence. It may therefore be said that normal tissue differentiation is essentially dependent upon the presence of an appropriately situated organizer or inductor on the one hand, and a specific responsiveness on the part of the tissue on the other, and that development consists of a progressive determination of embryonic parts to pursue fixed fates, the process being initiated by the primary organizer and carried on under the ægis of the secondary and tertiary organizing centres (Needham, 1942). The potential capacity inherent in most embryonic tissues to be thus regulated was formulated by Driesch (1929) in the concept of " the harmonic equipotential system ".

These organizers are elaborated in specific regions whence they spread by diffusion ; mechanical separation of this region from a specific tissue ordinarily responsive, whether it be by section (Spemann, 1912–38) or by the interposition of a layer of cellophane (McKeehan, 1951), stops the differentiation of the latter. The integrity of the cells concerned in the elaboration of the organizers, however, is not necessary for the inductive effect. They are non-living substances since cell-free extracts produce the same effects as the organizer cells ; crushing the cells, for example, has little or no deleterious effect upon this activity (Spemann, 1931) (Fig. 63), and the potency remains unimpaired after boiling, desiccation, freezing or treatment with alcohol

[1] Vol. VII, p. 35.

(Waddington, 1933–34 ; Luther, 1935 ; Lallier, 1950). It may indeed be that some degree of cellular destruction (morphogenetic degeneration) is an essential process in their liberation (Brachet, 1947).

Despite much work expended on their identification the chemical nature of these organizing substances is still in doubt.[1] They are, however, lipoidal and probably of a steroid nature having a structure similar to the corticosteroids and the bile acids (Needham, 1950) ; some œstrogenic hormones (dimethylphenanthrene) and certain carcinogenic substances (dibenzanthracene) possess organizing activity (Waddington and Needham, 1936 ; and others). In any event, it would seem that a variety of substances is involved, the inductors evoking the differentiation of mesoderm, for example, differing from those responsible for the production of neural tissue (Chuang, 1939). They are not, however, specific. Thus Spemann found that the evocator of the neural tissue of frogs when injected into newts, produced nerve tissue characteristic of the newt, not of the frog, a finding which indicates that the organizer produces nerve tissue in general while other factors determine its specific character.

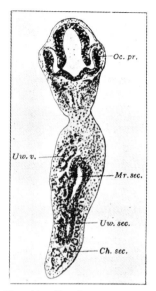

FIG. 63.—THE INDUCTION OF A SECONDARY EMBRYO BY THE IMPLANTATION OF CRUSHED ORGANIZER MATERIAL.

Oc. pr., host eye-cup ; *Mr. sec.*, induced neural tube ; *Uw. sec.*, induced somites ; *Ch. sec.*, induced notochord ; *Uw. v.*, accessory somite (Hans Spemann ; from Needham's *Biochemistry and Morphogenesis*, Cambridge Univ. Press).

It is interesting that the inductive process is associated with considerable metabolic as well as morphological activity. Anaerobic glycolysis becomes intense (Brachet, 1932–35 ; Stefanelli, 1937–41 ; Dalcq, 1954 ; de Vincentiis, 1957), substances blocking –SH activity act as inhibitors (Brachet, 1941), while the ribonucleic acid is increased out of all proportion to the normal content of the tissue (Brachet, 1941 ; Gallera, 1946 ; Needham, 1950 ; Rickenbacher, 1952 ; Töndury, 1954–55 ; and others).

Chemical stimulation and control, however, cannot alone explain all the facts of embryological development. *Genetic influences*, of course, are paramount, determining the gross differences between species and the more subtle differences between individuals of the same species. Embryonic differentiation is also determined by the complicated *interrelationships and interaction between the tissues* (Spemann, 1921 ; Waddington, 1932 ; Weiss, 1939) ; indeed, in the developing embryo its constituent parts must be regarded as dynamically interrelated and continuously reacting to each other

---

[1] Toivonen and Kuusi (1948), Toivonen (1949–51), Yamada (1950), Kuusi (1951), Hayashi (1956), Yamada and Takata (1956).

and to their environment, a relationship expressed by Needham (1942) in the concept of the *morphogenetic field*. In this respect the supreme importance of the role played by the third primary germ layer in embryogenesis was demonstrated by Holtfreter (1933) who found that if the mesoderm is experimentally prevented from taking up its normal position beneath the ectoderm, the latter is incapable of differentiation and merely develops into a mass of unspecialized epidermal cells. Similarly, in the sturgeon, without the surrounding mesenchyme the optic vesicle is incapable of forming pigmentary epithelium and develops entirely into sensory retinal tissue (Dabagian, 1959). As we have seen, the ectoderm possesses very wide potentialities of differentiation when exposed to suitable inductive stimuli, but although a cell responds to such a stimulus by differentiation in a certain direction and acquires the tendencies characteristic of this type, suitable environmental conditions provided by the formative influence of the surrounding tissues are necessary for these tendencies to be manifested and developed.

MECHANICAL FACTORS also play a part in the regulation of embryonic development. Thus, the moulding of the anterior part of the rudimentary central nervous system into the normal configuration of brain and bilaterally arranged eyes appears to be effected by the hydrostatic pressure generated within the neural tube resulting from the secretion of fluid from the ependymal cells lining its wall. It would appear that the association of the hydrostatic pressure on the inside of the tube with the restraint offered by the confining skull-capsule on the outside, modulates the continued enlargement of the brain and leads to a configuration which, depending on local conditions, is eventually manifested as the fissures and folds characteristic of the adult. Moreover, it has been shown by the Coulombres (1956–60) that the intra-ocular pressure exerts a considerable influence on the harmonious development of the globe of the eye, governing to some extent its rate of growth and the mutual spatial adjustment of its various parts ; if, for example, a capillary tube is inserted into the vitreous and the intra-ocular pressure is artificially reduced, the cornea and the ciliary processes fail in their normal development. This influence, however, is of secondary importance, merely translating the processes essentially determined by genetic and chemical factors and the mutually reacting influence of the surrounding tissues into specific spatial configurations (Weiss, 1950 ; Badtke, 1952).

The Determination of Embryogenesis

As would be expected, although descriptive embryology so far as human development is concerned is now on a reasonably secure basis, experimental embryology is largely based on the study of lower forms, particularly amphibians and birds, specimens of which are more readily obtained in a good state of preservation at any desired period, even at the early stages of development. Although many of our conceptions are thus based on experimental work carried out on the embryos of oviparous types, it seems likely that the preliminary stages of development in all vertebrates are so akin that the results obtained can reasonably be accepted as applicable by analogy in principle if not in detail.

The process and course of embryogenesis are determined at a very early stage, possibly at the time of fertilization. Even at the 2-cell stage it would seem that some difference exists between the future dorsal and ventral

FIGS. 64 and 65.—THE INDUCTION OF A SECONDARY EMBRYO BY
TRANSPLANTATION OF THE ORGANIZER.

(Needham's *Biochemistry and Morphogenesis*).

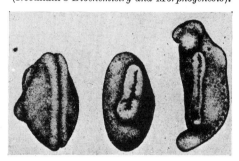

FIG. 64.—On the left, the host embryo from above ; in the centre, the host embryo from the side showing the induced neural folds ; on the right, the same at a later stage.

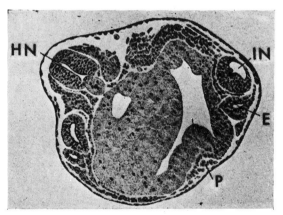

FIG. 65.—Transverse section showing the two medullary tubes. HN, host medullary tube ; IN, induced medullary tube ; E, induced otic vesicle ; P, pericardium. The fundamental experiment of Hans Spemann and H. Mangold.

aspects of the ovum ; one blastomere is usually larger and subdivides earlier than the other, and if the two are separated only one usually forms a complete embryo (Spemann, 1901–3 ; Mangold, 1920 ; Spemann and Mangold, 1924 ; Mangold and Seidel, 1927). The first accurate localization of organizing activity, however, was demonstrated by Spemann (1912) to lie in the region of *the dorsal lip of the blastopore* in the amphibian gastrula. If this region is removed the normal development of the embryo does not proceed (Lewis, 1904 ; Spemann, 1912) ; if all or parts of it are grafted into the undetermined tissue of another blastula or an early gastrula, the host tissues are stimulated to form, or to attempt to form, the tissues of a secondary embryo (Figs. 64 to 66) ; and if the part of the embryo cephalad to the blastopore is cut off, rotated through 90° and then replaced, development proceeds with

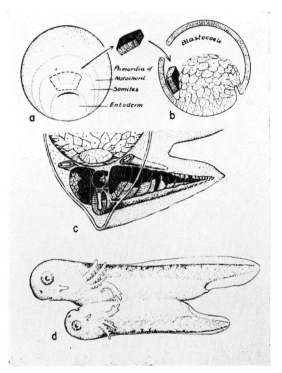

Fig. 66.—The Transplantation of the Upper Lip of the Blastopore into Another Gastrula.

In an amphibian. *a, b,* the transplantation of the upper lip of the blastopore into another gastrula. *c,* showing self-differentiations plus inductions of the graft. The tissues derived from the graft are shown in black and the induced tissues in white. *d,* shows the resultant fœtus (Holtfreter and Hamburger in *Analysis of Development* ; W. B. Saunders & Co.).

the axial structures in the meridian of the blastopore and not in the position which they would have occupied in the rotated segment. Similarly, in the developing chick, Waddington and Schmidt (1933) and Woodside (1937) showed that if a fragment of the primitive streak and the node of Hensen were grafted between the primary layers of another blastula, a secondary embryo with a new neural plate developed. In the higher vertebrates the same region is involved—the *chorda-mesoblast* which includes the notochord and the paraxial mesoderm developed from it which insinuates itself between the ectoderm and the endoderm.[1]

This organizing region has been shown to be responsible for the development of all the neural structures in the region of the head (including the optic vesicles). Other organizers are responsible for the development of the remainder of the body ; these *trunk-organizers* are developed by the chorda-mesoderm which invaginates at a later stage, but the difference between them and the *head-organizers* is probably quantitative and temporal rather than qualitative (Gallera, 1947 ; Dalcq and Lallier, 1948).

In the earlier stages the organizer acts upon ectodermal cells which are still undifferentiated and pluripotent, endowing them with the " potency " of forming an eye. Thus Spemann (1912) showed in amphibians that if two portions from two different embryos representing respectively a piece of the anterior part of the presumptive neural tube and a portion of presumptive abdominal skin, are removed at the stage before gastrulation is complete and are interchanged, development proceeds in a normal way so that the presumptive abdominal skin produces the optic vesicle. After the stage of gastrulation has passed, however, the capacity of the ectoderm to be thus induced is lost (Mangold, 1920–31 ; Mangold and von Woellwarth, 1950). The period during which induction of the ocular primordium can occur has been confirmed by the experimental production of monstrosities by the application of toxins to the developing embryo (Brachet, 1907–14 ; Leplat, 1922) ; if the lesion occurs during gastrulation (before the closure of the blastopore, that is, during the stage of *acrogenesis*), only the cells which eventually form the olfactory and visual apparatus will be interfered with, so that the resulting embryos are anophthalmic, showing no trace whatever of an eye ; if, on the other hand, interference is delayed until after the closure of the blastopore (that is, during the stage of *cephalogenesis*) various degrees of deformity of the eyes such as cyclopia, may be produced.

THE DETERMINATION OF THE HEAD

It would appear most probable that two mesodermal organizing centres control the development of the head-region in vertebrates (Marchesani, 1949 ; Hövels, 1953 ; Morlinghaus, 1955), but the relations between these are still obscure.

(1) An anterior PROSENCEPHALIC CENTRE, situated in the prechordal mesoblast lying in front of the anterior end of the notochord and Rathke's pouch, which induces the prosencephalon, the visual and the auditory apparatus. Disturbances of this centre result in gross ocular deformities such as cyclopia and arhinencephaly.

(2) A posterior RHOMBENCEPHALIC CENTRE, situated in the parachordal mesoblast in close relation to the cephalic part of the notochord, which induces the visceral skeleton of the face, the outer and middle ear, and the

---

[1] Mangold (1920–31), Lehmann (1928–37), Adelmann (1930–37), Holtfreter (1933), Töndury (1938), von Aufsess (1942), Pasteels (1945), Gallera (1949), and others.

subjacent endodermal foregut. Malformations of this centre result typically in anomalies affecting the first visceral arch and cleft, such as otocephaly and mandibulo-facial dysostosis.

The development of the eye from the optic primordium as a localized and discrete system provides one of the best examples of inductive activity. When the optic pits have been formed, however, the course of their further differentiation is not yet rigidly determined. To some extent they assume a limited power of working out their own development by themselves by secondary inductive processes ; thus in the salamander a small portion of the rudiment appears, under certain conditions, to be able to reproduce a perfect whole (Székely, 1957). Spemann (1921), for example, showed that if a portion of the neural tube containing the primordial eye were cut out, rotated through 180°, and then replaced, four small but complete eyes appeared, and not four halves, as might have been expected. It thus appears that, within limits, the optic pit always tends to form the normal organ no matter how much it is cut about (Petersen, 1923–4) ; although when very small parts are taken, clumps of pigmented cells only may develop. It seems, therefore, that not only the eye-primordium but any considerable portion of it becomes endowed with the potentiality of forming the entire adult eye.

The extent to which the eye is autonomous in this respect has excited some controversy. Several observations would suggest that it can develop as an isolated system, while there is much evidence that the optic primordium is a labile field subject to a considerable extent to the controlling influence of the underlying mesoderm. Thus, on the one hand, Lewis (1907) found that the primary optic vesicle grew and differentiated when grafted subcutaneously in abnormal positions such as the back or abdomen ; Hoadley (1924–25) showed that the ocular primordium of the embryonic fowl grew and developed readily on a graft upon the chorio-allantoic membrane ; while Strangeways and Fell (1926) and Spratt (1940) succeeded in cultivating explanted embryonic eyes of the fowl. On the other hand, several writers have confirmed that a large proportion (75 to 100%) of *Amblystoma* embryos develops gross ocular abnormalities following extirpation of the pre-chordal mesoderm (Mangold, 1931 ; Adelmann, 1937). Again, Holtfreter (1939) found that without this supporting mesenchyme the optic vesicles do not develop into the double layered optic cup and that eyes isolated *in vitro* and separated from the matrix of the mesenchyme which normally surrounds the developing vesicle attain only the most rudimentary level of organization. Holtfreter's work has served to expose perhaps better than any other the extreme limitation of the optic rudiment as an autogenous developmental unit and it may well be that the conflicting experimental evidence on the subject in the literature may be due to the fact that in transplantation experiments the optic vesicle has to some extent retained its normal environment so far as mesenchymal tissue is concerned (Twitty, 1955).

As differentiation proceeds, the plasticity of the ocular tissues is gradually lost, a process which can be exemplified in a number of instances. In the early stages of development during the process of the invagination of the optic vesicle, for example, the embryonic fissure may be induced to develop at any part of the vesicle. Thus in *Triton*, if the vesicle is rotated at an early stage of development through 180°, a secondary vesicle develops with a fissure in the normal ventral position ; if at a later stage, two fissures are formed, a principal ventral and an accessory dorsal ; at a still later stage, a principal dorsal and an accessory ventral (Sato, 1933 ; Barden, 1942 ; Woerdeman, 1950). Similarly, Stone (1948), studying the functional polarization of the retina in *Amblystoma punctatum*, found that up to the late tail-bud stages the eye could be rotated through 180° without normal vision being affected ; if, however, it were rotated at the developmental stage at which the first motor responses occur in the embryo, the subsequent visuo-motor reactions of the animal appear to become reversed and confused.

After the optic cup has been formed the orientation of the sensory layers may be changed up to the time when morphological differentiation begins. Thus, Eakin (1947) found that by reversing surgically the outer and inner surfaces of the inner layer of the optic cup prior to this stage, the retina developed with the normal arrangement of the percipient cells facing the pigment epithelium, while on reversal at a later stage the rods and cones remained facing towards the lens. It may be that induction not only by the pigment layer but also by the lens plays a part in the establishment of polarity within the inner layer of the cup.

Even when differentiation has proceeded to the stage of the formation of the optic cup, development does not proceed on a rigidly determined mosaic ; for a period a considerable degree of plasticity remains and it would appear that the assignment of specific roles to the constituent cells of the rudiment is controlled by morphogenetic influences which continue to operate throughout the period of the development of the retina, and in this respect the (relatively undifferentiated) outer layer of the cup (the pigment epithelium) is more potent than the more highly differentiated inner (sensory) layer. Several workers have shown that in some lower animals the retinal and pigmented layers of the optic cup may interchange prospective roles : small pieces of prospective retinal pigment epithelium and retinal sensory layers when transplanted separately can each form both pigmentary and nervous tissue (Dragomirow, 1932–36 ; Alexander, 1937 ; Dorris, 1938). Thus in *Triton*, small pieces of prospective pigment epithelium grafted between the lens and cornea and even to heterotopic positions elsewhere on the head will form small optic cups the walls of which are formed of both pigment and sensory layers ; while Detwiler and van Dyke (1953–54) have demonstrated that the part of the optic vesicle destined to become pigmented epithelium can differentiate into apparently normal retinal tissue if grafted into the acoustic primordium.

To some extent this problem is illustrated by experiments designed to explore the regenerative powers of adult retinæ, regarding which the most detailed work has been

FIGS. 67 to 72.—REGENERATION OF THE RETINA.

To show the regeneration of the retina of the adult *Triturus v. viridescens* from the pigmentary epithelium after removal of the original sensory retina (L. S. Stone, *J. exp. Zool.*).

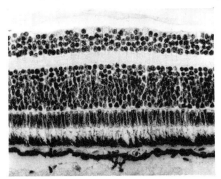

FIG. 67.—Normal retina.

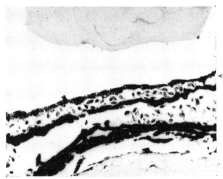

FIG. 68.—The pars optica retinæ removed, denuding the pigment epithelium (6 days later). The arrow indicates the pigment layer left *in situ* lying above the choroid.

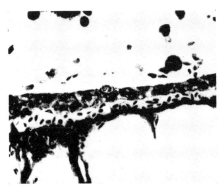

FIG. 69.—Ten days after removal. Proliferation of the pigment layer, some of the cells of which show mitotic figures.

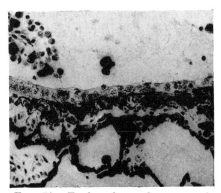

FIG. 70.—Twelve days after removal. Depigmented cells derived from the pigment epithelium forming a continuous layer.

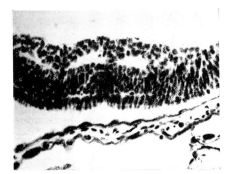

FIG. 71.—Thirty days after removal. The neural retina is regenerating and the differentiation of retinal layers is beginning in a limited area.

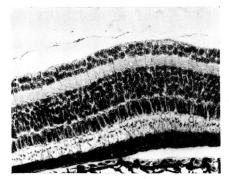

FIG. 72.—Fifty-seven days after removal. A fully regenerated functional retina has developed.

done by Stone and his colleagues (1940–60). If the eyes of adult urodeles are transplanted, the neural elements of the retina degenerate during the first three weeks and are then replaced by new neural tissue which later becomes functional ; regeneration followed by the return of vision can take place in the same eye even if it is repeatedly transplanted. The evidence seems conclusive that during regeneration the retinal pigment cells are the only source of origin of the new neural retina (Figs. 67 to 72), the sequence of events being the same whether the neural retina is eliminated by degeneration as in grafted eyes or is mechanically removed.

In the literature, however, reports are found of retinal regeneration arising from the pars iridica retinæ of grafted fragments of iris, and (in *Triton*) regeneration of the whole eye from a portion of iris transplanted to the region of the labyrinth is possible

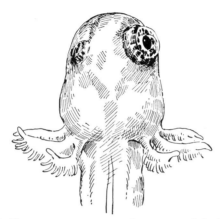

FIG. 73.—Larva of *Amblystoma punctatum* carrying an eye of the larger *tigrinum* species (Needham's *Biochemistry and Morphogenesis*, Cambridge Univ. Press).

(Wachs, 1914 ; Sato, 1930–33 ; Ikeda, 1934–37 ; Monroy, 1937–39). It may well be, however, as Stone (1950) insists, that a transplant of iris tissue alone never forms retinal tissue, and that these experimental results may be explained by the incomplete removal of the peripheral portion of the retina.

In these transplantation experiments, however, the grafted tissue does not act as an independent entity, but to some extent is subject to the regulatory control of the host. Thus in transplanting the developing eyes between *Amblystoma tigrinum* and *A. punctatum*, Heath (1957) found that the small eye exchanged heteroplastically to the larger host, after an initial post-operative period, grew at a sharply accelerated rate (Fig. 73). It would therefore seem that, as occurs in normal development, there is a considerable degree of reciprocity among all the tissues concerned.

Adelmann. *J. exp. Zool.*, **57**, 223 (1930) ; **67**, 217 (1934) ; **75**, 199 (1937).
Alexander. *J. exp. Zool.*, **75**, 41 (1937).
von Aufsess. *Arch. Entwickl.-Mech. Org.*, **141**, 248 (1942).
Badtke. *v. Graefes Arch. Ophthal.*, **152**, 671 (1952).
Barden. *J. exp. Zool.*, **90**, 479 (1942).
Brachet. *Arch. Biol.* (Liège), **23**, 165 (1907) ; **29**, 501 (1914) ; **46**, 25 (1935).
 C.R. Soc. Biol. (Paris), **110**, 562 (1932).
 Enzymol., **10**, 87 (1941).

Embryologie chimique, Paris (1944).
 Growth Symp., **11**, 309 (1947).
Chuang. *Arch. Entwickl.-Mech. Org.*, **139**, 556 (1939).
Coulombre, A. J. *J. exp. Zool.*, **133**, 211 (1956).
 Arch. Ophthal. (Chicago), **57**, 250 (1957).
Coulombre, A. J., and J. L. *Amer. J. Ophthal.*, **44** (2), 85 (1957).
 Arch. Ophthal. (Chicago), **59**, 502 (1958).
 Smelser's *The Structure of the Eye*, N.Y. 83 (1960).

Dabagian. *Dokl. Akad. Nauk.*, **125**, 938 (1959).

Dalcq. *Gaz. med. Port.*, **7**, 177 (1954).
Ann. Soc. Zool. Belg., **84**, 283 (1954).

Dalcq and Lallier. *C.R. Ass. Anat.*, **35**, 160 (1948).

Detwiler and van Dyke. *J. exp. Zool.*, **122**, 367 (1953) ; **126**, 135 (1954).

Dorris. *J. exp. Zool.*, **78**, 385 (1938).

Dragomirow. *Arch. Entwickl.-Mech. Org.*, **126**, 636 (1932) ; **129**, 522 (1933) ; **131**, 540 (1934) ; **134**, 716 (1936).

Driesch. *Z. wiss. Zool.*, **53**, 160 (1891).
The Science and Philosophy of the Organism, London (1908) ; 2nd ed. (1929).

Eakin. *Univ. Calif. Publ. Zool.*, **51**, 245 (1947).

Gallera. *C.R. Soc. Biol.* (Paris), **140**, 1155 (1946).
Arch. Biol. (Liège), **58**, 221 (1947).
C.R. Ass. Anat., **34**, 201 (1947) ; **36**, 353 (1947).

Glücksmann. *Biol. Rev.*, **26**, 59 (1951).

Hamburger. *Amer. J. Anat.*, **89**, 133 (1958).

Hamburger and Levi-Montalcini. *J. exp. Zool.*, **111**, 457 (1949).

Hayashi. *Embryologia*, **3**, 57 (1956).

Heath. *J. exp. Zool.*, **135**, 425 (1957).

Hoadley. *Biol. Bull.*, *Woods Hole*, **46**, 281 (1924).
J. exp. Zool., **42**, 163 (1925).

Hövels. *Z. Kinderheilk.*, **73**, 532 (1953).

Holtfreter. *Arch. Entwickl.-Mech. Org.*, **129**, 669 (1933) ; **134**, 466 (1936).
Arch. exp. Zellforsch., **23**, 169 (1939).

Hughes. *J. Embryol. exp. Morph.*, **7**, 22 (1959).

Ikeda. *Arb. Anat. Inst. Univ. Sendai*, **16**, 1, 47, 69 (1934) ; **17**, 11 (1935) ; **18**, 1, 17 (1936) ; **20**, 17 (1937).

Källén. *J. Anat.*, **89**, 153 (1955).

Kuusi. *Ann. Soc. Zool. Botan. Fenn. Vanamo*, **14**, 1 (1951).

Lallier. *Experientia* (Basel), **6**, 92 (1950).

Lehmann. *Arch. Entwickl.-Mech. Org.*, **113**, 123 (1928) ; **136**, 112 (1937).

Leplat. *C.R. Ass. Anat.*, **17**, 194 (1922).

Lewis. *Amer. J. Anat.*, **3**, 505 (1904) ; **6**, 473 (1906–7) ; **7**, 259 (1907).

Luther. *Biol. Zbl.*, **55**, 114 (1935).

McKeehan. *J. exp. Zool.*, **117**, 31 (1951).

Mangold. *Arch. Entwickl.-Mech. Org.*, **47**, 249 (1920) ; **100**, 198 (1923).
Ergebn. Biol., **7**, 193 (1931).

Mangold and Seidel. *Arch. Entwickl.-Mech. Org.*, **111**, 594 (1927).

Mangold and von Woellwarth. *Naturwissenschaften*, **37**, 365 (1950).

Marchesani. *Ber. dtsch. ophthal. Ges.*, **55**, 34 (1949).

Monroy. *Arch. Entwickl.-Mech. Org.*, **137**, 25 (1937) ; **139**, 536 (1939).

Morlinghaus. *Ueber multiple Missbildungen bei Fehlbildungen d. ersten Visceralbogens* (Thesis), Frankfurt (1955).

Needham. *Biochemistry and Morphogenesis*, Camb. (1942 ; 1950).

Pasteels. *Arch. Biol.* (Liège), **56**, 105 (1945).

Petersen. *Ergebn. Anat. Entwickl.*, **24**, 327 (1923) ; **25**, 623 (1924).

Raven. *Proc. Kon. Akad. Wet. Amst.*, **38**, 1107 (1935).
Arch. Entwickl.-Mech. Org., **132**, 509 (1935) ; **137**, 611 (1938).

Rickenbacher. *Arch. Entwickl.-Mech. Org.*, **145**, 387 (1952).

Sato. *Arch. Entwickl.-Mech. Org.*, **122**, 451 (1930) ; **128**, 342 ; **130**, 19 (1933).

Spemann. *Verhdl. Anat. Ges. Halle*, 61 (1901).
Arch. Entwickl.-Mech. Org., **12**, 224 (1901) ; **16**, 551 (1903) ; **48**, 533 (1921).
Zool. Jb., Abt. Zool. Physiol., **32**, 1 (1912) ; Suppl. 5, **34**, 129 (1931).
Embryonic Development and Induction, New Haven (1938).

Spemann and Geinitz. *Arch. Entwickl.-Mech. Org.*, **109**, 129 (1927).

Spemann and Mangold. *Arch. Entwickl.-Mech. Org.*, **100**, 599 (1924).

Spofforth. *J. exp. Zool.*, **99**, 35 (1948).

Spratt. *J. exp. Zool.*, **85**, 171 (1940).

Stefanelli. *J. exp. Biol.*, **14**, 171 (1937).
Boll. Soc. ital. Biol. sper., **12**, 284 (1937).
Arch. Sci. Biol., **27**, 74 (1941).

Stone. *Proc. Soc. exp. Biol.* (N.Y.), **44**, 639 (1940).
Arch. Ophthal. (Chicago), **35**, 135 (1946).
Trans. ophthal. Soc. U.K., **67**, 349 (1947).
Ann. N.Y. Acad. Sci., **49**, 856 (1948).
J. exp. Zool., **113**, 9 (1950).
Yale J. Biol. Med., **32**, 464 (1960).

Stone and Chace. *Anat. Rec.*, **79**, 333 (1941).

Stone and Farthing. *J. exp. Zool.*, **91**, 265 (1942).

Stone and Zaur. *J. exp. Zool.*, **85**, 243 (1940).

Strangeways and Fell. *Proc. roy. Soc. B*, **100**, 273 (1926).

Székely. *Arch. Entwickl.-Mech. Org.*, **150**, 48 (1957).

Töndury. *Arch. Entwickl.-Mech. Org.*, **137**, 510 (1938).
Ciba Symp., **2**, 138 (1954).
Naturwissenschaften, **42**, 312 (1955).
Münch. med. Wschr., **97**, 1009 (1955).

Toivonen. *Experientia* (Basel), **5**, 323 (1949).
Rev. suisse Zool., **57**, 41 (1950).
Arch. Soc. Zool. Botan. Fenn. Vanamo, **6**, 63 (1951).

Toivonen and Kuusi. *Ann. Soc. Zool. Botan. Fenn. Vanamo*, **13**, 1 (1948).

Twitty. In *Analysis of Development*, Phila., 404 (1955).

de Vincentiis. *Sui fattori che presiedono al differenziamento dell'abbozzo oculare con particolare riguardo alla morfogenesi del cristallino*, Torino (1957).

Wachs. *Arch. Entwickl.-Mech. Org.*, **39**, 384 (1914).

Waddington. *Phil. Trans. B*, **221**, 179 (1932).
Nature (Lond.), **131**, 275 (1933).
J. exp. Biol., **11**, 211 (1934).
Proc. roy. Soc. B, **125**, 365 (1938).

Waddington and Needham. *Proc. kon. Akad. wet. Amst.*, **39**, 887 (1936).

Waddington and Schmidt. *Arch. Entwickl.-Mech. Org.*, **128**, 522 (1933).

Weiss. *Principles of Development*, N.Y. (1939).
Quart. Rev. Biol., **25**, 177 (1950).

Woerdeman. *Ann. biol.* (Paris), **54**, 699 (1950).

Woodside. *J. exp. Zool.*, **75**, 259 (1937).

Yamada. *Embryologia*, **1**, 1 (1950).

Yamada and Takata. *Embryologia*, **3**, 69 (1956).

Secondary Inductions

After the determination of the neural ectoderm from the optic primordium the development of the remaining ocular tissues proceeds by a series of secondary inductions—the lens placode, the cornea and the lids essentially under the influence of the optic cup, the sclera under the influence of the retinal pigment epithelium.

THE INDUCTION OF THE LENS

Once the optic vesicle is formed from the neural ectoderm, the surface ectoderm with which it comes into contact contributes the dioptric apparatus. We have seen that a thickening in this region constitutes the forerunner of the lens, and there is little doubt that the lens plate formed in this way

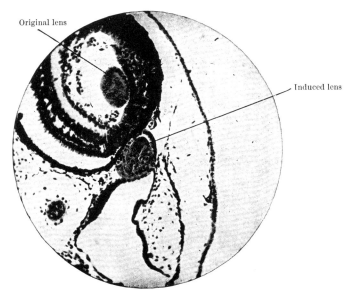

Original lens

Induced lens

Fig. 74.—INDUCTION OF LENS BY THE OPTIC CUP FROM THE WALL OF THE OTIC VESICLE. In an amphibian (Needham's *Biochemistry and Morphogenesis*, Cambridge Univ. Press).

results primarily from chemical induction from the underlying neural tissue. Thus, in amphibians if the optic vesicle is removed or is too small to reach the surface layer, differentiation of the latter into a lens does not occur (Lewis, 1903–7 ; Harrison, 1920) ; nor does it occur unless the contact

between the two epithelial layers has been intimate since their separation by
the interpolation of mesodermal tissue (Weiss, 1950) or a thin sheet of cellophane (McKeehan, 1951) or a membrane of high porosity (de Vincentiis,
1957) inhibits the formation of the lens plate. It is interesting that in
Leplat's (1913–40) work on artificially produced monsters, in no case did he
find a lens apart from contact with an optic vesicle, although in 60% of
cases in one series an abnormal optic vesicle was present without a lens. This
phenomenon of lens-induction can act over a considerable time so that
repeated extirpation of the specialized ectoderm may be followed by successive regenerations (seven times in succession, Nikitenko, 1937). It would
seem, however, that the chemical stimulant may eventually become exhausted
since Manuilova (1935–38) found that the third lens of such a series was ill-

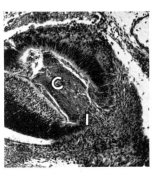 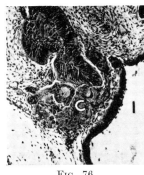 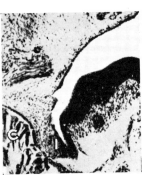

FIG. 75.   FIG. 76.   FIG. 77.

FIGS. 75 to 77.—THE DEPENDENCE OF THE DIFFERENTIATION OF THE IRIS ON THE LENS.

In fœtal rats subjected to folic acid deficiency. In the resulting microphthalmic eyes
the differentiation of the iris (I) is limited to the region where contact can be made between
the optic cup and the lens (C). In Fig. 76, where the lens is in contiguity with the surface
epithelium, this is transformed into iris tissue (A. Giroud).

developed whereafter the power of further lens regeneration was lost, to
return only after an interval. The period during which induction can occur,
however, is limited ; thus in the frog and *Amblystoma*, Liedke (1942–51)
noted that the ectoderm retained the " competence " of lens-formation
only while the neural canal remained opened. It should be noted, however,
that the optic vesicle is not the only tissue which may induce the surface
ectoderm to lens-formation ; Okada and Mikami (1937) found that a
similar response could be elicited by the olfactory primordium, the otic
vesicle and brain tissue (Fig. 74).

It is also probable that the final differentiation of the lens is to some
extent dependent on the influence of the neighbouring mesoderm (Jacobson,
1955) ; in this respect an analogy with the development of the otic placode
is suggestive for it seems clear that both ectodermal and mesodermal tissue
participate in the induction of the labyrinth. This reciprocity in inductive

processes so that the whole of development is coordinated is seen in the reciprocal influence of the lens on the developing retina. Thus in *Amblystoma*, Beckwith (1927) found that the removal of the lens vesicle resulted in failure of the closure of the embryonic cleft, an anomaly which did not occur if a lens were regenerated from the iris.[1] The findings of Reyer (1950-4) were comparable—that removal of the lens led to thickening and folding of the retina, reduction of the vitreous, and absence of the anterior chamber as well as failure of invagination of the optic vesicle—while Giroud (1957) showed experimentally in rats that the development of the iris was dependent upon contiguity with the lens (Figs. 75 to 77). All this evidence seems to suggest that chemical induction from the developing lens is a necessary factor in the normal development of the neural ectoderm and the mesodermal elements of the eye.

Induction being a chemical process stimulating and directing metabolism, it is not surprising that it can be inhibited by chemical agents ; thus the formation of the lens does not occur after treatment with chemicals such as urea (Jenkinson, 1906), chloretone or trichlorobutylalcohol (Lehmann, 1934-36), phlorizine (Tamini, 1943), lithium chloride or sodium sulphocyanide (de Vincentiis, 1957), or after modifications of the temperature (Lehmann, 1936) or ultra-violet radiation (A. Dürken, 1950).

It would appear that a fleeting contact of the neural and surface ectoderm is all that is necessary to initiate the process of lens induction (24 hours, Filatov, 1934 ; Woerdeman, 1950) ; and, indeed, the general polarity of the tissue by which the direction of the growth of the fibres is determined, is laid down at an early stage. Thus (in amphibians) Woerdeman (1934-50) found that by rotating the presumptive lens ectoderm through 90° at various stages of development, the posterior horizontal suture was in a labile condition before the elevation of the neural folds but was fixed and determined just before the neural folds closed. Nevertheless, the longer the two epithelial layers remain in contact, the better is the final differentiation of the lens the tissues of which (in amphibians) require the continued stimulation of the neural ectoderm for their full and normal development (LeCron, 1907 ; Liedke, 1951-55) ; moreover, if the retina fails to differentiate, the lens may also be abnormal (Figs. 78 and 79) (Giroud, 1957). A reflection of this may well be seen in man in the occurrence of localized lenticular opacities in the region of colobomata of the optic cup (Wessely, 1910 ; Danchakoff, 1926 ; Mann, 1934 ; and others).

Whether the development of the lens-plate is specific and inherent in the surface ectoderm of the region wherein it is normally formed, or whether it occurs in undifferentiated ectoderm merely as a response to the inductive chemical stimulus from the primary optic vesicle, is a question which has given rise to some controversy (see Reyer, 1954). It may be of significance that the specific lenticular proteins are normally found only in the epidermal

[1] p. 69.

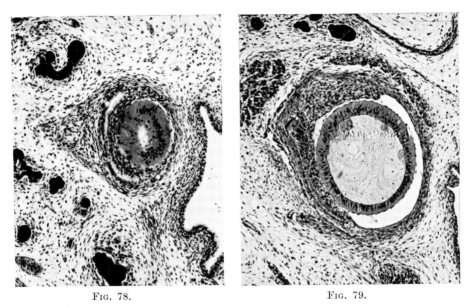

Fɪɢ. 78.   Fɪɢ. 79.

Fɪɢs. 78 and 79.—Lᴇɴs Iɴᴅᴜᴄᴛɪᴏɴ.

Fœtal rats of 21 days rendered microphthalmic by hypervitaminosis A. In each case the retina is represented merely by two undifferentiated layers. In consequence the lens vesicle is ill-formed without polar differentiation (Fig. 78) or is filled with acidophil cells (Fig. 79) (A. Giroud).

cells superficial to the optic vesicle (Flickinger *et al.*, 1955 ; de Vincentiis, 1957) ; but this, of course, does not preclude their enzymic induction else-where.

Indeed, that undifferentiated ectodermal tissue can be thus induced has been shown by a number of experimental observations. Lewis (1903), for example, found that in the early stages of the development of amphibian embryos, transplanted optic vesicles could give rise to the formation of lens thickenings in any area of the surface ectoderm ; but there would appear to be a gradient of competence since the lenses induced by such implants are smaller in the trunk than in the head (Becker, 1960). These experimental results were confirmed by Adelmann (1928) who found that portions of the retina and the upper border of the iris had the same inductive effect. Conversely, it is equally clear that if surface ectoderm from the head or body is transplanted over the optic cup in amphibians, development of the lens proceeds (Lewis, 1907 ; Popov, 1938–39 ; Stone and Dinnean, 1940). In these exchanges in some species the surface ectoderm seems to be dominated by the neural ; thus Popov and his associates (1937) showed that if the optic vesicle of one species of amphibian were transplanted under the surface ectoderm of another, the lens characteristic of the former was always formed. In other species the surface ectoderm seems to retain its own genetic characteristics and does not conform with those of the host (*Triturus cristatus* and *T. tœniatus*, Rotmann, 1939), a conservatism seen if the entire developing eye is exchanged between *Amblystoma tigrinum* and *A. punctatum* (Harrison, 1924 ; Twitty and Schwind, 1931) (Fig. 73). Although induction of the lens in this way does not occur in ectodermal grafts in all species (*Amblystoma*, Beckwith, 1927), these experimental results would seem to indicate that in certain amphibians the optic vesicle is capable of exercising a strong stimulus to lens-formation on any ectodermal structure in its neighbourhood.

Although experiments on species other than amphibians have been rare, the same conclusions have been reached. In chick embryos the optic anlage transplanted at a sufficiently early stage (up to 4 somites) will give rise to lens-formation in the ectoderm of any part of the body (head, neck or trunk), while at a slightly later stage a lens or lentoid will appear only in the head and neck (Alexander, 1937) ; in this species the transplanted optic vesicle, or a portion of it, will induce lens-formation in ectopic regions of the ectoderm up to the 5th day of incubation (Amprino, 1949 ; McKeehan, 1951). Similar induction can be obtained in mammalian embryos, although the resultant lens may be small and ill-formed (Giroud and Boisselot, 1948 ; Giroud, 1957).

There is, however, a considerable amount of evidence that in some species the ectoderm in this region has some independent power of self-determination and that the possibility of lens-formation is to some extent inherent in it. The homologous position of the olfactory and optic anlages suggested first to Sharp (1885) that the anlage of the lens arose as an independent organ derived from an ectodermal placode of the epibranchial series, a view elaborated by Jelgersma (1906), Studnicka (1918) and Schimkewitsch (1921). Thus Mencl (1903) showed that the lens could develop spontaneously in *Salmo*, Stockard (1910) found in artificially produced abnormal fish embryos (anophthalmic, cyclopean, etc.) that a lens thickening may appear on the surface of the head in regions where there has been no contact with the optic vesicle, and Spemann (1912) confirmed this in certain cases in frogs. The last investigator therefore concluded that whilst in some species the formation of the lens is entirely dependent upon the influence of the optic vesicle, in others the presumptive lens area possesses the power of differentiation independent of the vesicle, a finding confirmed (in *Taricha*) by Jacobson (1959). The contrast is well shown in Figs. 80 and 81 ; after excision of the optic cup whereas a lens is shown without an eye-cup in the embryo of *Rana esculenta*, there is complete absence of a lens in an embryo of *R. bombinator*.

The paradox may possibly be explained in several ways ; either the optic primordium even while still undifferentiated from the anterior part of the neural plate possesses a lens-inducing power in certain species, or the inducing stimulus may in some species escape from the optic cup into the surrounding mesoderm so that removal of the former need not completely eliminate the inducing stimulus ; in either event, the later development of the lens would give the impression that it was self-differentiated (Needham, 1942). Evidence confirming the latter theory has been brought forward by von Ubisch (1927) and Perri (1934) who cultivated the presumptive ectoderm of *Rana esculenta* and *R. bombinator* in true isolation from an early stage ; in these circumstances no lens appeared, a finding which strongly suggests that a chemical stimulus is necessary for the differentiation of this tissue.

A possible alternative explanation may lie in the effect of temperature on the conditions of the laboratory. The experiments of Ten Cate (1946) on the effect of

FIGS. 80 and 81.—THE VARIATION IN THE DEVELOPMENT OF THE LENS AFTER REMOVAL OF THE OPTIC CUP.

(From Hans Spemann; Needham's *Biochemistry and Morphogenesis*, Cambridge Univ. Press.)

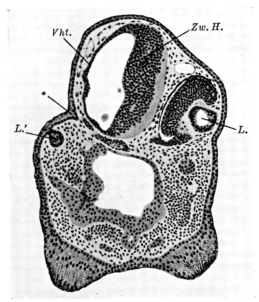

FIG. 80.—Development of the lens without the inductive effect of the optic cup in *Rana esculenta*.

Vht., site of excision on the operated side ; *Zw. H.*, midbrain ; *L*, lens of normal side ; *L'*, lens of operated side.

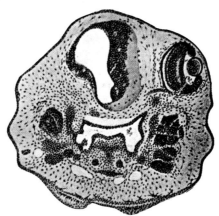

FIG. 81.—Absence of lens on the operated side after removal of the optic cup in *Bombinator pachypus*.

temperature on development indicate that the level of differentiation can be considerably altered thereby. It may be that while lens-formation is normally induced by the action of two mutually reinforcing inductors, the mesoderm of the head and the retinal anlage, at low temperatures the surface ectoderm may become sufficiently mature and responsive to react to the stimulus of mesoderm alone (Twitty, 1930–56 ; Woerdeman, 1950 ; Liedke, 1951). Indeed, there is much evidence to show that the time at which induction of the overlying ectoderm by the optic vesicle is initiated and the period over which induction extends vary in different species of amphibians ; the stage of development of the embryo influences the distribution and the extent of the areas of ectoderm capable of forming a lens, progressive localization of the lens-forming capacity occurring with increasing age of the ectoderm (see Werber, 1918 ; Mangold, 1931 ; Koch, 1933 ; Perri, 1934 ; Spemann, 1938 ; Woerdeman, 1950). In certain circumstances, however, it would appear that the lens can be formed apart altogether from the surface ectoderm. Thus in amphibians, on cultivating *in vitro* a large segment of the medullary plate which had been denuded of the anlage of the lens, Jolly (1947) found that a small head resulted possessing two eyes each equipped with a lens.

After the optic vesicle has developed not only is it capable of inducing a lens in the surface ectoderm, but in the embryos of certain species it possesses the power of re-forming a lens from its own tissues if the lens derived from the surface layer had previously been removed. This interesting phenomenon, first noted by Colucci (1891) and adequately described by Wolff (1894–1904) in the triton, is frequently referred to as *Wolffian regeneration* and has attracted much study[1] (Figs. 82 to 89). While this phenomenon undoubtedly occurs in the *Triturus* group of salamanders, there is some evidence that it is largely if not exclusively restricted among the vertebrates to this species in which the lens appears to be less resistant to injury than in other forms, and it has been contended that reports of regeneration occurring in most other species may be attributable to incomplete removal of the original structure (Stone and Dinnean, 1940 ; Reyer, 1956).

The regeneration habitually occurs from the dorsal segment of the iris, but even when the entire iris had been removed from the eye of *Triturus viridescens*, regeneration of the iris from the retinal pigment epithelium was followed by regeneration of a normal lens ; it would seem, therefore, that the potency to regenerate the lens extends into the dorsal portion of the pigment epithelium (Stone, 1950–7 ; Sato, 1951), and it may be significant that lens antigen is found in these two tissues (Langman and Prescott, 1959).[2] The developmental stages occurring in the regeneration of the lens from the dorsal iris of *Triturus* have been traced most extensively by Stone and Dinnean (1940–3). The first sign of regeneration appears on the 5th day as a thickening of the dorsal part of the iris and 24 days after the extirpation of the original lens the regenerating lens is filled with fibre-cells and shows a well-developed epithelial capsule (Figs. 82 to 89). The same phenomenon has been claimed to occur in the chick embryo (Fig. 90).

---

[1] Colucci (1891), Wolff (1894–1904), Müller (1896), Fischel (1898–1921), Wachs (1914), Ogawa (1921), Beckwith (1927), Sato (1930–33), Törö (1932), Dinnean (1942), Reyer (1950–54), Stone (1950–59), Stone and Steinitz (1957), Takano *et al.* (1957–8), Hasegawa (1958), Takano (1959), in salamanders ; Kochs (1897), Alberti (1922), Perri (1934–42), in anurans ; Grochmalicki (1908) and Alberti (1923) in fishes ; and Barfurth (1902) and Amprino (1949) in the chick.

[2] It may perhaps be relevant to note in this context that a lentoid growth from the ciliary body has been observed in a human microphthalmic eye by Fischer (1929).

FIGS. 82 to 89.—REGENERATION OF THE LENS FROM THE DORSAL PORTION OF THE IRIS.
Occurring in *Triturus torosus* after removal of the lens (× 150) (F. L. Dinnean, *J. exp. Zool.*).

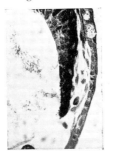 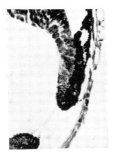 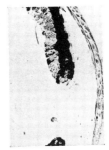

FIG. 82.—Four days after removal of the lens. The heavily pigmented dorsal portion of the iris near the pupillary margin appears normal.

FIG. 83.—Seven days after removal. The iris becomes thicker and depigmented near the margin. The cells of the inner layer are increasing in height and contain only scattered pigment granules.

FIG. 84.—Nine days after removal of the lens. Complete depigmentation of the inner layer and definite demarcation between the inner and outer layers of the dorsal portion of the iris.

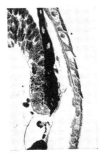 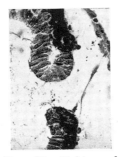 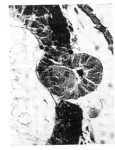

FIG. 85.—Fourteen days after operation. Complete depigmentation has proceeded towards the pupillary edge of the dorsal portion of the iris.

FIG. 86.—Eighteen days after operation. Proliferation of the unpigmented cells beyond the pupillary edge of the dorsal iris to form an early lens vesicle with a cavity in the centre.

FIG. 87.—Twenty-one days after operation. There is a well defined fibre-pole within the lens vesicle which is still attached to its source of origin.

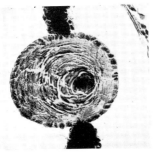 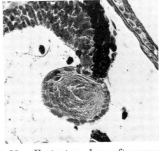

FIG. 88.—Twenty-four days after operation. The lens is solidly filled with fibres and shows an epithelial capsule. It is now isolated from the source of origin.

FIG. 89.—Forty-two days after removal of the lens. The development of a fully-formed lens in the pupillary margin.

Not only may regeneration of the lens occur after removal of the original structure, but fragments of iris or ectoderm inserted into the anterior chamber may be induced to form well-formed lenses, particularly if the fragment is implanted into the site of the normal lens (Wachs, 1914 ; Sato, 1930 ; Nikitenko, 1937 ; Mikami, 1937). This takes place more effectively if the lens had previously been removed as if its presence inhibited the formation of the new structure, while the injection of cysteine inhibits and of cystine accelerates the process (Dinnean, 1942 ; Takano, 1959).

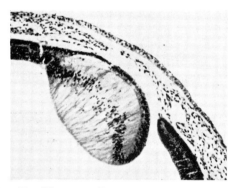

FIG. 90.—WOLFFIAN REGENERATION OF THE LENS.
From the anterior rim of the optic cup in the chick embryo (Genis Gálvez).

That the process of regeneration of the lens is not necessarily confined to embryonic life has long been known and, indeed, the possibility of the new formation of lens fibres if the lens substance were removed from the capsule was recognized by ophthalmologists a century and a half ago (Buchner, 1801 ; Cocteau and Leroy d'Etiolles, 1827 ; Backhauser, 1827 ; Day, 1828 ; Middlemore, 1832 ; Löwenhardt, 1841 ; Valentin, 1842 ; Ivanov, 1867 ; Milliot, 1868–72 ; Randolph, 1900 ; and others). We have already seen that the process of organogenesis is usually associated with some cytolysis, suggesting that the destruction of the organizing cells liberated the required organizing stimulus in quantity.[1] It may well be that the inclusion of degenerating epitrichial cells of the epidermis in the developing lens vesicle[2] may exert a similar influence, and it would appear that the process of regeneration of the lens can be similarly stimulated. Thus after removal of the lens in frogs and tadpoles, only the earliest stages of regeneration occur (Schwalb, 1954), but if a piece of degenerating epidermis is implanted into the posterior chamber, regeneration may proceed to the formation of a well-formed lens with good optical properties (Sicharulidze, 1954). The same phenomenon is seen in the adult animal. If cytolysed fœtal tissues are injected into the cavity of the capsule after discission of the lens in the rabbit, a well-formed lens may develop (Sicharulidze, 1956), while Chanturishvili (1958), Stewart and 'Espinasse (1959) and Stewart (1960) have shown in mice and rabbits that if the lens is rendered cataractous, the injection of minced brain or embryonic epidermal tissue (conserved at 30° C for 7 days) may lead to the same result (Figs. 91 and 92). On the other hand, Binder and his colleagues (1961–2) failed to find any advantage in the injection of cytolysing embryonic material in the process of regeneration ; indeed, they concluded that the

[1] p. 51.   [2] p. 130.

FIGS. 91 and 92.—REGENERATION OF THE LENS (Chanturishvili).

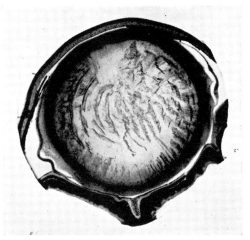

FIG. 91.—The eye of the mouse 160 days after the extracapsular evacuation of a cataractous lens and the implantation of conserved minced brain tissue. A large normal lens fills up the whole eye.

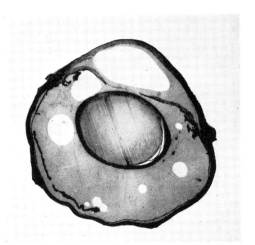

FIG. 92.—The eye of a rabbit 420 days after the replacement of normal lens tissue by conserved epidermis taken from the embryo of a rabbit from the region of the commissure between the upper and lower lids.

implantation of such material sometimes led to the development of intra-ocular monstrosities. The possible clinical implications of these observations have not yet been assessed.

INDUCTION OF THE CORNEA

The differentiation of the cornea is also dependent upon the presence of the developing eye for no cornea is formed when the eye is missing. In amphibian embryos if the optic vesicle is removed at an early stage, the over-lying surface ectoderm remains undifferentiated (Spemann, 1901 ; Lewis, 1903–7; Mangold, 1931; Koch, 1933); if the lens and optic cup are removed in the early larval stages, the corneal epithelium is transformed into ordinary epidermis (Lewis, 1903–7 ; B. Dürken, 1913; Groll, 1924) ; while if the cornea is replaced by epidermis from another region of the body, the grafted tissue will be histologically transformed into typical corneal epithelium. Conversely, if the optic vesicle is transplanted elsewhere, or even if an emulsion of retinal or iridic tissue is injected beneath the surface layer, the overlying epithelium at the heterotopic site takes on the characteristics of a cornea, a transition, however, which is inhibited by the interposition of mesodermal tissue (Fischel, 1919 ; Adelmann, 1928 ; Pasquini, 1932 ; Amprino, 1949 ; Neufach, 1950).

It would thus appear that the differentiation of the cornea depends essentially upon induction by the optic vesicle ; but there is evidence that the stimulatory process is shared by other elements of the developing eye (Popov, 1936) ; indeed, as was shown by Werber (1918), differentiation of the ectoderm may occur over an isolated lens, while in the absence of the lens, corneal differentiation is rarely complete (Reyer, 1950). Mechanical factors also enter into the question since after incision of the globe in the chick embryo, corneal differentiation is abnormal (Amprino, 1949). That the essential stimulus, however, is chemical in nature and not mechanical is seen in the fact that the implantation of a glass ball (Cole, 1922), or wax (Baurmann, 1922) under the skin may cause some thinning of the overlying epidermis, whereas no change occurs when a flat piece of glass is introduced.

THE INDUCTION OF THE SCLERA AND CHOROID

It would seem clear that the development of the mesodermal tissue around the optic vesicle is induced by the pigmentary epithelium (Gruenwald, 1944) ; where the outer layer of the optic vesicle has been partially destroyed or replaced, as by toxic chemicals, the choroid and sclera do not differentiate (Giroud *et al.*, 1954 ; Giroud, 1957) (Figs. 93 and 94), and the same lapse occurs where this layer is lacking in cyclopia (Gartner, 1947). It is significant that the development of the choriocapillaris occurs in step with the appearance of the pigment in this ectodermal layer (Mann, 1949). As occurs in other situations, however, mechanical factors influence the full differentiation of the mesoblast ; if the ocular tension of the developing globe is reduced mechanically by incision (Amprino, 1949) or if the full cellular proliferation in the retinal and lenticular vesicles is inhibited by antimitotic agents (Sentein, 1949), the surrounding mesoblast remains massive and abundant.

THE INDUCTION OF THE EXTRA-OCULAR MUSCLES AND ORBITAL STRUCTURES

It has been shown that in amphibians (Twitty, 1932), birds (Amprino, 1949–50) and mammals (Wessely, 1920 ; Lefebvres, 1951) the extrinsic

FIGS. 93 and 94.—INDUCTION OF THE CHOROID.

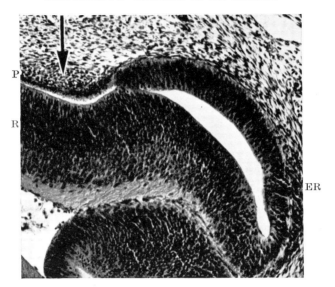

FIG. 93.

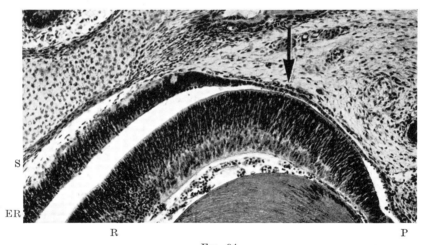

FIG. 94.

To show the dependence of the development of the choroid on the pigment epithelium. Fœtal rats subjected to folic acid deficiency. The embryonic fissure has not closed and the neural layer of the retina is everted around the fissure so that it is orientated with the visual cells internally and the nerve-fibre layer externally. In this region no choroid develops, but it does develop immediately the neural tissue gives place to pigment epithelium (arrowed) (× 130) (A. Giroud).

ER. Everted retina.   R. Normal retina.
P. Pigment epithelium.   S. Sclera.

ocular muscles and the skeletal structures associated with the eye develop in large measure independently of the optic or lenticular vesicle ; this occurs in embryos rendered anophthalmic by chemicals or when the optic vesicle has been mechanically damaged (Figs. 95 and 96). The muscle bellies are usually smaller than normal and may suffer some abnormal arrangement, but they become normally innervated and remain contractile even when they are attached merely to the surrounding mesoderm. This same inde-

FIGS. 95 and 96.—THE INDEPENDENCE OF THE DEVELOPMENT OF THE OCULAR ADNEXA (A. Giroud).

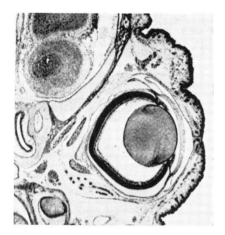

FIG. 95.—The eye of a normal fœtal rat.

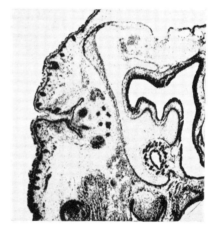

FIG. 96.—A fœtal rat of the same age rendered anophthalmic by deficiency of pantothenic acid. All the adnexa—lids, palpebral fissure, lacrimal gland and ocular muscles—are present, despite the absence of the globe.

pendent differentiation of the musculature with, however, a partial dependence on mechanical factors is seen in the human microphthalmic or (apparently) anophthalmic orbit. The lacrimal glands and passages similarly develop independently, and although the lids of the chick may remain rudimentary in the absence of the eye (Amprino, 1949), this dependence does not seem to be present in mammals (Redslob, 1932 ; Sédan, 1956).

Adelmann. *Arch. Entwickl.-Mech. Org.*, **113**, 704 (1928).
Alberti. *Arch. Entwickl.-Mech. Org.*, **50**, 355 (1922).
  Arch. mikr. Anat., **98**, 496 (1923).
Alexander. *J. exp. Zool.*, **75**, 41 (1937).
Amprino. *C.R. Ass. Anat.*, **36**, 3 (1949).
  Accad. dei Lincei., **6**, 645 (1949).
  Arch. Entwickl.-Mech. Org., **144**, 71, 81 (1949).
  Acta anat. (Basel), **10**, 38 (1950).

Backhauser. *De regeneratione lentis*, Berlin (1827).
Barfurth. *Anat. Anz.*, **21**, Erg., 185 (1902).
Baurmann. *Klin. Mbl. Augenheilk.*, **68**, 73 (1922)
Becker. *Arch. Entwickl.-Mech. Org.*, **152**, 339 (1960).
Beckwith. *J. exp. Zool.*, **49**, 217 (1927).
Binder, H. F., Binder, R. F., Wells and Katz. *Amer. J. Ophthal.*, **52**, 919 (1961).
  Brit. J. Ophthal., **46**, 416 (1962).

Buchner. *Waarneming von eene entbinding der crystalvogten*, Amsterdam (1801).

Chanturishvili. *Trans. ophthal. Soc. U.K.*, **78**, 411 (1958).

Cocteau and Leroy d'Etiolles. *J. Physiol. exp.* (Paris), **7**, 30 (1827).

Cole. *J. exp. Zool.*, **35**, 353 (1922).

Colucci. *Mem. real. Accad. Bologna, Sez. Sci. nat.*, **1**, 167, 593 (1891).

Danchakoff. *Contrib. Embryol. Carneg. Instn.*, **18**, 63 (1926).

Day. *Lancet*, **2**, 212 (1828).

Dinnean. *J. exp. Zool.*, **90**, 461 (1942).

Dürken, A. *Arch. Entwickl.-Mech. Org.*, **144**, 278 (1950).

Dürken, B. *Z. wiss. Zool.*, **105**, 192 (1913).

Filatov. *Biochem. Z.*, *U.R.S.S.*, **3**, 261 (1934).

Fischel. *Anat. Anz.*, **14**, 373 (1898).
　Arch. Entwickl.-Mech. Org., **15**, 1 (1902) ; **42**, 1 (1916) ; **49**, 383 (1921).
　Klin. Mbl. Augenheilk., **62**, 1 (1919).

Fischer. *Z. Augenheilk.*, **69**, 30 (1929).

Flickinger, Levi and Smith. *Physiol. Zool.*, **28**, 79 (1955).

Gartner. *Arch. Ophthal.* (Chicago), **37**, 220 (1947).

Giroud. *Acta anat.* (Basel), **30**, 297 (1957).

Giroud and Boisselot. *Arch. Anat. micr.*, **37**, 168 (1948).

Giroud, Delmas, Lefebvres and Prost. *Arch. Anat. micr.*, **43**, 21 (1954).

Grochmalicki. *Z. wiss. Zool.*, **89**, 164 (1908).

Groll. *Arch. Entwickl.-Mech. Org.*, **100**, 385 (1924).

Gruenwald. *Anat. Rec.*, **88**, 67 (1944).
　Amer. J. Anat., **74**, 217 (1944).

Harrison. *Proc. Soc. exp. Biol. Med.*, **17**, 199 (1920).
　Proc. nat. Acad. Sci. Wash., **10**, 69 (1924).

Hasegawa. *Embryologia* (Nagoya), **4**, 1 (1958).

Ivanov. *Medit. Vestn.*, **23**, 217 (1867).

Jacobson. *Proc. nat. Acad. Sci. Wash.*, **41**, 522 (1955).
　J. exp. Zool., **139**, 525 (1959).

Jelgersma. *Morph. Jb.*, **35**, 377 (1906).

Jenkinson. *Arch. Entwickl.-Mech. Org.*, **21**, 367 (1906).

Jolly. *Acta anat.* (Basel), **4**, 149 (1947).

Koch, C. *Boll. Fac. Med. Padova*, **2**, 5 (1933).

Kochs. *Arch. mikr. Anat.*, **49**, 441 (1897).

Langman and Prescott. *J. Embryol. exp. Morph.*, **7**, 549 (1959).

LeCron. *Amer. J. Anat.*, **2**, 245 (1907).

Lefebvres. *Ann. Méd.*, **52**, 225 (1951).

Lehmann. *Arch. Entwickl.-Mech. Org.*, **131**, 333 (1934) ; **134**, 166 (1936).
　Naturwissenschaften, **24**, 401 (1936).

Leplat. *Ann. Soc. Med. Gand*, **4**, 230 (1913).
　Anat. Anz., **46**, 280 (1914).
　Arch. Biol. (Liège), **30**, 231 (1919).
　Bull. Soc. belge Ophtal., No. 79, 6 (1940).

Lewis. *Amer. J. Anat.*, **3**, 505 (1903–4) ; **6**, 473 (1906–7) ; **7**, 259 (1907).

Liedke. *J. exp. Zool.*, **90**, 331 (1942) ; **117**, 573 (1951) ; **130**, 353 (1955).

Löwenhardt. *Neue Notizen usw. von Froriep*, **19**, 344 (1841).

McKeehan. *J. exp. Zool.*, **117**, 31 (1951).

Mangold. *Ergebn. Biol.*, **7**, 193 (1931).

Mann. *Arch. Ophthal.* (Chicago), **11**, 174 (1934).
　Development of the Human Eye, 2nd ed., London (1949).

Manuilova. *C.R. Acad. Sci.* (U.R.S.S.), **14**, 504 (1935) ; **18**, 689 (1938).

Mencl. *Arch. Entwickl.-Mech. Org.*, **16**, 328 (1903).

Middlemore. *Lond. med. Gaz.*, **10**, 344 (1832).

Mikami. *Bot. Zool. Jap.*, **5**, 45 (1937).

Milliot. *Experiments of the Restoration of a normal Crystalline Lens in some Mammals after its Removal*, St. Petersburg (1868).
　J. Anat. Physiol., **8**, 1 (1872).

Müller, E. *Arch. mikr. Anat.*, **48**, 23 (1896).

Needham. *Biochemistry and Morphogenesis*, Camb. (1942 ; 1950).

Neufach. *Dokl. Akad. Nauk.*, S.S.S.R., **75**, 141 (1950).

Nikitenko. *C.R. Acad. Sci.* (U.R.S.S.), **16**, 477 (1937).

Ogawa. *J. exp. Zool.*, **33**, 395 (1921).

Okada and Mikami. *Proc. imp. Acad. Tokyo*, **13**, 283 (1937).

Pasquini. *J. exp. Zool.*, **61**, 45 (1932).

Perri. *Arch. Entwickl.-Mech. Org.*, **131**, 113, (1934).
　Arch. ital. Anat. Embriol., **47**, 673 (1942).

Popov. *C.R. Acad. Sci.*, U.R.S.S., **11**, 347 (1936) ; **25**, 262 (1939).
　Bull. Biol. Med. exp., U.R.S.S., **2**, 245 (1936).
　Biol. Zh., U.R.S.S., **7**, 483 (1938).
　Acta néerl. Morph., **3**, 81 (1939).

Popov, Kislow, Nikitenko and Chanturishvili. *C.R. Acad. Sci.*, U.R.S.S., **16**, 245 (1937).

Randolph. *Johns Hopk. Hosp. Rep.*, **9**, 237 (1900).

Redslob. *Ann. Oculist.* (Paris), **169**, 433 (1932).

Reyer. *J. exp. Zool.*, **113**, 317 (1950) ; **125**, 1 (1954) ; **133**, 145 (1956).
　Quart. Rev. Biol., **1**, 29 (1954).

Rotmann. *Arch. Entwickl.-Mech. Org.*, **139**, 1 (1939).

Sato. *Arch. Entwickl.-Mech. Org.*, **122**, 451 (1930) ; **128**, 342 ; **130**, 19 (1933).
　Embriologia, **1**, 21 (1951).

Schimkewitsch. *Lhb. d. vergl. Anat. d. Wirbeltiere*, Stuttgart (1921).

Schwalb. *J. Bioch. Chark. Un.*, **19**, 103 (1954).

Sédan. *Ann. Oculist.* (Paris), **189**, 392 (1956).

Sentein. *C.R. Ass. Anat.*, **36**, 10 (1949).

Sharp. *Proc. Acad. nat. Sci.* (Phila.), 300 (1885).

Sicharulidze. *C.R. Acad. Sci.* (U.R.S.S.), **95**, 901 (1954).
　Bull. Acad. Sci., Georgia S.S.R., **14**, 337 (1956).

Spemann. *Verhdl. Anat. Ges. Halle*, 61 (1901).
Zool. Jb., Abt. Zool. Physiol., **32,** 1 (1912).
Embryonic Development and Induction, New Haven (1938).
Stewart. *Trans. ophthal. Soc. U.K.*, **80,** 357 (1960).
Stewart and 'Espinasse. *Nature* (Lond.), **183,** 1815 (1959).
Stockard. *Amer. J. Anat.*, **10,** 369, 393 (1910).
Stone. *Zoologica, N.Y.*, **35,** 23 (1950).
Anat. Rec., **120,** 599 (1954).
J. exp. Zool., **129,** 505 (1955) ; **136,** 17, 75 (1957).
Trans. ophthal. Soc. U.K., **79,** 471 (1959).
Yale J. Biol. Med., **32,** 464 (1960).
Stone and Chace. *Anat. Rec.*, **79,** 333 (1941).
Stone and Dinnean. *Proc. Soc. exp. Biol. (N.Y.)*, **45,** 183 (1940) ; **49,** 232 (1942).
J. exp. Zool., **83,** 95 (1940).
Yale J. Biol. Med., **16,** 31 (1943).
Stone and Steinitz. *J. exp. Zool.*, **135,** 301 (1957).
Studnicka. *Zool. Jb., Abt. Anat.*, **40,** 1 (1918).
Takano. *Mie med. J.*, **8,** 385 (1959).
Takano, Yamanaka and Mikami. *Mie med. J.*, **8,** 177 (1958).
Takano, Yoshida, Ohashi, Ogasawara, *et al. Mie med. J.*, **7,** 257 (1957).

Tamini. *Arch. Entwickl.-Mech. Org.*, **142,** 455 (1943).
Ten Cate. *Ned. T. Geneesk.*, **90,** 1695 (1946).
Törö. *Arch. Entwickl.-Mech. Org.*, **126,** 185 (1932).
Twitty. *J. exp. Zool.*, **55,** 43 (1930) ; **61,** 333 (1932).
In *Analysis of Development*, Phila., 404 (1956).
Twitty and Schwind. *J. exp. Zool.*, **59,** 61 (1931).
von Ubisch. *Z. wiss. Zool.*, **129,** 213 (1927).
Valentin. *Z. rat. Med.*, **1,** 227 (1842).
de Vincentiis. *Sui fattori che presiedono al differenziamento dell'abbozzo oculare*, Torino (1957).
Wachs. *Arch. Entwickl.-Mech. Org.*, **39,** 384 (1914).
Weiss. *Quart. Rev. Biol.*, **25,** 177 (1950).
Werber. *Biol. Bull.*, **34,** 219 (1918).
Wessely. *Arch. Augenheilk.*, **65,** 295 (1910).
Z. Augenheilk., **43,** 654 (1920).
Woerdeman. *Z. mikr.-Anat. Forsch.*, **36,** 600 (1934).
Ann. biol. (Paris), **54,** 699 (1950).
Wolff. *Biol. Zbl.*, **14,** 609 (1894).
Arch. Entwickl.-Mech. Org., **1,** 380 (1895) ; **12,** 307 (1901).
Arch. mikr. Anat., **63,** 1 (1904).

SECTION II

EMBRYOLOGY OF THE EYE

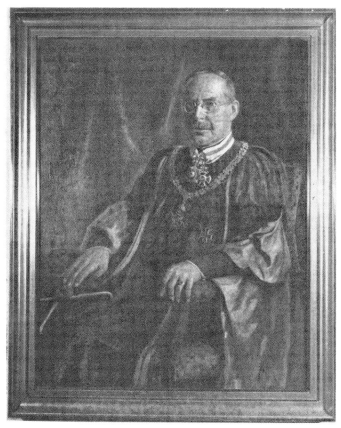

FIG. 97.—RICHARD SEEFELDER
[1875–1949].
A portrait painted when Rector of the University of Innsbruck.

CHAPTER IV

THE DIFFERENTIATION OF THE NEURAL ECTODERM

WE have already seen that as the primary optic vesicle invaginates to form the optic cup, the distal portion of the vesicle gradually approaches the proximal portion until the two ectodermal layers are separated by a potential space only. The outer layer remains largely undifferentiated as the pigment epithelium, appearing as a single row of cells throughout life ; the inner layer, which suffers invagination, becomes polystratified and highly specialized to form the sensory retina proper or pars optica retinæ, while the anterior portions of both layers develop at a considerably later stage into the double-layered epithelium of the ciliary body and iris as well as the musculature associated with the latter. At the same time the neural ectoderm of the optic stalk gives rise to the neuroglial supporting tissue of the optic nerve, the nerve fibres of which are derived from retinal cells.

The initial researches made on the development of the retina concerned the lower vertebrates (Huschke, 1832 ; Schöler, 1848 ; Remak, 1855) and in these the false conclusion was reached that the visual elements arose in the external layers of the optic cup. It was not until the work of Rudolf von Kölliker (1861),[1] the great anatomist of Würzburg, that it was established that this layer furnished the single stratum of pigmented epithelium, an observation supplemented by Babuchin (1863) who showed in embryos of the frog, chicken and rabbit that the visual elements and the ganglion cells arose from the inner layer of the cup. These findings were confirmed for the first time in the human embryo by Karl Ritter (1864), the anatomist of Bremen, who traced in a general way the development of the various retinal layers. Twenty years later these studies were further elaborated by von Kölliker (1883), Chievitz (1887), who made a particular study of the region of the posterior pole, and Rochon-Duvigneaud (1895), the director of the laboratory at the Hôtel Dieu in Paris.[2] The 20th century saw a progressively detailed elaboration of these early studies by Magitot (1910) and Seefelder (1910–30), and the somewhat intricate story was coordinated and shaped by Ida Mann (1928–49)[3] into the form still recognized today.

From among these workers we have chosen to introduce this chapter with the photograph of RICHARD SEEFELDER [1875–1949] on whose classical researches our ideas of the development of this tissue were essentially founded (Fig. 97). Born in Nesselbach in Bavaria, he received his medical education in Erlangen and Munich and thereafter went to Leipzig where he was converted to ophthalmology by Hubert Sattler. He immediately applied himself with unusual energy and enthusiasm to the study of the embryology of the eye and the histology of congenital deformities to which he contributed so greatly that he was made a titular professor at Leipzig in 1914, the year in which his classical and magnificent *Atlas zur Entwicklungsgeschichte des menschlichen Auges*, written in association with Ludwig Bach of Marburg, appeared. After the First World War, in 1919, he was elected to the chair of ophthalmology at Innsbruck to succeed Josef Meller, where he remained until 4 years before his death, all the time interesting himself in his chosen aspect of our speciality.

[1] See Vol. II, p. 227.   [2] See Vol. I, p. 332.   [3] p. 157.

Central Nervous Differentiation

Since the eye originates as an outgrowth of the prosencephalon, it is to be expected that its neural basis should conform to the same pattern as that shown by the area of the central nervous system from which it is derived. In its earliest stages this system consists of a single layer of primitive medullary epithelial cells lining the central neural tube. As these proliferate into a stratum several cells thick, they may be divided histogenetically into three types (Figs. 98 to 100) : (1) *ependymal cells* remaining attached to the internal

Figs. 98 to 100.—The Development of Elements in the Wall of the Neural Tube (modified from Harrison).

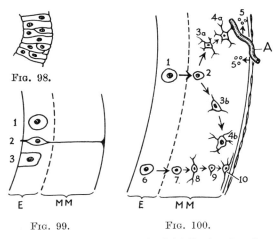

Fig. 98.

Fig. 99.   Fig. 100.

Fig. 98.—The single layer of columnar cells initially forming the neural (medullary) epithelium.

Fig. 99.—The grouping of the nuclei near the central canal to form an inner nucleated germinal (ependymal) layer (*E*), and an outer non-nucleated cytoplasmic layer which eventually becomes the mantle and marginal zones (*MM*).

1, undifferentiated germinal cell ; 2, spongioblast attached by cytoplasmic processes to the external and internal limiting membranes of the neural tube ; 3, ependymal cell.

Fig. 100.—1, germinal cell giving rise to glial elements :—2, medulloblast, differentiating either into 3*a*, an astrocytoblast, and eventually to 4*a*, an astrocyte which sends a process to the artery (*A*) ; or into 3*b*, an oligodendroblast, and then into 4*b*, an oligodendrocyte ;

5, microglia ;

6, a germinal cell developing into neural elements :—7, an apolar neuroblast, to 8, a bipolar neuroblast, to 9, a unipolar neuroblast, and eventually to 10, a multipolar neuroblast.

limiting membrane lining the central canal as a single layer ; (2) *spongio-blasts* developing into astroblasts and eventually astrocytes with a sustentacular and nutritive function ; and (3) *germinal cells* showing intense mitotic activity developing in one of two ways, forming either (i) *medulloblasts*, sustentacular in nature, giving rise to *astrocytes* and *oligodendrocytes* (with a myelinating function) or (ii) *neuroblasts*, the essential nerve cells. The remaining element in the system is the *microglia* of mesodermal origin and

PLATE I
THE DEVELOPMENT OF THE CENTRAL NERVOUS SYSTEM.

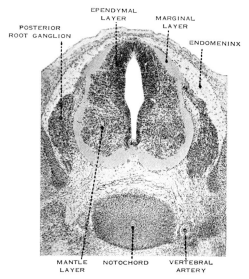

As seen in the spinal cord of a 17 mm. human embryo (Hamilton, Boyd and Mossman, *Human Embryology*, Heffer and Sons, Camb.).

[To face p. 82.

phagocytic function which at a later stage buds out from the adventitia of the blood vessels.

At an early stage of neural differentiation, this complex structure becomes arranged in three basic zones (Plate I) : (1) an epithelial or *ependymal zone* surrounding the lumen of the neural tube, the cells of which show marked mitotic activity (the *germinative layer of His*) ; (2) the *mantle zone* of cells which, migrating towards the periphery of the tube, give origin to neuroblasts and glioblasts ; and (3) outside this an acellular stratum into which the expansions of the neuroblasts subsequently grow constituting

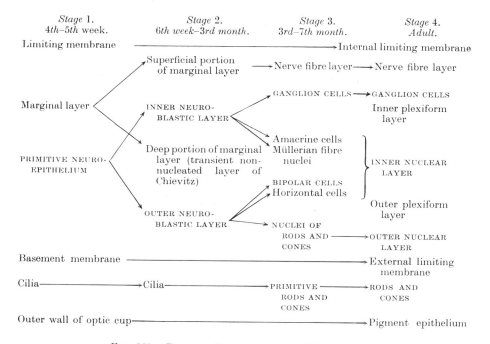

Fig. 101.—Retinal Differentiation (Mann 1928).

an external nerve-fibre layer (the *marginal zone*). The pars optica of the retina in its turn undergoes the same type of differentiation. The epithelial or ependymal layer of the neural tube probably determines the neuro-epithelial layer of the retina, the mantle layer of the brain is analogous to the cellular and synaptic layers of the retina, and the cerebral marginal layer finds a parallel in the nerve-fibre layer of the retina (Haden, 1945 ; da Costa, 1947) (Fig. 101).

Meantime, from the specialized strip of cells of the neural crest developing outside the central nervous system the ganglion cells of the autonomic and posterior root ganglia are formed (Fig. 26). Since they are not included within the central complex, they cannot obtain their myelin from oligodendrocytes ; this is produced by the neurilemmal cells of Schwann, also originating in the neural crest. It is interesting that these play a very important part in the regeneration of the peripheral nerves, a facility therefore denied to fibres within the central nervous system.

The details of this very complex process of specialization have long been recognized and have attracted a considerable literature. For the histogenesis of the central nervous system, see Harrison (1910), del Rio Hortega (1921), Bailey and Cushing (1926), Penfield (1932), Bailey (1933), Windle (1956), Bensted et al. (1957), de Robertis et al. (1958), Rowbotham et al. (1959). For the development and stratification of the retina, see M. Schultze (1867), Loewe (1878), Chievitz (1887–88), Falchi (1888), Cajal (1896), Bernard (1903), Tornatola (1905), Magitot (1910), Bach and Seefelder (1914), Cattaneo (1922), Mann (1928), Seefelder (1930), Barber (1955), Hervouët (1958).

THE SENSORY RETINA

THE EARLY DEVELOPMENT

No detailed histological studies are available in man concerning the earliest changes in that part of the neural tube which is destined to become the retina, but in the embryos of animals the region of the optic pit, on its appearance at the 2 to 2·4 mm. stage, can be differentiated from the surrounding neural ectoderm by its greater thickness ; the columnar cells are elongated, the nuclei sink to a deeper position and mitotic figures are obvious (Froriep, 1906). In the human eye this proliferative activity is evident in the distal portion of the optic vesicle (the presumptive sensory retina). Initially arranged as a single layer of columnar cells this area undergoes a progressive thickening and enlargement when the process of invagination commences (4·5 mm. stage), a process which continues until the 20 mm. stage by which time it has attained its adult thickness ; it is interesting that thereafter growth occurs in area only (Mann, 1949). For descriptive purposes the progressive differentiation of the tissue is conveniently divided into four stages (Figs. 102 to 112) :

Stage I.   The initial differentiation into zones (4 to 10 mm.).
Stage II. The differentiation into temporary layers (10 to 68 mm.; 6th week to 3rd month).
Stage III. The migration and differentiation of cells (65 to 230 mm. ; 3rd to 7th month).
Stage IV. The final organization of layers (7th to 13th month).

The first phase of regional development occupies the relatively short period of 2 weeks (4 to 10 mm. stage), during which the wall of the optic vesicle differentiates in a manner similar to the rest of the central nervous system. The prospective retina at this stage is represented by a neuro-epithelium of which the cells next to the cavity of the vesicle are rapidly dividing (the proliferating ependymal layer), superimposed on which is a number of rows of primitive cells. The cells are undifferentiated with oval

FIGS. 102 to 112.—THE DEVELOPMENT OF THE RETINA (Ida Mann).

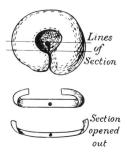

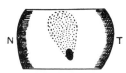

FIG. 103.—12 mm. embryo
(× 38).

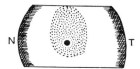

FIG. 104.—13 mm. embryo
(× 38).

FIG. 102.—The method of
reconstruction ; a thick horizontal section is taken from
the region of the optic disc
and spread out flat.

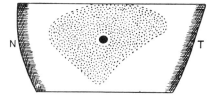

FIG. 105.—16 mm. embryo (× 38).

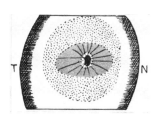

FIG. 106.—17 mm. embryo
(× 38).

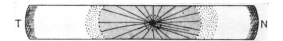

FIG. 107.—21 mm. embryo (× 38).

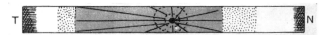

FIG. 108.—30 mm. embryo (× 38).

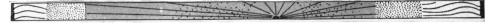

FIG. 109.—48 mm. foetus (× 26).

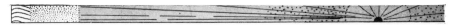

FIG. 110.—65 mm. fœtus (× 13).

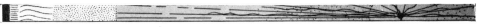

FIG. 111.—5 months' fœtus (× 13).

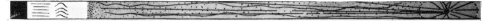

FIG. 112.—7 months' fœtus (× 6).

In Figs. 103 to 112 the black area shows initially the epithelial papilla and eventually
the optic disc ; the dotted area, the region over which migration of nuclei into the marginal
layer is taking place ; the blank area, the region over which the marginal layer is free from
nuclei ; the shaded band, the area where the margin of the optic cup has the character of
simple neuro-epithelium ; the shaded area marked with radiating lines, the area over which
nerve fibres can be recognized. The wavy lines represent the ciliary processes, the parallel
lines the iris, and the vertically shaded area the sphincter muscle of the pupil. N, nasal ;
T, temporal.

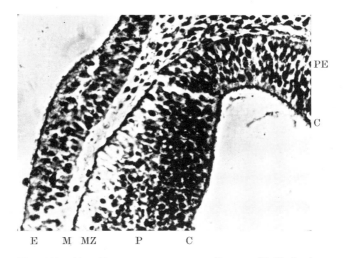

FIG. 113.—THE DEVELOPMENT OF THE RETINA (F. Vrabec).

At an early stage (5 mm.). E, surface ectoderm showing the thickening of the lens plate ;
M, fibrillar substance with mesodermal elements separating the surface ectoderm from the
neural ectoderm of the optic vesicle ; MZ, marginal zone of the optic vesicle (without nuclei) ;
P, primitive zone of neuro-epithelium ; C, ciliated basement membrane bordering the cavity
of the primary optic vesicle ; PE, outer layer of optic vesicle (presumptive pigment epithelium).
(Phase contrast.)

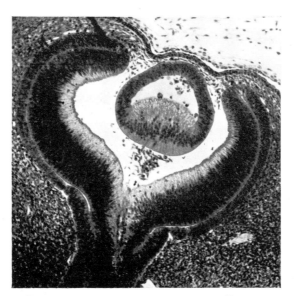

FIG. 114.—THE DEVELOPMENT OF THE RETINA.

In an embryo of 10 mm. The invagination of the optic cup is now completed and its two
walls are in contact throughout. The two retinal zones, primitive and marginal, are well
differentiated and the migration of cells from the former to the latter is still scanty (A. N.
Barber, *Embryology of the Human Eye*).

nuclei containing a darkly staining nucleolus and a prominent chromatin net, and side by side with mitotic activity in some, the opposite process of morphogenetic degeneration[1] is evident in others. At about the 4 mm. stage the tissue can be differentiated into two zones (Fig. 113):

(1) the PRIMITIVE ZONE of neuro-epithelium, initially lying deeply (and, after invagination, lying outermost), containing a mass of oval nuclei arranged in 8 or 9 rows showing many mitotic figures ; the greatest activity is in the layer of cells next the cavity of the vesicle (the ependymal layer) ; at this stage this nucleated zone occupies $\frac{9}{10}$ of the thickness of the retina ; and (2) the thin MARGINAL ZONE, initially situated superficially (and, after

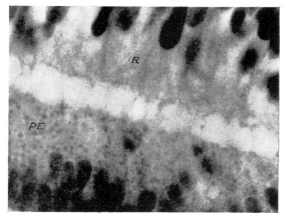

FIG. 115.—THE CILIATED BASEMENT MEMBRANE.

The deep surface of the optic cup bordering the cavity of the primary optic vesicle is clothed by a basement membrane provided with fine cilia extending from the outer surface of the retina (R) to the pigment epithelium (PE) (A. N. Barber, *Embryology of the Human Eye*).

invagination, lying innermost), remaining free from nuclei until it is eventually invaded by cells migrating from the primitive layer (Fig. 114).

At this early stage the deep surface which borders the cavity of the primary optic vesicle is covered by a basement membrane clothed by numerous fine cilia similar to those which persist in the central canal of the spinal cord, and as the two walls of the vesicle become approximated to form the optic cup during the process of invagination (at the 10 mm. stage), protoplasmic processes can be seen in histological sections to extend between them, apparently linking both layers together (Fig. 115). Somewhat similarly, on the distal surface which is relatively free from nuclei, a multitude of cone-shaped processes appears to branch outwards making contact with similar filaments projecting inwards from the surface layer of ectodermal cells immediately superficial (Fig. 113). With these are associated processes

[1] p. 51.

derived from mesodermal cells at this stage massing at the lower margin of
the optic vesicle, so that a network is formed wherein an apparent continuity
is established between the three layers of cells—the neural and the surface
ectoderm   and   the   mesoderm   (von   Szily,   1903–8 ;   Magitot,   1910 ;
v. Lenhossek, 1911).

The nature of these interconnecting filaments seen in histological sections is
unknown. Practically everyone has assumed that they are protoplasmic filaments
secreted by the neighbouring cells, ectodermal or mesodermal.   On the other hand,
others (such as Redslob, 1935) have suggested that they merely represent coagula of
the protein-rich fluid of the embryonic cavity determined artificially by fixation of the
specimen. Either view may be right, most probably the latter ; we do not know.[1]

At an early stage when invagination is proceeding (6 mm.) an interesting phase of
vascularity develops as a transient phenomenon. As also occurs throughout the whole
central nervous system, the superficial part of the wall of the vesicle becomes vascularized by the invasion of fine capillaries from the surrounding mesoderm, the vessels
being abundant in the distal and lower parts which invaginate, and scarce in the upper
and proximal parts which are destined to form the outer layer of the optic cup. In the
brain this capillary network gives rise to the definitive system of cerebral vessels,[2] but
in the optic vesicle the vascularization is transient and disappears entirely (at the
7 mm. stage), leaving the developing retina completely avascular until the 100 mm.
stage. It would appear that such a capillary system is seen only in the mammalian
retina (Mann, 1928).   Mawas and Magitot (1912) considered that this mesodermal
invasion was of specific import, giving rise to the primitive vitreous by its disintegration ; but the observations of Bach and Seefelder (1914) and Mann (1928) suggest that
the vessels form part of the general vascularity which pervades the whole of the central
nervous system at this period, the need for which is evident in the retina at the time
when unusually active growth is commencing.

By the 10 mm. stage the first period of development may be considered
to have passed, and a process of differentiation into layers becomes evident.
In general, throughout the whole central nervous system this process is
accomplished by a division and proliferation of the cells near the inner surface
and their migration outwards ; in the invaginated portion of the retina the
orientation is, of course, reversed so that the cells of the outer layer of
nuclei proliferate and migrate inwards.   Moreover, as occurs from the
earliest stage of development, the changes always proceed most rapidly and
therefore are more advanced in the region of the posterior pole, and are most
retarded anteriorly and in the region of the embryonic fissure.

During this second stage, which lasts from the 6th week to the 3rd
month, the neuro-epithelium of the primitive zone continues to proliferate
and divides to give rise to two layers of cells, the innermost of which
migrates into the acellular marginal zone which becomes increased in width
to accommodate it.   The original zone of primitive cells thus becomes
divided into two, the INNER and OUTER NEUROBLASTIC LAYERS, leaving
between them a narrow zone devoid of nuclei—the TRANSIENT FIBRE LAYER

---

[1] For further discussion, see p. 131 et seq.   [2] Vol. II, p. 690.

The division of the primary neuro-epithelium into inner and outer neuroblastic layers (A. N. Barber, *Embryology of the Human Eye*).

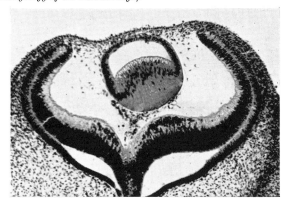

FIG. 116.—At the 13 mm. stage the process is evident at the posterior pole.

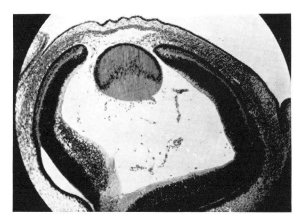

FIG. 117.—At the 26 mm. stage the process reaches to the equator.

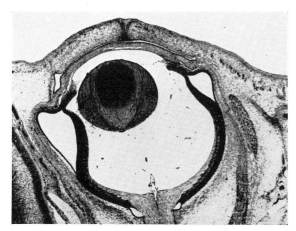

FIG. 118.—At the 65 mm. stage the process extends to the region of the future ora serrata.

(of Chievitz, 1887–88) (Fig. 119). This fibre layer does not persist into adult life ; but from the two neuroblastic layers the complex structure of the retina is evolved by a gradual process of differentiation which proceeds from the inner to the outer surface, that is, in the reverse direction of the ultimate path of visual impulses, the ganglion cells being the first of the definitive retinal elements to appear, and the rods and cones the last. The time involved is considerable for although differentiation of the neuroblastic layers is evident at the posterior pole at the 13 mm. stage, it has not developed beyond the equator at the 20 mm. stage (Figs. 116 and 117) and it is not until the latter part of the third month (65 mm. stage) that the formation of both layers extends to the region of the future ora serrata (Fig. 118).

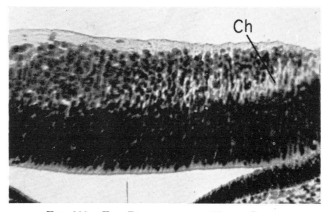

FIG. 119.—THE RETINA AT THE 26 MM. STAGE.

High-power view of the retina near the posterior pole showing the inner and outer (above) neuroblastic layers separated by the transient fibre layer of Chievitz (Ch) (A. N. Barber, *Embryology of the Human Eye*).

THE SUSTENTACULAR STRUCTURES

In the development of neural tissues it is a general rule that the supporting elements appear early and form a scaffolding around which the more highly specialized nervous elements may be built. As would be expected, therefore, the sustentacular cells of Müller can be distinguished at a very early stage from the deeper cells of the inner neuroblastic layer, being recognizable in the posterior region from the 10 to 13 mm. stage. These cells become elongated with their long axes at right angles to the plane of the retina and from them processes extend both internally and externally towards the inner and outer surfaces of the retina which they reach during the third month. The development of astrocytes is similar.

There has been much controversy, however, regarding the origin of the two *limiting membranes* of the retina. In the classical view, advocated by Schwalbe (1874) and Greeff (1899), both were considered as a continuous layer formed by the apposition of the terminal expansions of Müller's fibres, an opinion supported by many subsequent writers (Mann, 1928 ; Menner, 1930 ; Redslob, 1939). It has been established, however, that although both are of a glial nature, the limiting membranes do not invariably stain in an identical manner with Müller's cells (for example, with Mallory's triple stain, Wolff, 1937 ; with Laidlaw's stain, Hervouët, 1958). Moreover, the membranes are formed before the terminal expansions of Müller's cells reach the surfaces of the retina, a process which is not complete until the 3rd month of development (Leboucq, 1909 ; Magitot, 1910 ; Seefelder, 1930). Some embryologists, therefore, considered that the external membrane merely represented the borders of the marginal cells associated with the intercellular cement substance between them (Leboucq, 1909 ; Seefelder, 1930). It would seem more probable, however, that both structures represent the limiting membranes of the layer of cells which forms the primary optic vesicle, corresponding to the similar membranes which surround the neural tube.

The *external limiting membrane* can thus most reasonably be regarded as the internal limiting membrane of the primary optic vesicle corresponding to the similar structure which lines the ependymal epithelium of the brain and spinal cord. When the vesicle invaginates to form the optic cup, the proximal half of the membrane continues to line the cells of the pigment epithelium while the distal half forms the external limiting membrane of the retina ; between the two portions (which are continuous) lies the cavity of the optic vesicle and as it becomes fenestrated at a later stage, the processes of the pigment cells and the rods and cones project through it into the potential cavity of the vesicle (the *inter-retinal space*). At the optic disc the two membranes are anatomically continuous (Verhoeff, 1903 ; Wolff, 1940), and anteriorly they blend with the cement substance between the pigmented and unpigmented ciliary epithelium (Wolfrum, 1908).

The *internal limiting membrane* was described by Retzius (1871–1904) as a double contour, a view not generally accepted (Pedler, 1961). Lining the vitreal face of the retina is a thin acellular structure forming the true limiting membrane, extending from the optic disc which it covers with the exception of the site of the hyaloid artery to the region of the ora serrata, where it is continued forwards at a later stage as an extremely tenuous layer on the inner (posterior) surface of the prolongation of the retinal epithelium which forms the ciliary body and iris (Salzmann, 1912 ; Tousimis and Fine, 1959). On its outer surface (towards the retina) and independent of the true membrane are splayed out the expanded polygonal inner ends of Müller's fibres when these structures reach the retinal margin. The membrane and its relation to the footplates of the radial fibres of Müller are, in this view, exactly comparable to that lining the external surface of the primitive central nervous system and its relation to the feet of the bipolar spongio-blasts in that system (Strong and Elwyn, 1953 ; Pedler, 1961).

THE FORMATION OF THE RETINAL LAYERS

The third stage of retinal development is marked by the commencement of cellular specialization in the inner neuroblastic layer, while the outer neuroblastic layer remains at first comparatively unchanged. The most internal cells of the inner layer assume the characteristics of ganglion cells, a transformation evident at the 17 mm. stage. At first consisting of small cells with deeply staining nuclei and little protoplasm, they gradually enlarge and their nuclei stain less deeply ; then, migrating inwards towards the vitreal surface of the retina, they send out processes which run centripetally in the optic stalk towards the brain, forming in so doing the nerve-fibre layer of the retina and the fibres of the optic nerve (Figs. 120 to 122) ; they eventually form the first individual layer of the retina to be completely established (130 mm.). When their migration has occurred the portion of the marginal zone they have traversed appears as an acellular strip separating the ganglion cells from the main mass of the cells of the inner neuroblastic layer, thus constituting the inner plexiform layer. While these changes are proceeding the rest of the inner neuroblastic cells, apart from the Müllerian nuclei, remains undifferentiated for some time ; they are destined to become the amacrine cells at a later period (48 mm. stage).

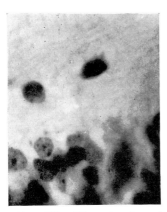

FIG. 120.—The migration of the ganglion cells from the inner neuroblastic layer at the 65 mm. stage (A. N. Barber, *Embryology of the Human Eye*).

Retinal differentiation during the 4th and 5th months is characterized by the formation of the inner nuclear layer from elements of both neuroblastic strata. This process is initiated by the inward migration of the innermost 7 or 8 rows of cells of the outer neuroblastic layer (the prospective bipolar and horizontal cells), to merge with the Müllerian and amacrine cells of the inner neuroblastic layer (130 mm.) (Figs. 121 to 124). The result of this migration is to cause the gradual obliteration of the transient layer of Chievitz which originally separated the two primitive neuroblastic layers, a process which is long delayed in the region of the macula[1] ; it also necessarily leads to the development of an acellular zone (the outer plexiform layer) separating this mass of closely packed nuclei from the remaining cells of the outer neuroblastic layer. These latter are destined to constitute the cell-bodies of the rods and cones (Fig. 121).

It has long been accepted that the cell-bodies of the rods and cones which form the outer nuclear layer are differentiated late, but it would seem that their precursors in the outer neuroblastic layer may be distinguished from their neighbours at a very early stage, even before the separation of the ganglion cells, in so far as they alone show well-marked staining properties with the use of the Unna-Pappenheim methyl pyronin green stain (da Costa, 1947). The first morphological evidence of this layer, however, occurs at the

[1] p. 96.

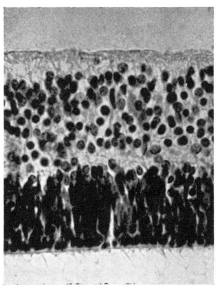

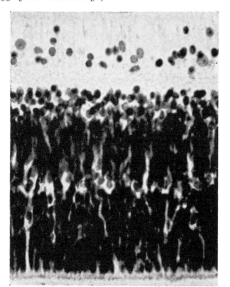

FIG. 121.—At the 65 mm. stage (3rd month). The two neuroblastic layers are seen and the outermost row of nuclei (at the bottom) which determine the rods and cones can be distinguished from the rest of the outer neuroblastic layer.

FIG. 122.—At the 130 mm. stage (5th month). The ganglion cells form the layer separated from the inner neuroblastic layer by the inner plexiform layer. Bipolar and horizontal cells are beginning to migrate from the outer neuroblastic layer into the inner nuclear layer.

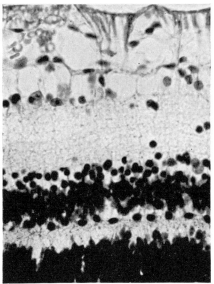

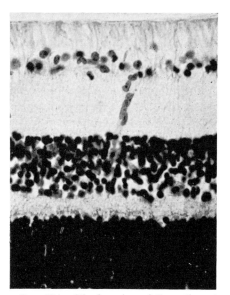

FIG. 123.—At the 180 mm. stage (6th month). The bipolar and horizontal cells merge with the nuclei of the fibres of Müller and the amacrine cells to form the inner nuclear layer, separated from the nuclei of the rods and cones by the outer plexiform layer.

FIG. 124.—The layering of the retina at birth.

48 mm. stage when the cells of the outermost row of the outer neuroblastic layer become kidney-shaped ; by the 65 mm. stage they are recognizable as a discrete row of nuclei lying just underneath the outer limiting membrane, the precursors of the cone nuclei (Fig. 121). Thereafter the inner cells of the primitive outer neuroblastic layer migrate inwards separating themselves from the remainder of the layer, destined to become rod-cells, by an acellular zone (the outer plexiform layer) ; a zone of nuclei next to the external surface of the retina is thus left as an isolated stratum (the outer nuclear layer). This separation is completed at the 170 mm. stage ($5\frac{1}{2}$ months), when all the layers of the adult retina are thus formed (Figs. 122 and 124). At the 250 mm. stage (8 months) vascularization has spread throughout the inner retinal layers and any changes which occur subsequently are incidental. After birth there seems to be little division of cells ; as the eye grows to adult dimensions the increase of retinal area is attained by a thinning and spreading out of the layers of nuclei, the total thickness of the tissue being maintained by a corresponding increase of the fibre layers.

About the time of birth, however, there appears to be a marked change in the metabolism of the retina which would seem to reach biochemical maturity only when fully developed and functioning. Thus in the rat at about the time at which the eyes first open (12–13 days after birth) there is a dramatic increase both of the aerobic and the anaerobic glycolytic metabolism (Graymore, 1959).

THE PERCIPIENT ELEMENTS

We have seen that the inner surface of the optic vesicle, as occurs throughout the inner surface of the whole central nervous system, was originally covered with a basement membrane provided with minute cilia (Fig. 113). It seems possible, although it is not certain, that these cilia develop into the outer limbs of the rods and cones, suffering, in so doing, a reduction of their number and an increase in their size. In any event, at the 17 mm. stage, when the vesicle has invaginated to form the optic cup, the cilia have disappeared and long protoplasmic processes are found to be stretched across the potential cavity of the primary optic vesicle and to become adherent to the pigment epithelium (Fig. 115). Their attachment here is definite, and they frequently remain adherent to the pigment cells if the two walls of the cup are artificially separated. At a later stage (80 mm.) when the nuclei of the prospective rod and cone cells become oval or kidney-shaped, the outer portions of the cytoplasm of the cells bulge through the basement membrane rendering it fenestrated, each cone-shaped protrusion being capped by the original filamentous process, at the base of which appear two darkly staining diplosomes. It is probable that this large conical protuberance of cellular protoplasm forms the inner limb of the cone, while the more attenuated cilium capping it forms the outer limb (Figs. 125 to 129). The rods develop in the same way at a somewhat later stage (7th month, Magitot, 1910 ; 5th month, Barber, 1955), but they remain smaller and thinner and their nuclei are derived from more deeply situated nuclei in the outer retinal layer of cells. It is interesting that Tansley (1933) found in the retina of the developing rat that visual purple could not be recognized until the first appearance of the outer limbs of the rods.

FIGS. 125 to 129.—THE DEVELOPMENT OF THE RODS AND CONES (after Seefelder).

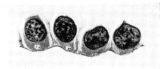

FIG. 125.—Cone cells in the central area of the retina (65 mm. stage).

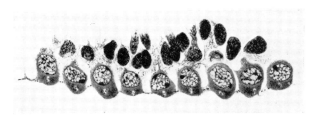

FIG. 126.—Cone cells in the centre of the retina (80 mm. stage).

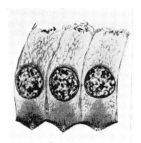 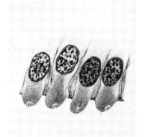 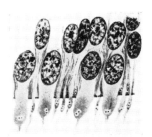

FIG. 127.—Cone cells in the centre of the retina (345 mm. stage). | FIG. 128.—Cone cells in the paracentral area of the retina (345 mm. stage). | FIG. 129.—Cone and rod cells in the paracentral area of the retina (345 mm. stage) (Held staining ; × 750).

While this is the view generally held today, the origin of the rods and cones has long remained a matter of dispute. Ever since the time of Schwalbe (1874) they had been generally considered as neuro-epithelium. It is true that Krause (1875) originally put forward the suggestion that they were derived from the ciliated ependymal cells lining the neural tube, the cilia eventually forming the outer segments of the visual cells, a view, however, which he quickly withdrew to conform with that advocated by his colleague. The vast authority of those two pioneers in the histology of the visual organs long remained unchallenged, but the suggestion that this layer of cells might be ependymal in origin, the receptor end being phylogenetically homologous with the single cilium of an ependymal cell, was revived by Leboucq (1909) ; this theory was elaborated with great persuasiveness by Studnicka (1912–18), and subsequently supported by Walls (1939) and Willmer (1953).

Such a development would not be unique since modified flagellated cells of this type are also seen in other sensory organs such as the olfactory cells, the hair cells of the labyrinth, the cells of the taste-buds and lateral line organs ; and it is to be remembered that there is a considerable amount of evidence that the ependymal cells in the diencephalic region retain some photo-sensory properties in several species of vertebrates[1] (von Frisch, 1911 ; Scharrer, 1928 ; Nowikoff, 1934 ; Young, 1935 ; Benoit, 1937 ; and others). In this view the phylogenetic homologue of the vertebrate retina may be assumed to be the infundibular organ of *Amphioxus*[2] ; but it must be remembered that any convincing phylogenetic sequence connecting the two is lacking.

Agreement on the ependymal origin of the visual receptors is, however, by no means universal and many investigators, following Schwalbe, believe that they are endoneural (Boveri, 1904 ; Parker, 1908–9 ; Tretjakoff, 1913 ; Hescheler and Boveri, 1923 ; Nowikoff, 1932). It could be assumed that these cells became orientated in a regular manner towards the central canal of the neural tube and then were carried towards the skin in company with paired lateral diverticuli which formed the optic vesicles (Fig. 35). It is to be noted that by this hypothesis the inversion of the retina and the position of the pigmentary epithelium are also well explained. In this view a phylogenetic homologue would be the ganglion-like cells of Hesse in an Amphioxus-like ancestor.[3] Although objections have been raised to this conception, the theory is undoubtedly ingenious and the question must be left open.

THE MACULA

In its development the region of the macula shows highly specialized features. Here, in common with the rest of the posterior region, differentiation is rapid and precocious until the 3rd month of fœtal life ; thereafter the central area lags behind the rest of the retina in its development, and a state of retardation persists until the 8th month. Subsequently differentiation proceeds apace along characteristic lines, and, although the rest of the retina has almost attained its final arrangement by the 9th month, the central region continues to differentiate until at least 16 weeks after birth. The main characteristics of the period of retardation are (1) the persistence of the acellular layer of Chievitz, which attains its maximum width in the central region at the 8th month and can still just be recognized in this region 4 months after birth (Mann, 1928), (2) an increase in the number of ganglion cells which, by the 6th month, may be 8 to 9 rows deep in the centre of the macula, (3) the development of cones to the exclusion of rods, and (4) a failure of this region to conform to the usual tendency to increase in area by a thinning and spreading out of the nucleated layers (Chievitz, 1890).

It follows from these peculiarities that the general configuration of the macular area differs considerably from the rest of the retina. At the 6th month it is thicker than the surrounding retina and appears as a heaped-up elevation instead of a depression (Fig. 130). During the 7th and 8th months, however, the thinning process becomes evident, and the fovea is formed largely by a gradual but progressive spreading out of the ganglion cells away

---

[1] Vol. I, p. 537.   [2] Vol. I, p. 229.   [3] Vol. I, p. 230.

Figs. 130 to 135.—Diagrammatic Scheme of the Development of the Macula (after R. Seefelder).

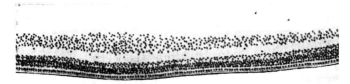

Fig. 130.—In a fœtus of 5 to 6 months.

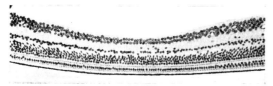

Fig. 131.—In a fœtus of 8 months.

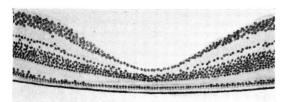

Fig. 132.—In a new-born child.

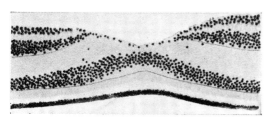

Fig. 133.—In an adult.

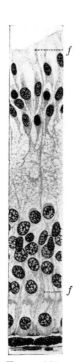

Fig. 134.—The structure of the fovea centralis in a 345 mm. fœtus.

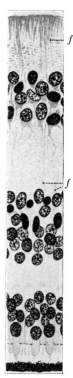

Fig. 135.—The structure of the parafoveal region in a 345 mm. fœtus. *f*, fibres of Müller.

from the central area (Fig. 131). At birth the layer of Chievitz has almost disappeared, and the ganglion cells at the fovea are reduced to a single row, although in the immediately surrounding area the ganglion cell layer remains thicker than elsewhere. The inner nuclear layer is also thinner, the outer

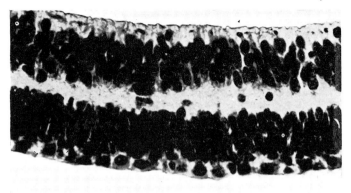

FIG. 136.—In a 62 mm. human fœtus. The retinal cones form a single row close to the external limiting membrane.

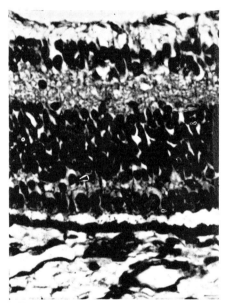

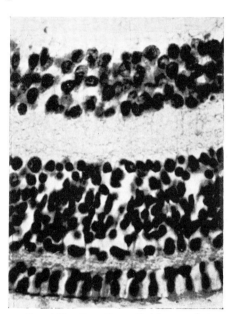

FIG. 137.—In a 3 months' human fœtus, slightly older than that of Fig. 136. The cones begin to show differentiation.

FIG. 138.—In a 6 months' human fœtus. The cones are now developing.

nuclear layer remains as a single layer of cone cells in the central region although the nuclei have increased to two and sometimes three rows at the periphery of the macula (Figs. 132, 134 to 138). The cones themselves are short and ill-developed, a circumstance which helps to explain the absence of fixation at birth. The nerve-fibre and inner plexiform layers are almost absent but the width of the outer plexiform layer has markedly increased at the fovea. Four months after birth the layer of Chievitz has practically disappeared, while the ganglion cells and the bipolars have shared a similar fate, being represented only by a few scattered cells lying upon the cone nuclei ; their absence is essentially responsible for the hollow of the fovea (Fig. 133). At this time, however, the cone nuclei have increased in number and the cones themselves have increased in length so that the external limiting membrane is curved to accommodate them, forming as it does so the fovea externa.

It will thus be seen that the differentiation of the retina is a complicated process in which three progressive factors interact—*the differentiation and migration of cells from without inwards, the differentiation of layers from within outwards, and the progressive evolution of differentiation from the posterior pole forwards*, apart from its retardation in the region of the embryonic fissure, while the fovea is not completely differentiated until the 13th month after fertilization.

THE RETINAL PIGMENT EPITHELIUM

As has already been noted, the pigment epithelium of the retina is formed by the proximal portion of the optic vesicle and the outer layer of the optic cup. In contrast to the sensory layer of the retina it remains largely undifferentiated as a single row of cells which, originally columnar in type, eventually become shortened and more cuboid in shape. Apart from this change of shape, the acquirement of pigment and the duplication necessary to cover the increase in area, the layer remains unaltered throughout life.[1]

In the first few weeks of development cellular division is rapid and intense so that the cells become crowded together and their nuclei, showing much mitotic activity, seem on section to be arranged in several rows, an appearance, however, due merely to differences in their level (Fig. 139). At the 9 to 12 mm. stage there are thus 2 or 3 rows of nuclei and the mitotic activity is intensively maintained until about the end of the eighth week (30 mm.), whereafter it begins to slow down and the cells become less crowded together, spreading out to assume the adult appearance of a single row.

From the earliest stage the inner surface of the cells is covered by a basement membrane and numerous fine cilia identical with those lining the neural tube, similar to those covering the corresponding surface of the presumptive sensory retina, but differing from the latter in the important respect that they disappear by the 10 mm. stage. From the outer surface of the cells a cuticular lamina is secreted, developing at a variable period usually between the 14 and 18 mm. stage into the ectodermal inner layer of Bruch's membrane ; the time of its appearance is disputed (6·5 mm., Seefelder, 1910 ; 3 months, Nordmann, 1947), but it is fully formed during

[1] For development see von Kölliker (1861), Rochon-Duvigneaud (1895), Kruckmann (1899), Raehlmann (1907), Lauber (1908), Seefelder (1910), Magitot (1910).

Figs. 139 and 140.—The Development of the Retinal Pigment Epithelium
(F. Vrabec).

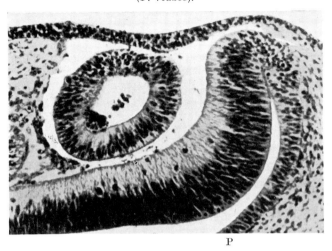

P

Fig. 139.—At the 8 mm. stage. Section through the anterior margin of the optic cup. The single outer layer of presumptive pigment epithelium, P, appears on section as if arranged in several rows owing to the differences in the level of the nuclei. There is little or no pigment present.

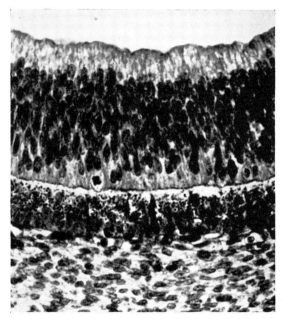

Fig. 140.—At the 30 mm. stage. There is a dense matting of pigment granules and the underlying choriocapillaris is well developed. Note the mitotic figures in the outer cellular layer of the retina.

the 4th month. By the 5th month the dual nature of Bruch's membrane has become apparent, the two layers (the ectodermal and the mesodermal) are separated from each other by a narrow space traversed by fine collagenous fibres (Wolfrum, 1908 ; Komai, 1937 ; Wolter, 1955), and by the 6th month the two portions become closely associated and the pigment epithelium is closely bound to the choroid (Barber, 1955). On the inner surface, however, the association with the sensory retina remains permanently loose ; between the two layers (the pigment epithelium and the sensory cells) a mucopoly-saccharide material was identified in the embryos of mice by Zimmerman and Eastham (1959), which may act as a cement substance or, alternatively may be concerned with the biochemistry of melanin.

Initially the cells of this layer contain no pigment, nor does this appear

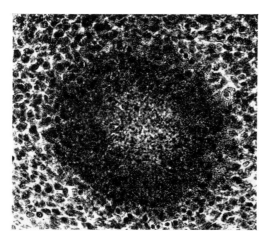

FIG. 141.—TANGENTIAL SECTION THROUGH THE PIGMENT EPITIHELIUM
IN AN EMBRYO OF 8 MM. (G. Renard).

until development is advanced to about the 5th week,[1] when small brown granules begin to make their appearance at the time when vascularization of the surrounding mesoderm commences ; it would appear that the proximity of capillaries is essential for the elaboration of pigment (Redslob, 1925). There is some doubt where the pigmentation first appears—at the equator (Lauber, 1908), whence it spreads posteriorly and anteriorly ; in the upper part of the cup anteriorly (Seefelder, 1910) ; or diffusely all over (Hervouët, 1958)—but once it has appeared pigmentation of the cells proceeds rapidly and is widespread by the 6th week (10 mm. stage) (Fig. 141). Initially, during the 2nd month, the granules are condensed in the outer half of the cells when a narrow brown line appears ; at the 23 mm. stage a similar line becomes evident in the inner parts of the cell so that for some time the central nuclei

[1] 5 to 6 mm., Barber 1955 ; 6·5 mm., Seefelder, 1910 ; 7 mm., Lauber, 1908 ; 7–8·5 mm., Magitot, 1910, Kolmer, 1936.

lie in a clear zone ; but by the 3rd month the pigment has become diffuse and the nuclei and all cellular structures have become obscured by the dense mass of pigment granules (Fig. 140).

THE CILIO-IRIDIC RETINA

Some time after the embryonic fissure has closed and the optic cup is thus fully formed, the cells comprising its anterior lip commence to proliferate rapidly and to grow forwards (48 mm. stage). The changes thus involved were extensively studied by Angelucci (1881), Schön (1895), O. Schultze (1902), von Lenhossek (1911), and others. At first the cavity of the optic vesicle persists separating its two walls, and, just as we have seen to occur at

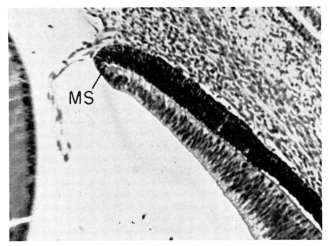

FIG. 142.—THE MARGIN OF THE OPTIC CUP AT THE 48 MM. STAGE.
The marginal sinus, MS, is beginning to develop at the tip of the growing margin
(A. N. Barber, *Embryology of the Human Eye*).

the upper part of the embryonic fissure, the inner wall shows the more rapid growth and everts itself over the edge so that the outer pigmented layer does not reach the margin (Fig. 139). Ultimately, however, both layers adhere except at the anterior growing edge where the cavity of the primary vesicle remains patent for a long time (Fig. 142).

Meantime, a number of radial folds appears round the circumference of the cup, at first involving the inner layer alone but eventually complicating both layers (65–75 mm. stage), and as the growing edge of the cup advances to form the ectodermal part of the iris, the folds, 70 to 75 in number, are left behind each to form a single CILIARY PROCESS (Fig. 143). Each fold is formed of the two fused layers of neural epithelium, the outer pigmented like the pigmented epithelium of the retina from which it is derived, and the inner composed of non-pigmented short columnar cells which retain all the characteristics of the primitive sensory retina of the 4 mm. stage. These folds increase slowly in size and depth, and into each projects a mesodermal core destined to become the ciliary muscle, carrying with it vascular elements. From the 5th to the 9th month, in accordance with the progressive increase in the size of the eye, they gradually move farther forwards, leaving behind a smooth region composed of the two fused epithelial layers (the pars plana) between the ciliary folds and the periphery· of the retina (Fig. 144). It is interesting that at the end of the 6th month the ora serrata lies on a level with the anterior border of the ciliary muscle, by the 8th month it lies approximately in its middle, and by the 9th month it reaches the posterior border of the muscle (Barber, 1955).

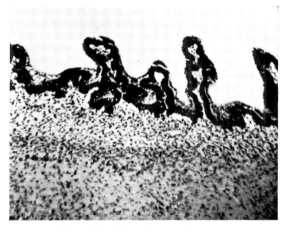

FIG. 143.—THE CILIARY REGION.

Cross-section of the ciliary processes at the 130 mm. stage. Both epithelial layers are composed of a single row of columnar cells, the outer being pigmented and the inner non-pigmented. Each process contains a core of mesodermal stroma (A. N. Barber, *Embryology of the Human Eye*).

The time at which the ciliary epithelium begins to secrete aqueous humour has been determined in the rabbit by Kinsey and his colleagues (1945) by studies of the hydrodynamics of the intra-ocular fluid, particularly concerning the initial secretion of ascorbic acid ; they found that this function began between the 7th and 9th day after birth. This can be correlated with structural changes occurring about the same time. In the basal cells the nuclei are situated apically until the 5th day but by the 30th day assume the basal position characteristic of the adult rabbit (Holmberg, 1959), while about the 7th day the complex interdigitations of the cell membranes usually associated with the development of a secretory function make their appearance and thereafter become progressively more complex (Pappas *et al.*, 1959).

As the margin of the optic cup grows forwards it curves inwards and insinuates itself in front of the lens and behind the mesoderm which separates it from the surface ectoderm ; with the posterior leaf of this mesoderm, which eventually forms the iris stroma, it remains closely associated and its anterior

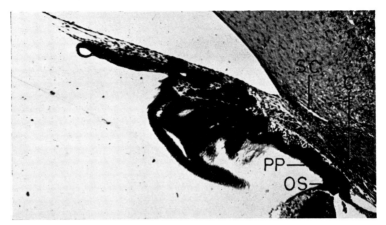

FIG. 144.—THE DEVELOPMENT OF THE CILIARY REGION.

At the 210 mm. stage (7th month). The marginal sinus of the iris is well seen. The ciliary region is divided into its two sections, the ciliary processes anteriorly and the pars plana, PP, posteriorly, running between the former and the ora serrata, OS. SC, Schlemm's canal ; C, ciliary muscle (A. N. Barber, *Embryology of the Human Eye*).

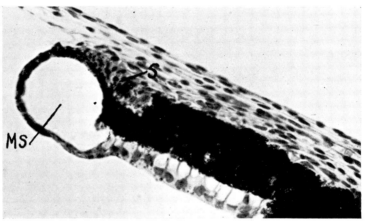

FIG. 145.—THE DEVELOPMENT OF THE IRIS.

At the 130 mm. stage. The marginal sinus, MS, has reached its maximum size. The unpigmented cells appearing on the lateral side of the anterior wall of the sinus are the sphincter muscle, S. The two epithelial layers of the iris are well seen. The unpigmented layer is below and the pigmented layer above, while the mesodermal stroma lies on top (A. N. Barber, *Embryology of the Human Eye*).

free border eventually forms the pupil. As it grows forwards the inner wall continues to show the more rapid growth and the same process of adhesion between its two constituent layers occurs as took place in the ciliary region so that the cavity of the vesicle is gradually obliterated. This process takes place from behind forwards until the cavity remains patent only at the

FIGS. 146 and 147.—THE DEVELOPMENT OF THE IRIS
(A. N. Barber, *Embryology of the Human Eye*).

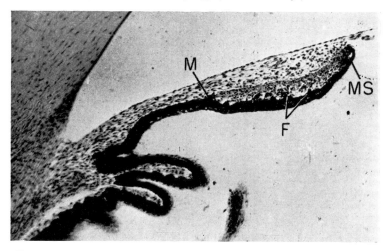

FIG. 146.—An unbleached specimen showing the marginal sinus, MS, reduced to a minute canal at the border of the iris. The sphincter muscle is well developed, demarcated proximally by von Michel's pigmented spur (M), while the posterior surface of the muscle is indented by the small groups of pigmented cells which constitute Fuchs's spurs (F). 230 mm. stage.

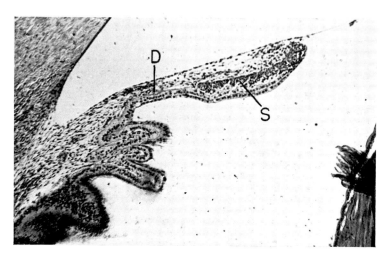

Fig. 147.—The same specimen as Fig. 146 bleached. The sphincter muscle (S) is seen to be divided into bundles of fibres by septa of connective tissue and it is separated from the underlying iris epithelium by a capillary plexus. The nuclei in the epithelial cells of the anterior layer near the periphery of the iris show the earliest signs of the formation of the dilatator muscle (D) by their migration to the posterior portion of the cells.

anterior extremity to form the MARGINAL (or RING) SINUS of von Szily (Figs. 144 and 145). As the ectodermal portion of the iris grows forward, this sinus enlarges and reaches its maximum size at 5 months, whereafter it slowly becomes smaller and disappears after the 7th month. It has been suggested by Mann (1949) that the persistence of this sinus probably depends on a lack of cohesion between the two layers owing to the rapid proliferative changes occurring in the growing lip of the optic cup. During its forward growth the inner (now the posterior) layer of columnar cells is originally unpigmented, but during the 5th month pigmentation gradually extends round from the outer (anterior) wall of the marginal sinus and proceeds along the posterior layer and extends backwards towards the ciliary region, a point which is reached by the 7th month. Apart from becoming more cuboid in shape, the posterior layer shows no further changes.

The anterior columnar layer, on the other hand, becomes differentiated to form the sphincter and dilatator pupillæ muscles. The SPHINCTER MUSCLE begins to become evident at the 65 mm. stage. In the small cubical cells lining the anterior wall of the marginal sinus, fine myofibrils make their appearance, and a compact mass of muscle cells is developed, gradually increasing in area down the anterior wall of the sinus as the growth of the iris proceeds (Fig. 145). These cells are non-pigmented, and thus the peripheral limit of the muscle is marked off by a projecting spur of pigment at the level where the epithelium retains its original character (von Michel's spur, 1890) (Fig. 146). At first the muscle forms a compact mass of fibres lying in close apposition with the anterior surface of the ectodermal layer, but at the 6 months' stage capillaries and connective tissue begin to grow into it, dividing it into bundles and finally separating it from the parent epithelium except at the pupillary border, where the two remain permanently associated (8th month) (Figs. 146 and 147).

The DILATATOR MUSCLE does not make its appearance until the 6th month, at which time in the anterior layer of the epithelium peripheral to von Michel's spur fine longitudinal fibrillations appear in the most anterior part of the cells, while the nuclei and pigment are posteriorly displaced (Figs. 147 and 148). The contractile muscle thus represents a direct transformation of the cytoplasm of the epithelial cells, to form, so to say, a myoepithelial unit. Although, unlike the sphincter, the dilatator is not fully formed or actively functional until after birth, it thus retains its embryonic nature practically unchanged throughout life ; it is not invaded by mesoderm nor is it vascularized and it remains permanently in close association with the epithelium of which it remains an integral part.

The ectodermal origin of these muscles is of great interest, for they are comparable in some measure to the primitive contractile cells in the body-wall of very lowly creatures such as the cœlenterates.[1] This primitive origin explains the fact that although in adult life they are ordinarily controlled by a nervous mechanism, they retain to some

[1] Vol. I, p. 513.

extent their ability to respond to the most primitive stimulus—the direct reaction to light. The only other muscular tissues in man which are not of mesodermal origin are the erectores pilorum and the myo-epithelial cells of the mammary glands, both of which are developed from the surface ectoderm of the skin. A further example of this embryological rarity is the origin of the retractor lentis muscle of teleosteans from the ectoderm of the lips of the embryonic fissure (von Szily, 1922)[1] ; while the contractility of the same layer of ectoderm under the same stimulus is seen in the phototactic movements of the cones.

So anomalous, indeed, are the origin and appearance of the dilatator muscle that, as we have already noted,[2] a controversy continued for long as to whether it existed as a muscle at all (Grünhagen, 1863–93 ; Fuchs, 1885 ; and others). The question was largely settled through the embryological researches of Grynfeltt (1898–9), Nussbaum

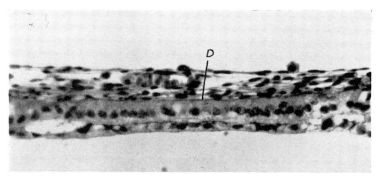

FIG. 148.—THE DILATATOR MUSCLE.

Bleached specimen at the 200 mm. stage. The nuclei of the anterior layer of epithelium have migrated to the posterior two-thirds of the cell and myofibrillæ running parallel to the surface of the iris form a discrete layer of dilatator fibres (D) in the anterior portion of the cells (A. N. Barber, *Embryology of the Human Eye*).

(1899–1901), Heerfordt (1900), von Szily (1901–2), Herzog (1902), and Vollaro (1908), and it has been amply confirmed by the subsequent work of Jusélius (1908), Speciale-Cirincione (1922), Wolfrum (1926), Mann (1928), Seefelder (1930), and Kolmer (1936).

At the same time it should be noted that the ectodermal origin of the muscle has not been completely accepted, and the original view put forward by von Kölliker (1867–98) and advocated by Bruch (1844), Dogiel (1870–86), and Vialleton (1897), that, like most muscles, it was formed from the mesodermal stroma of the iris, still has adherents (Redslob, 1928–53 ; Sondermann, 1932). Although the last word has perhaps not been said regarding the problem, it would seem, however, that the great mass of evidence supports the ectodermal origin of this somewhat anomalous muscle.

Angelucci. *Arch. mikr. Anat.*, **19** (2), 152 (1881).
Babuchin. *Würzburg. naturwiss. Z.*, **4**, 71 (1863).
Bach and Seefelder. *Atlas z. Entwicklungsgeschichte d. mensch. Auges*, Leipzig (1911–14).
Bailey. *Intracranial Tumours*, Springfield (1933).

Bailey and Cushing. *A Classification of Tumours of the Glioma Group on a Histogenic Basis*, Phila. (1926).
Barber. *Embryology of the Human Eye*, St. Louis (1955).
Benoit. *Bull. Biol.*, **71** (4), 393 (1937).
Bensted, Dobbing, Morgan, Reid and Wright. *J. Embryol. exp. Morph.*, **5**, 428 (1957).
Bernard. *Quart. J. micr. Sci.*, **44**, 25 (1903).

[1] Vol. I, p. 302.

[2] Vol. II, p. 178.

Boveri. *Zool. Jb., Suppl.* 7, 409 (1904).
Bruch. *Untersuch. z. Kenntniss d. körnigen Pigmentes d. Wirbelthiere*, Zürich (1844).
Cajal. *J. Anat. Physiol.* (Paris), **32**, 481 (1896).
Cattaneo. *Ann. Ottal.*, **50**, 349 (1922).
Chievitz. *Int. Mschr. Anat. Physiol.*, **4**, 201 (1887).
    Anat. Anz., **3**, 579 (1888).
    Arch. Anat. Entwickl., 332 (1890).
da Costa. *Acta anat.* (Basel), **4**, 79 (1947).
Dogiel. *Arch. mikr. Anat.*, **6**, 89 (1870) ; **27**, 403 (1886).
Falchi. *v. Graefes Arch. Ophthal.*, **34** (2), 67 (1888).
von Frisch. *Pflügers Arch. ges. Physiol.*, **138**, 319 (1911).
Froriep. *Hb. d. vergl. u. exper. Entwicklungslehre d. Wirbeltiere*, Jena, **2** (1906).
    Anat. Anz., **29**, 145 (1906).
Fuchs, E. *v. Graefes Arch. Ophthal.*, **21** (3), 39 (1885).
Graymore. *Brit. J. Ophthal.*, **43**, 34 (1959).
Greeff. *Graefe-Saemisch Hb. d. ges. Augenheilk.*, 2nd ed., Leipzig, **1** (2), Chap. 5 (1899).
Grünhagen. *Zbl. med. Wiss.*, 577 (1863).
    Z. rat. Med., **28**, 177 (1866).
    Pflügers Arch. ges. Physiol., **3**, 440 (1870) ; **33**, 59 (1884) ; **40**, 65 (1887) ; **53**, 348 (1892–3).
Grynfeltt. *C.R. Acad. Sci.* (Paris), **127**, 966 (1898).
    Ann. Oculist. (Paris), **121**, 122, 331 (1899).
Haden. *Amer. J. Ophthal.*, **28**, 943 (1945).
Harrison. *J. exp. Zool.*, **9**, 787 (1910).
Heerfordt. *Anat. Hefte*, **46**, 487 ; **49**, 721 (1900).
Hervouët. Dejean, Hervouët and Leplat's *L'embryologie de l'œil et sa tératologie*, Paris, 53 (1958).
Herzog. *Z. Augenheilk.*, **7**, 47 (1902).
    Arch. mikr. Anat., **60**, 517 (1902).
Hescheler and Boveri. *Vjschr. naturf. Ges.* Zürich, **68**, 398 (1923).
Holmberg. *Arch. Ophthal.* (Chicago), **62**, 935 (1959).
Huschke. *Arch. Anat. Physiol.*, **6**, 1 (1832).
Jusélius. *Klin. Mbl. Augenheilk.*, **46** (2), 19 (1908).
Kinsey, Jackson and Terry. *Arch. Ophthal.* (Chicago), **34**, 415 (1945).
von Kölliker. *Entwicklungsgeschichte d. Menschen*, Leipzig (1861).
    Hb. d. Gewebelehre d. Menschen, 5th ed., Leipzig, 667 (1867).
    Vhdl. phys.-med. Ges. Würzburg, **17**, 1 (1883).
    Anat. Anz., **14**, 200 (1897) ; Erg., 154 (1898).
Kolmer. *Hb. d. mikr. Anat. d. Menschen*, Berlin, **3** (2), 623 (1936).
Komai. *Acta Soc. ophthal. jap.*, **41**, 1891 (1937).
Krause, W. *Arch. mikr. Anat.*, **11**, 216 (1875).
Kruckmann. *v. Graefes Arch. Ophthal.*, **47** (3), 644 (1899).

Lauber. *v. Graefes Arch. Ophthal.*, **68**, 1 (1908).
Leboucq. *Arch. Anat. micr.*, **10**, 555 (1909).
von Lenhossek. *Anat. Anz.*, **38**, Erg., 81 (1911).
Loewe. *Arch. mikr. Anat.*, **15**, 596 (1878).
Magitot. *Ann. Oculist.* (Paris), **143**, 241 (1910).
Mann. *Amer. J. Ophthal.*, **11**, 515 (1928).
    Brit. J. Ophthal., **6**, 145 (1922) ; **12**, 449 (1928).
    Development of the Human Eye, Camb. (1928) ; 2nd ed. (1949).
    Trans. ophthal. Soc. U.K., **49**, 202 (1929).
Mawas and Magitot. *Arch. Anat. micr.*, **14**, 41 (1912).
Menner. *Z. Zellforsch.*, **11**, 415 (1930).
von Michel. *Lhb. d. Augenheilk.*, 2nd ed., Wiesbaden, 309 (1890).
Nordmann. *Bull. Histol. Techn. micr.*, **24**, 97 (1947).
Nowikoff. *Biol. Zbl.*, **52**, 548 (1932).
    Z. Morph. Oekol. Tiere, **29**, 374 (1934).
Nussbaum. *S. B. Niederrhein Ges. Natur.-Heilk.*, Bonn, 4 (1899).
    Arch. mikr. Anat., **58**, 199 (1901).
Pappas, Smelser and Brandt. *Arch. Ophthal.* (Chicago), **62**, 959 (1959).
Parker. *Amer. Nat.*, **42**, 601 (1908).
    Amer. J. Physiol., **25**, 77 (1909).
Pedler. *Brit. J. Ophthal.*, **45**, 423 (1961).
Penfield. Cowdry's *Special Cytology*, N.Y., **3** (1932).
Raehlmann. *Z. Augenheilk.*, **17**, 1 (1907).
Redslob. *Ann. Oculist.* (Paris), **162**, 368 (1925) ; **186**, 289 (1953).
    Bull. Soc. franç. Ophtal., **41**, 3 (1928) ; **43**, 206 (1930).
    Arch. Anat. (Strasbourg), **19**, 135 (1935).
    Traité d'Ophtal., Paris, **1**, 382 (1939).
Remak. *Untersuch. ü. d. Entwickl. d. Wirbelthiere*, Berlin (1855).
Retzius. *Nord. Med. Ark.*, **3**, 1 (1871).
    Biol. Untersuch., **11**, 82 (1904).
del Rio Hortega. *Mem. Spec. esp. Hist. Nat.*, **11**, 213 (1921).
Ritter. *v. Graefes Arch. Ophthal.*, **10** (1), 61 ; (2), 60, 142 (1864).
de Robertis, Gerschenfeld and Wald. *J. biophys. biochem. Cytol.*, **2**, 531 (1958).
Rochon-Duvigneaud. *Précis iconographique d'anatomie normale de l'œil*, Paris (1895).
Rowbotham, Haigh and Leslie. *Lancet*, **1**, 12 (1959).
Salzmann. *Anat. u. Histol. d. mensch. Augapfels*, Leipzig (1912).
Scharrer. *Z. vergl. Physiol.*, **7**, 1 (1928).
Schöler. *De oculi evolutione in embryonibus gallinaceis* (Diss.), Dorpat (1848).
Schön. *Arch. Anat. Entwickl.*, 417 (1895).
Schultze, M. *Arch. mikr. Anat.*, **3**, 215 (1867).
Schultze, O. *Verhdl. phys.-med. Ges. Würzburg*, **34**, 131 (1902).
Schwalbe. *Graefe-Saemisch Hb. d. ges. Augenheilk.*, 1st ed., Leipzig, **1**, 351 (1874).

Seefelder. *v. Graefes Arch. Ophthal.*, **73**, 419
(1910) ; **111**, 82 (1923).
  Anat. Hefte, **48**, 453 (1913).
  Kurzes Hb. d. Ophthal., Berlin, **1**, 476
(1930).
Sondermann. *Ber. dtsch. ophthal. Ges.*, **49**,
413 (1932).
Speciale-Cirincione. *Ann. Ottal.*, **50**, 5 (1922).
Strong and Elwyn. *Human Neuroanatomy*,
3rd ed., Baltimore, 51 (1953).
Studnicka. *Anat. Anz.*, **41**, 561 (1912) ; **44**,
273 (1913).
  Zool. Jb., Abt. Anat., **40**, 1 (1918).
von Szily. *Anat. Anz.*, **20**, 161 (1901) ; **24**,
417 (1903).
  v. Graefes Arch. Ophthal., **53**, 459 (1902) ;
109, 3 (1922).
  Anat. Hefte, **35**, 649 (1908).
Tansley. *Proc. roy. Soc. B.*, **114**, 79 (1933).
Tornatola. *Atti real. Accad. Peloritana*, **20**,
1 (1905).
Tousimis and Fine. *Amer. J. Ophthal.*, **48**
(2), 397 (1959).

Tretjakoff. *Z. wiss. Zool.*, **105**, 537 (1913).
Verhoeff. *Roy. Lond. ophthal. Hosp. Rep.*, **15**,
309 (1903).
Vialleton. *Arch. Anat. micr.*, **1**, 374 (1897).
Vollaro. *Ann. Ottal.*, **37**, 301 (1908).
Walls. *Arch. Ophthal.* (Chicago), **22**, 452
(1939).
Willmer. *Symposia Soc. exp. Biol.*, **7**, 377
(1953).
Windle. *Physiol. Rev.*, **36**, 427 (1956).
Wolff. *Trans. ophthal. Soc. U.K.*, **57**, 186
(1937) ; **60**, 61 (1940).
Wolfrum. *v. Graefes Arch. Ophthal.*, **69**, 145
(1908).
  Graefe-Saemisch Hb. d. ges. Augenheilk.,
2nd ed., Leipzig, **1** (2) (1926).
Wolter. *Arch. Ophthal.* (Chicago), **53**, 208
(1955).
Young. *J. exp. Biol.*, **12**, 254 (1935).
Zimmerman and Eastham. *Amer. J. Ophthal.*,
47 (2), 488 (1959).

THE LOWER VISUAL PATHWAY

THE OPTIC NERVE

The short optic stalk, which connects the optic vesicle to the forebrain, is originally (4 mm. stage) freely open to both cavities with a wide circular lumen, its walls being composed of a single layer of undifferentiated epithelial cells (Figs. 43 and 44 ; 149). We have seen that when the optic vesicle invaginates, the stalk shares in the process and a shallow depression appears along its ventral aspect. As the distance between brain and surface ectoderm increases, however, elongation of the stalk occurs but the invaginated portion does not extend proximally so that eventually (17 mm. stage) a gradually deepening groove near the eye divides the stalk into two regions, a distal invaginated segment which on section is crescent-shaped, and a proximal circular segment (Figs. 150 and 151). As the stalk lengthens it becomes thinner and the lumen progressively diminishes.

During this time nerve fibres are growing from the ganglion cells of the retina (15 mm.) and in the meantime the embryonic cleft is in the process of closing. As it does so the inner (retinal) wall of the optic cup at its proximal part, having folded around the hyaloid artery, is initially in direct continuity with the rest of the retina. As the first axons of the ganglion cells reach this point on their journey towards the brain, they turn at right angles and traverse the retinal layer to reach the optic stalk (Figs. 153 to 155). As this occurs all round the rim of the stalk some retinal cells are cut off from the main body and become sequestrated as a small clump of glial cells in the centre of the presumptive optic disc (Fig. 154). This cone-shaped mass of cells is known as the PRIMITIVE EPITHELIAL PAPILLA (of Bergmeister, 1877) and, as it is vascularized by the hyaloid artery, its cells form the sheath of this vessel and its branches (Figs. 154 and 155) (Jacoby, 1905 ; Wolfrum, 1907 ;

Seefelder, 1910 ; von Szily, 1921–22). When the main vessel disappears before birth the papilla atrophies simultaneously, the degree of atrophy determining the depth of the physiological cup of the disc, but some of its elements persist in the glial sheaths of the arteries ultimately supplying the retina (Versari, 1903–23 ; Krückmann, 1906 ; Seefelder, 1910).

Entering the optic stalk, the nerve fibres invade its invaginating (inner) layer and run towards the brain on its infero-nasal aspect (Cameron, 1905 ; von Szily, 1912 ; Barber *et al.*, 1954). This process proceeds gradually, many

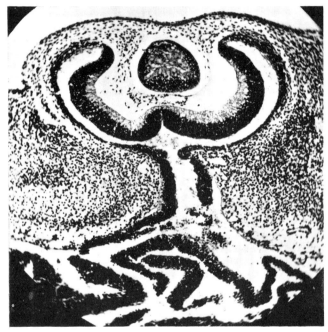

Fig. 149.—The Optic Pathways.
To show the continuity between the invaginated optic vesicle, the optic nerve and the forebrain ; in an embryo of 10 mm. (Henry Haden).

of the invaded cells becoming vacuolated and disappearing, until by the 19 mm. stage the lumen has been almost entirely filled in with nerve fibres (Fig. 152) ; at 25 mm. the whole of the stalk is thus occupied.[1] Some of the cells of the invaginated layer persist, however, and become transformed into star-like cells with anastomotic processes through the meshes of which the nerve fibres run. These cells, derived from the primitive epithelium of the optic stalk, form the glial supporting framework of the optic nerve (Lundberg, 1939 ; Haden, 1947). Initially they are scattered irregularly throughout the

---

[1] For the progress of development of the optic nerve fibres in the chick embryo, see Rogers (1957).

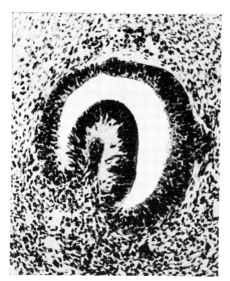

FIG. 150.—SECTION THROUGH THE DISTAL END OF THE OPTIC NERVE
IN A 14 MM. EMBRYO.

The invagination of the ventral wall is very obvious, reducing the lumen to a crescentic
shape. Inferiorly the ventral groove is filled with the mesodermal elements of the hyaloid
vessels. Around the nerve the beginning of the condensation of the sheaths is seen (F. Vrabec).

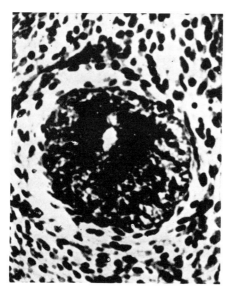

FIG. 151.—THE PROXIMAL PART OF THE OPTIC STALK IN A 20 MM. EMBRYO.
A small circular lumen near the centre represents the remains of the cavity (Henry Haden).

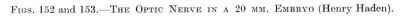
FIGS. 152 and 153.—THE OPTIC NERVE IN A 20 MM. EMBRYO (Henry Haden).

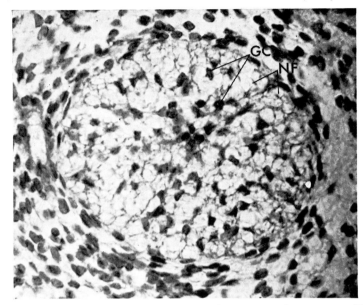

FIG. 152.—Cross-section showing glial cells with anastomosing processes, GC, and nerve fibres, NF.

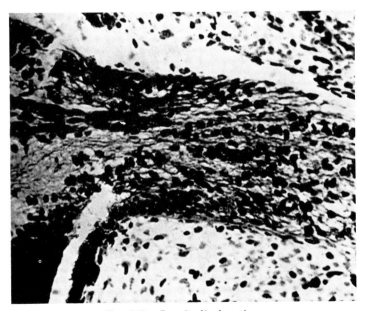

FIG. 153.—Longitudinal section.

FIGS. 154 and 155.—THE DEVELOPMENT OF THE OPTIC NERVE (Henry Haden).

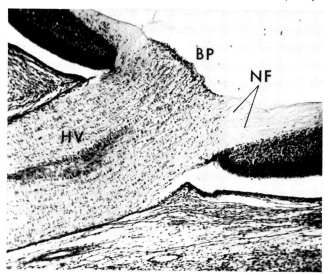

FIG. 154.—In a 45 mm. fœtus. BP, Bergmeister's papilla ; HV, hyaloid vessels ; NF, nerve fibres.

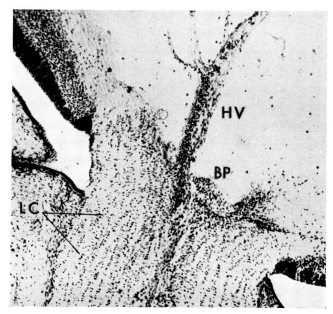

FIG. 155.—In a 67 mm. fœtus. The septa are rudimentary at this stage. LC, marks the anlage of the lamina cribrosa ; HV, hyaloid vessels continuing the central artery ; BP, tissues of Bergmeister's papilla.

FIGS. 156 and 157—THE DEVELOPMENT OF THE OPTIC NERVE (Henry Haden).

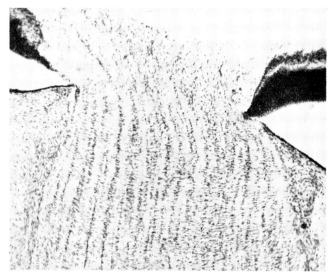

FIG. 156.—In a 97 mm. fœtus. Longitudinal section showing the development of septa and fibrous connective tissue.

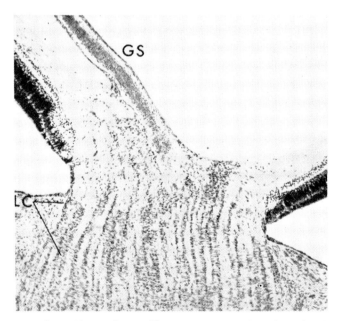

FIG. 157.—In a 160 mm. fœtus. The septa are more fully formed. The hyaloid artery has a marked glial sheath, GS.

nerve but by the 45 mm. stage they show an increasing tendency to assume an ordered arrangement and lie in longitudinal rows between the bundles of nerve fibres (Figs. 154 and 155). At this period the original epithelial cells forming the outer surface of the optic stalk, a layer of cells continuous with the pigment epithelium of the retina, are similarly transformed into the peripheral glial mantle surrounding the nerve ; these send processes into the substance of the nerve, but no mesodermal tissue other than that entering with the hyaloid artery[1] is present in the nerve at this stage (Haden, 1947) (Figs. 154 to 156). In the second half of the 2nd month a dense feltwork of these

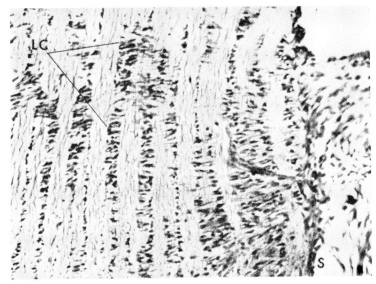

Fig. 158.—Development of the Optic Nerve in a 5 Month Fœtus.

High-power view to show the external glial mantle and the glia consolidating to form the lamina cribrosa (LC). Some capillaries are penetrating into the nerve from the periphery. S, the intervaginal space (F. Vrabec).

cells at the distal part of the nerve becomes orientated perpendicular to the nerve fibres to constitute the first elements of the lamina cribrosa, at this period wholly neuroglial in its constitution, composed entirely of astrocytes (Redslob, 1956) (Fig. 155). During the 4th month astrocytes and oligo-dendrocytes have begun to differentiate in the glial framework throughout the nerve (Marchesani, 1926 ; Lundberg, 1939) (Fig. 158).

As this development proceeds, from the 25 mm. stage onwards, the cavity of the optic vesicle thus no longer communicates with that of the forebrain ; only the recessus opticus in the floor of the third ventricle is left to mark the cerebral end of the original wide connection between the two. In the meantime, the lips of the distal part of the embryonic cleft have fused so

[1] p. 163.

8—2

Figs. 159 to 161.—The Formation of the Optic Nerve Sheaths.

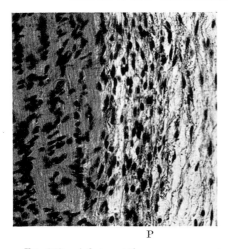 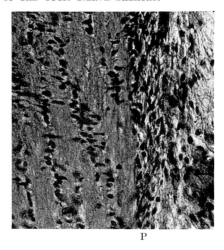

P   P

Fig. 159.—A fœtus at the commencement | Fig. 160.—At the end of the third month.
of the third month. The cells of the pial | The cells of the pial sheath (P) are becoming
sheath (P) are loosely arranged (G. Renard). | condensed (F. Hervouët).

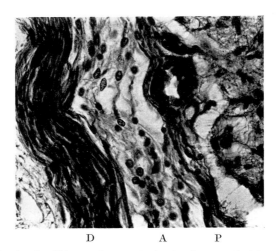

D   A   P

Fig. 161.—At the fifth month.   Both the dural (D) and pial sheaths (P) are
evident ; between them lie the presumptive cells of the arachnoid sheath (A)   (F.
Hervouët).

that the hyaloid artery, which eventually becomes the intraneural portion
of the central retinal artery,[1] after entering at the extreme proximal end of
the fissure with its accompanying mesoderm, becomes buried in the midst of
the nerve fibres (Figs. 155 and 157).   From the surrounding mesoderm, blood
vessels also invade the periphery of the nerve—starting proximally (65 mm.

[1] p. 204.

stage) and extending distally—taking with them mesodermal elements, primarily elastic tissue, and these, together with the mesoderm associated with the hyaloid vessels, eventually complete the septal system (Wilczek, 1947) (Fig. 158).

The surrounding tissue also develops layers of condensation, a process which begins to be apparent as early as the 10 mm. stage (Barber, 1955) ; by the 17 mm. stage a single compact coat begins to form, and at the 45 to 50 mm. stage the pial sheath is defined (Figs. 159 and 160); by the 5th month the dura is distinguishable, and last of all (6th and 7th months) the arachnoid sheath becomes differentiated between the two (Fig. 161). Although formerly

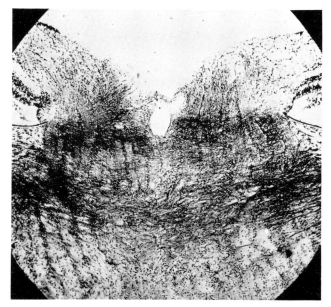

Fig. 162.—The Lamina Cribrosa in a Child of 2 Months (Henry Haden).

considered to be of mesodermal origin, it has been more recently shown that both the pia and arachnoid are largely ectodermal in nature, derived from neuroglial elements from the neural crests which migrate to the periphery (Harvey and Burr, 1926 ; Sensenig, 1951 ; Hervouët, 1958).

During the 8th and 9th months the architecture of the nerve is complete in all its essentials, and the fibres are enveloped in their sheathing of astrocytes and oligodendrocytes, the mesodermal elements of the septa have consolidated, while towards the end of this period the mesodermal microglia has made its appearance. The LAMINA CRIBROSA is the last part of the framework to be fully differentiated. Here mesodermal elements begin to reinforce the original glial basis ; they are discernible at the end of the 5th month and are well in evidence by the 7th month (Maggiore, 1923 ; Redslob, 1956 ;

Hervouët, 1958) (Fig. 158). During the 8th month the lamina becomes permeated by collagenous fibres from the sclera, the choroid, the dural sheath and the central core of connective tissue associated with the hyaloid vessels, a process which will be considered at a later stage (Wilczek, 1947 ; Redslob, 1956). Even at the end of the 9th month, however, this structure is quite supple and is not fully consolidated until some time after birth (Fig. 162).

During this period the nerve increases both in girth and length ; the most rapid increase occurs during the 5th month, the period when the dural sheath is being consolidated, during which time its length changes from 3 to 7 or 8 mm. (Hervouët, 1958). At birth its diameter is some 2·0 mm. and its length 24 mm. ; largely owing to the increase in the thickness of the myelin sheaths its diameter has increased to 2·4 mm. during the 3rd month after birth ; about the 6th month it lengthens considerably to accommodate the growth of the orbit and the brain, until at puberty its diameter is 3 to 4 mm. and its length averages 40 mm. (Keeney, 1951).

THE CHIASMA AND OPTIC TRACT

After the 25 mm. stage no fundamental alteration occurs in the optic nerve itself apart from its gradual increase in girth as the nerve fibres multiply, and its increase in length. At this stage the nerve appears as an elongated strand attached to the optic recess at the ventro-lateral angle of the diencephalon. As development proceeds the fibres gradually grow proximally into the central nervous system : at the 18 mm. stage they have left the ventral aspect of the stalk and have penetrated the marginal zone of the neural tube at the lateral angle of the optic recess on the under surface of the forebrain in front of the pituitary region, and enter the structures of the floor of the third ventricle near the junction of the telencephalon and the diencephalon ; by the 22 mm. stage (7 weeks) their decussation has given rise to the chiasma ; thereafter the fibres partially encircle the lateral aspect of the diencephalon where they approach and attach themselves to a peripheral collection of cells which differentiate from the dorso-lateral part of the mantle layer of the thalamus to form the dorsal nucleus of the lateral geniculate body (30 mm., Gilbert, 1935 ; Cooper, 1945) (Fig. 166). By the 48 mm. stage the optic tract has been formed and the lower visual pathway is completed (Fig. 163). Initially the anlage of the chiasma occupies a large portion of the floor of the third ventricle, but as it becomes increasingly enlarged by the addition of more nerve fibres, it dissociates itself from the floor of the ventricle and protrudes outwards so that the adult chiasma is related to the ventricle only on a small portion of its posterior aspect. Immediately above it is the optic recess, the permanent remnant of the proximal end of the cavity of the optic vesicle.

It is interesting that in the early stages of human development the primitive phylogenetic arrangement of a complete decussation of the nerve fibres occurs at the chiasma.[1] It is not until the 11th week (59 mm. stage) that uncrossed fibres begin to appear ; by the 13th week (80 mm.) the arrangement of a partial decussation similar to the adult condition has become established (Sakamoto, 1952).

Myelination. After the complete pathway has been laid down, medullation of the nerve fibres occurs in the reverse direction to their growth. At first very thin and composed of fine droplets of myelin, the medullated

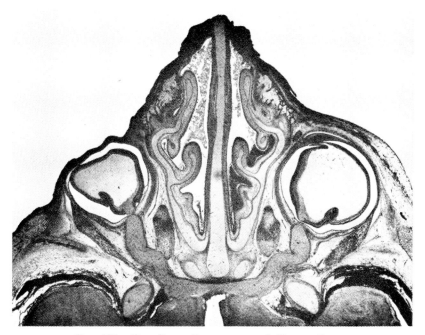

FIG. 163.—THE OPTIC CHIASMA IN A 3 MONTH FŒTUS.
Showing the completion of the lower visual pathways (G. Renard).

sheaths gradually become thickened, the droplets becoming larger and aggregated, a process which depends on the glial oligodendrocytes. There is no evidence of this process until about the 5th month when myelination is evident in the geniculate bodies and some time during the 6th month it is recognizable in the tract : at about the 6th or 7th month medullation has reached the chiasma, at the 8th month it is usually apparent in the optic nerve, and it slowly extends distally to reach the level of the lamina cribrosa at birth or some weeks thereafter, at which point the process normally ceases (Sattler, 1915 ; Beauvieux, 1926–47 ; Keeney, 1951).

Nothing is known of the development of the centrifugal fibres in the optic nerve although they may be seen as early as the 2nd month.

[1] Vol. I, p. 487.

THE CENTRAL VISUAL SYSTEM

In a book of this specialized type it is only desirable to outline the development of those parts of the brain which are particularly associated with vision and that in the most general manner. The following summary may, however, be useful from the ophthalmological point of view. We are concerned merely with the anterior part of the neural tube—that portion which forms the mesencephalon which is associated with visual functions in the lower vertebrates and the photostatic reflexes and visuo-motor system in the higher, and the prosencephalon within which are contained the visual pathways of the higher mammals (Fig. 164).[1] Below this level

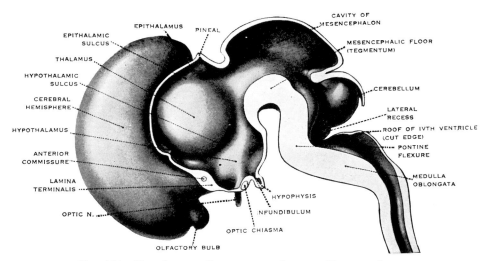

FIG. 164.—THE CRANIAL PART OF THE CENTRAL NERVOUS SYSTEM
IN A HUMAN FŒTUS.

Reconstruction of the medial surface of the right half of the cranial part of the central nervous system in a 43 mm. fœtus (× c. 6) (Hamilton, Boyd and Mossman's *Human Embryology*, W. Heffer, Cambridge).

the VIth, VIIth and VIIIth nerves (which are of ophthalmic interest) are developed at the junction of the metencephalon and the myelencephalon.

The MESENCEPHALON is developed from the walls of the mesencephalic vesicle as it constricts to form the narrow aqueduct of Sylvius. Dorsal to the aqueduct the roof of the neural tube becomes the *tectum*. Here two longitudinal elevations appear and these, subsequently developing a transverse constriction, evolve into the corpora quadrigemina, of which the superior colliculi are concerned with the visual reflexes, the inferior with the auditory ; as occurs throughout the nervous system both of them are formed by the migration of cells of the mantle zone into the marginal zone. From the floor of the mesencephalon ventral to the aqueduct (the *tegmentum*) are

[1] Vol. I, p. 530; see Figs. 30–32.

similarly developed the red nucleus and the substantia nigra as well as (probably) the somatic efferent nuclei of the 3rd and 4th cranial nerves. At a later stage, also in the floor, are developed several tracts interconnecting various parts of the brain—first the medial longitudinal fasciculus linking a number of cranial nerve nuclei ; at a later stage the lemnisci, both medial and lateral, the former bearing sensory (including trigeminal) impulses up to the thalamus, the latter associating the cochlea and cerebellum with the red nucleus and the inferior colliculi ; and finally, at a still later stage, the centrifugal pyramidal fibres.

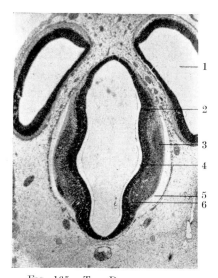

Fig. 165.—The Diencephalon.

In a 16 mm. embryo (× 30) (E. R. A. Cooper).

1, the cerebral vesicle ;	2, pars dorsalis thalami ;
3, pars ventralis thalami ;	4, hypothalamic sulcus ;
5, subthalamic nucleus ;	6, hypothalamus.

The PROSENCEPHALON, the most anterior part of the neural tube, becomes divided at an early stage (11 mm.) into two components, the diencephalon proximally and the paired vesicles of the telencephalon distally.

From the DIENCEPHALON which surrounds the cavity of the neural canal dilated to form the third ventricle, a number of structures of the visual system is developed (Fig. 165). At the 8·5 mm. stage (5 weeks) it is an oval tube from the anterior and ventral parts of which the hollow optic vesicles emerge and from the floor immediately behind these the minute hypophysial evagination is seen. At the 13 mm. stage (6 weeks) the cellular content of the lateral wall increases, and shortly thereafter (16 mm.) two sulci are evident, dividing the wall into three areas which bulge inwards towards the cavity of the ventricle—the thalamus centrally, the hypothalamus below and the epithalamus above (Gilbert, 1935 ; Cooper, 1945–50). From the mantle zone of these three areas is formed a large number of nuclear masses which bulge into the cavity of the third ventricle reducing it to a mere slit—the many nuclei of the thalamus (Figs. 166 and 167), the lateral constituents of the complex nuclear system of the hypothalamus, and (from the epithalamic region) the habenular nuclei.[1]

FIGS. 166 and 167.—THE DIENCEPHALON (E. R. A. Cooper).

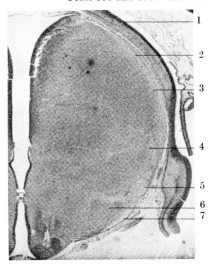
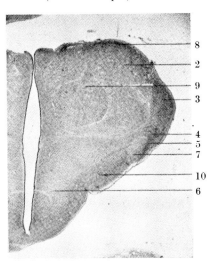

FIG. 166.—In a 35 mm. embryo (× 15).   FIG. 167.—In a 130 mm. fœtus (× 7).

1, wall of cerebral hemisphere ; 2, lateral thalamic nucleus ; 3, dorsal nucleus of lateral geniculate body ; 4, ventral nucleus of lateral geniculate body ; 5, fibres of optic tract ; 6, subthalamic nucleus ; 7, crus cerebri ; 8, pulvinar ; 9, dorso-median thalamic nucleus ; 10, substantia nigra.

Of these nuclei the most interesting from our point of view and the first to appear is the LATERAL GENICULATE BODY. The dorsal nucleus is recognizable in the 22 mm. embryo in the lateral part of the dorsal thalamus at a time when the remainder of the thalamus is still undifferentiated, its formation coinciding with the arrival of the optic nerve fibres in this region. The ventral nucleus of the geniculate appears somewhat later, being first apparent at the 35 mm. stage in the subthalamic region (Fig. 166). At this time there is no lamination within the nucleus, nor does this become evident until the 6th month of gestation when six U-shaped laminæ appear with their convex aspects orientated ventro-laterally to receive the fibres of the optic tract (Figs. 168 and 169) ; from their concavities, directed dorso-medially, issue the fibres of the optic radiations (Cooper, 1945).

From the roof-plate of the diencephalon are developed the tela choroidea, the paraphysis (which disappears in human embryos but develops into the

[1] See Kuhlenbeck (1930), Clark (1932), Crouch (1934), Walker (1938), Cooper (1945–50), Krieg (1948), and others.

FIGS. 168 and 169.—THE LATERAL GENICULATE BODY (E. R. A. Cooper).

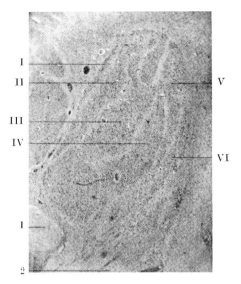

FIG. 168.—In a 6½ months' fœtus (× 20).

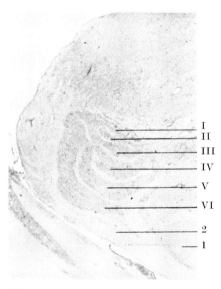

FIG. 169.—In a full-term fœtus (× 12).

I to VI, the laminæ of the geniculate body ; 1, crus cerebri ; 2, fibres of optic tract.

parietal gland of reptiles[1]) and the pineal body. In the floor lie the medial hypothalamic nuclei, anterior to which is a diverticulum (the infundibulum) from which the stalk and the pars nervosa of the hypophysis develop, and immediately cephalad is the thickening into which the optic nerve fibres travel to form the chiasma.

The development of the HYPOPHYSIS is composite. The *pars nervosa* is composed of the modified neuroglial cells of the floor of the diencephalon which, as we have seen, forms a diverticulum extending ventrally. The anterior lobe is determined by an ectodermal diverticulum (Rathke's pouch) which extends upwards from the roof of the stomatodæum in front of the tip of the notochord towards the floor of the diencephalic portion of the neural tube. The two come into contact at the 14 mm. stage ; Rathke's pouch loses its connection with the stomatodæum, the cells of its anterior wall proliferate so actively as to reduce its lumen to a narrow cleft, thus forming the *pars anterior* of the gland, while the posterior wall develops but poorly and remains as the *pars intermedia*.

The TELENCEPHALON appears at about the 9 mm. stage as bilateral evaginations from the most anterior portion of the prosencephalon, the walls forming the cerebral hemispheres, and the cavities (lateral ventricles) retaining connection with the axial neural canal through the interventricular foramina. The basal part of the wall of each hemisphere becomes thickened to form a *striatal* portion within which the nuclei of the corpus striatum are developed ; above this the wall remains relatively thin as the *pallium*, the primordium of the cerebral cortex. The part lateral to the developing corpus striatum—the *palæo-pallium* (the sole representation of the cortex in cyclostomes and selachian fishes[2])—forms the pyriform cortex which is associated with olfactory impulses. More centrally, encircling the median and lateral ventricles, is the *archipallium* (appearing phylogenetically in teleostean fishes and ontogenetically at the 12 mm. stage) : this determines the hippocampal formation with which is associated a ring of primitive gyri, the *mesopallium*, both of which are concerned with olfactory and autonomic functions. The remainder of the telencephalon forms the *neopallium*, the enormous growth of which pushes aside the other components of the cortex so that eventually they occupy a relatively insignificant area mainly on the medial surface of the hemisphere. Throughout this region the neuroblasts of the mantle zone proliferate peripherally to the marginal zone to form the grey matter of the cerebral cortex, to which afferent (including visual) impulses are relayed from the diencephalic nuclei, from which motor impulses are sent out, and within which a complex system of associations is formed to coordinate the incoming and outgoing messages and to mediate the higher intellectual functions.

The first step in cortical differentiation is, as usual in neural development, a migration of cells from the mantle zone into the marginal zone to form a superficial cortical layer, a process occurring first in the lateral portion

[1] Vol. I, p. 715.   [2] Vol. II, p. 807.

of the cerebral wall in the parietal area (30 mm. stage) and extending rapidly into the roof and medial wall. This migration does not occur in the frontal and occipital lobes until later, but at the 50 mm. stage it has extended over the entire hemisphere. The main somatic sensory receptive area thus takes precedence over the visual area in development, both, of course, being secondary to the olfactory mechanism. Stratification of the cortex is achieved slowly, partly by the breaking up of the primary superficial layer and partly by the arrival of successive waves of migration from the mantle layer.

Myelination of the tracts of the central nervous system occurs at various times ; indeed, it was owing to this observation that Paul Flechsig (1874–1927) of Leipzig was able first to delineate accurately many of the fibre-tracts in the central nervous system, including the optic radiations.[1] The first of these to show myelination is the medial longitudinal bundle (6th month) but it is rapidly followed by several tracts in the midbrain. Cerebellar and thalamic connections are myelinated about the 8th month ; and in the cerebral cortex the process occurs in projection systems before association tracts. Of the former the upper visual pathways are the first to be implicated and begin to be myelinated about the time of birth, the process proceeding centrifugally from the occipital centre ; at the end of the 4th month after birth all the main fibre-tracts have similarly developed.

Flechsig (1876) originally thought that myelination could be correlated with functional activity, a suggestion, however, disproved by Langworthy (1929) who demonstrated that fibres can be myelinated and yet not function, and others function although not yet myelinated. Magitot (1909), for example, established the functional activity of the lower visual pathway at the 6th month by demonstrating the photo-motor reflex in premature infants—that is, at a stage long before myelination of the fibres is complete. It may, however, be that the pupillomotor fibres are medullated before the visual fibres (Beauvieux, 1947). It is thus dangerous to attribute functional ocular defects, such as amblyopia or strabismus in infants, to delayed myelination (Beauvieux, 1947 ; Keeney, 1951).

Barber. *Embryology of the Human Eye*, St. Louis (1955).
Barber, Rowstrom and Muelling. *Amer. J. Ophthal.*, **52**, 447 (1954).
Beauvieux. *Ann. Oculist.* (Paris), **163**, 881 (1926).
   Arch. Ophtal. (Paris), **7**, 241 (1947).
Bergmeister. *Mitt. embryol. Inst. Wien, Heft.* 1, 63 (1877).
Cameron. *J. Anat. Physiol.*, **39**, 135, 332, 471 (1905).
Clark. *Brain*, **55**, 406 (1932).
Cooper. *Brain*, **68**, 222 (1945) ; **69**, 45 (1946). *Acta anat.* (Basel), **9**, 201 (1950).
Crouch. *J. comp. Neurol.*, **59**, 431, 451 (1934).
Flechsig. *Allg. Z. Psychiat.*, **30**, 112 (1874).

Die Leitungsbahnen im Gehirn u. Rücken-mark d. Menschen, Leipzig (1876).
Meine myelogenetische Hirnlehre, Berlin (1927).
Gilbert. *J. comp. Neurol.*, **62**, 81 (1935).
Haden. *Amer. J. Ophthal.*, **30**, 1205 (1947).
Harvey and Burr. *Arch. Neurol. Psychiat.* (Chicago), **15**, 545 (1926).
Hervouët. Dejean, Hervouët and Leplat's *L'embryologie de l'œil et sa tératologie*, Paris, 171 (1958).
Jacoby. *Klin. Mbl. Augenheilk.*, **43** (1), 129 (1905).
Keeney. *Chronology of Ophthalmic Development*, Springfield (1951).
Krieg. *J. comp. Neurol.*, **88**, 1 (1948).

---

[1] Vol. II, p. 65.

Krückmann. *Klin. Mbl. Augenheilk.*, **44** (1),
      162 (1906).
Kuhlenbeck. *Anat. Anz.*, **70**, 122 (1930).
Langworthy. *Contrib. Embryol. Carn. Instn.*,
      20, 127 (1929).
Lundberg. *Acta ophthal.* (Kbh.), **17**, 259
      (1939).
Maggiore. *Ann. Ottal.*, **51**, 727 (1923).
Magitot. *Ann. Oculist.* (Paris), **141**, 161 (1909).
Marchesani. *v. Graefes Arch. Ophthal.*, **117**,
      575 (1926).
Redslob. *Ann. Oculist.* (Paris), **189**, 749
      (1956).
Rogers. *Anat. Rec.*, **127**, 97 (1957).
Sakamoto. *Acta Soc. ophthal. jap.*, **56**, 1355
      (1952) ; **57**, 146 (1953).
Sattler. *v. Graefes Arch. Ophthal.*, **90**, 271
      (1915).

Seefelder. *v. Graefes Arch. Ophthal.*, **73**, 419
      (1910).
Sensenig. *Contrib. Embryol. Carn. Instn.*, **34**,
      147 (1951).
von Szily. *v. Graefes Arch. Ophthal.*, **81**, 67
      (1912) ; **106**, 195 (1921) ; **107**, 317 ; **109**,
      3 (1922).
Versari. *Ric. Lab. Anat. Univ. Roma*, **10**, 1
      (1903).
      Anat. Anz., **35**, 105 (1909).
      Ric. Morfol., **3**, 1 (1923).
Vrabec. *Csl. Ofthal.*, **11**, 213 (1955).
Walker. *The Primate Thalamus*, Chicago
      (1938).
Wilczek. *Brit. J. Ophthal.*, **31**, 551 (1947).
Wolfrum. *v. Graefes Arch. Ophthal.*, **65**, 220
      (1907).

CHAPTER V

THE DEVELOPMENT OF THE SURFACE ECTODERM

WE are introducing this chapter with a portrait of CARL RABL [1853–1917] (Fig. 170), one of the greatest zoologists and anatomists at the turn of the century. Born in Wels in Austria, he studied medicine in Vienna, Leipzig and Jena under such masters as Ernst Haeckel and Ernst Brücke. In 1886 he was appointed professor in the Anatomical Institute in Prague and during the year 1903–4 he became Rector of that university. Thereafter he went to Leipzig to occupy the chair in the Anatomical Institute after Wilhelm His. His early fundamental work concerned the minute structure of cells, their organization and differentiation, but in his later years he spent much time on embryology. The process of gastrulation was considerably clarified by his researches and he also contributed to such difficult problems as the role of the mesoderm in development and the metamerism of the head. He always maintained an interest in the embryology of the eye, particularly of the vitreous, but his greatest contribution in this respect was undoubtedly the classical study he made of the development and morphology of the lens throughout the animal kingdom. It is interesting that the last paper he wrote was on the bilateral and naso-temporal symmetry of the eyes of vertebrates.

At a very early stage in embryonic life there is nothing to differentiate the surface ectoderm in the region of the future eye ; the whole of the ecto-dermal covering is uniformly composed of a single layer of cubical cells. As soon as the optic vesicle approximates the surface, however, changes begin to occur in the ectoderm, which, as we have seen,[1] are presumably determined by a chemical inductive stimulus from the vesicle itself. These changes involve a thickening of the epithelium to form the lens plate and its invagination into the lens vesicle from which the lens is ultimately evolved ; while the surface epithelium, closing up once more over the invaginated vesicle, remains to form the epithelium of the cornea.

THE LENS

The story of the development of the lens has long been known ; imperfectly told in the writings (among others) of Huschke (1832), von Baer (1837) (both of whom considered it to be a coagulum formed within the optic vesicle), Valentin (1835) (who demonstrated its origin from ectodermal cells), Schwann (1839), Meyer (1851), Kessler (1877), His (1880), von Kölliker (1887), and Cirincione (1897), the sequence of events was finally established in its true perspective by the classical work of Rabl (1898–1900) on the developing lenses of all types of vertebrates.

The development of the lens may be divided into two stages : the formation of the lens vesicle, and the development of the lens fibres with the evolution of the nuclei.

Up to the 4 mm. stage the surface ectoderm is composed of a single layer

---

[1] p. 63.

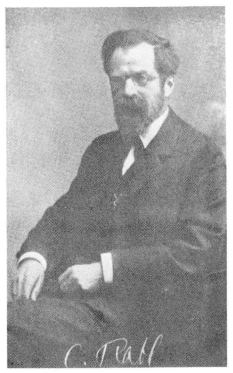

FIG. 170.—CARL RABL
[1853–1917].

of cubical cells and is entirely undifferentiated, but as soon as the optic vesicle approaches it (about the 4·5 mm. stage), the surface cells immediately overlying the vesicle, while still remaining arranged in a single row, assume a columnar form and undergo mitotic division, so that their nuclei become arranged unevenly and appear on section to lie in several rows. In this way

FIGS. 171 to 174.—THE DEVELOPMENT OF THE LENS
(R. O'Rahilly, Carnegie Institution of Washington, Baltimore).

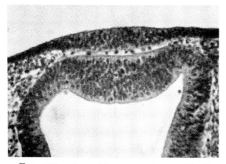

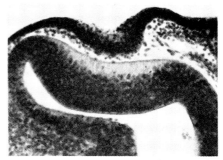

FIG. 171.—In a 4·8 mm. embryo. The lens plate is seen as a thickening of the surface epithelium overlying the neuro-epithelium of the presumptive retina just beginning to thicken and invaginate.

FIG. 172.—In a 5·3 mm. embryo. The beginnings of the invagination of the lens plate to form the lens pit.

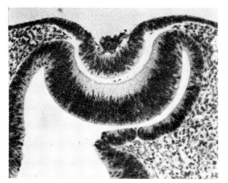

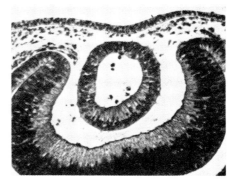

FIG. 173.—In a 6·3 mm. embryo. The lens pit deepens to form the beginnings of the lens vesicle. Note the epitrichial cells in the depths of the pit.

FIG. 174.—In an 8·8 mm. embryo. The lens pit has invaginated to form the lens vesicle containing a few epitrichial cells in its cavity.

a thickening of the epithelium is formed: the LENS PLATE (Fig. 171). It is interesting that immediately after the optic vesicle contacts the surface ectoderm and before morphological differentiation occurs to form the lens plate, specific antigens are found in the surface ectodermal cells (Langman, 1959 ; Koniukhov and Lishtvan, 1959).

Shortly after its appearance (about the 5 mm. stage) the lens plate begins to invaginate, making a depression on the surface towards the lower part of the plate: the LENS PIT, a formation first demonstrated by Kessler (1877) (Figs. 172 and 173). The walls of the pit are still composed of cells arranged in a single row, although the nuclei still lie at different levels. This pit rapidly deepens by cellular multiplication, and as invagination progresses it remains open to the exterior by an ever-narrowing stalk until at the 7 mm. stage the lumen of the stalk disappears and the LENS VESICLE separates itself from the surface ectoderm (Fig. 174). At the 10 mm. stage it has become a hollow sphere the wall of which remains as a single layer of epithelium, but it has now become separated from the surface by the ingrowth of mesodermal cells which not only insinuate themselves between the surface ectoderm and the lens vesicle but also invade the interior of the optic cup. As the process of invagination and vesicle-formation proceeds, the primary optic vesicle is similarly invaginating to form the optic cup,[1] and as the lens vesicle retreats from the surface it enters the cup and initially almost completely fills its cavity (Fig. 174). At the same time the separation of the three ectodermal layers appears on histological sections not to be complete, for the lens vesicle remains connected for some time both to the surface ectoderm and to the underlying neural ectoderm as it invaginates to form the optic cup by fine strands or filaments in the composition of which the mesodermal cells also appear to participate (the anterior vitreous).[2] Classically these connecting strands have been interpreted as protoplasmic bridges, but it has been suggested by some workers that these bridges are in fact artefacts induced by fixatives in a protein-rich fluid (Dejean, 1958) (see Fig. 195) ; their histological appearance is undoubtedly due to coagulation, but that some protoplasmic continuity exists seems possible.

In most vertebrates the lens is formed in this way as an invaginated vesicle ; but in selachians the vesicle is formed secondarily from a solid mass of cells which separates from the surface.

At an early stage the surface epithelium differentiates into two layers : (1) the primitive layer of cubical cells, and (2) a superficial epitrichial layer of flat cells lying upon them, the precursors of the squamous cells which will eventually cover the whole body of the embryo. When the lens pit is formed a mass of these superficial cells lies within it (Fig. 173), and when the lens pit closes to form a vesicle, some of these cells are shut up inside (Fig. 175), but soon degenerate and disappear (16 mm. stage). Their presence is thus purely fortuitous and they take no share in the development of the lens, a circumstance which is seen more clearly in lower forms. Thus in Sauropsidæ the superficial layer does not become differentiated until after the closure of the vesicle, in which case no epitrichial cells are ever associated with it, and in most fishes (other than selachians) and some amphibians, wherein the lens is formed after the differentiation of the ectoderm is complete, it is developed from an invagination of the deep layer only (Mann, 1928).

Once the vesicle is formed, the second stage of development proceeds apace. The cells of the anterior wall, which were derived from the periphery

[1] p. 32.   [2] p. 153.

of the lens plate, divide in one plane only but otherwise remain unchanged and appear all through life as a single layer of cubical cells under the anterior capsule. The cells of the posterior wall and the equatorial region of the vesicle, on the other hand, undergo marked differentiation, and from these is

FIGS. 175 to 178.—THE DEVELOPMENT OF THE LENS.

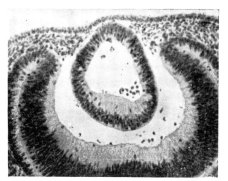

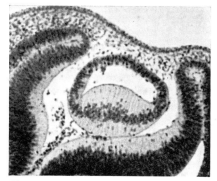

FIG. 175.—In a 9·0 mm. embryo. The commencement of growth in the cells of the posterior aspect of the lens vesicle.

FIG. 176.—In a 13·2 mm. embryo. The growth of the posterior epithelium is diminishing the cavity of the lens vesicle to a crescent.

(Figs. 175 and 176, R. O'Rahilly, Carnegie Institution of Washington.)

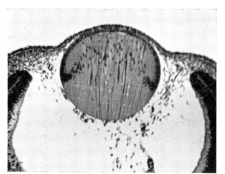

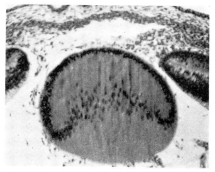

FIG. 177.—In an 18 mm. embryo. The cavity of the lens vesicle is practically closed.

FIG. 178.—In a 26 mm. embryo. The nuclei of the fibres have orientated themselves to form a lens bow.

(Figs. 177 and 178, A. N. Barber.)

formed the whole of the adult lens. At the 9 to 10 mm. stage the most central cells of the posterior wall (which were derived from the central area of the lens plate) differentiate first, becoming elongated and columnar ; the more peripheral cells of the posterior wall of the vesicle rapidly follow suit with a resulting encroachment upon the cavity of the vesicle so that it becomes crescentic instead of circular (Figs. 175 and 176) ; ultimately they reach the anterior wall and thus completely obliterate the cavity (18 mm. stage :

Figs. 177 and 178) ; simultaneously the cell nuclei initially migrate anteriorly to form a curved line (the *nuclear bow*) (20 to 22 mm.) but thereafter they gradually disappear in the centre.   These constitute the *primary lens fibres* which remain unchanged throughout life, ultimately occupying the central area of the lens ; here they form the optically clear embryonic nucleus in which the central elongated lens fibres run in a direct antero-posterior course while the shorter peripheral fibres show a curve concave towards the equator.   At a relatively early period, however, they lose all evidence of the

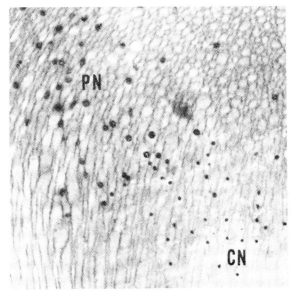

FIG. 179.—PARA-SAGITTAL SECTION THROUGH THE LENS.
In a 3 month fœtus. Showing normal nuclei in the periphery (PN) and nuclei of the central fibres undergoing pyknotic changes (CN) (F. Vrabec).

capacity for metabolic activity, their nuclei becoming pyknotic and their mitochondria granular and eventually disappearing (Stroeva, 1959) (Fig. 179).

Meantime, cellular division and growth are proceeding at the region of the equator, where the cubical cells lining the lateral part of the vesicle rapidly multiply and elongate to form *secondary fibres*.   Their mode of growth is peculiar and regular : the anterior end of each passes forwards towards the anterior pole of the lens, insinuating itself underneath the anterior epithelium, while the posterior end passes backwards towards the posterior pole running deep to the hyaline capsule (Fig. 180).   In this way new fibres are formed, layer upon layer, encircling the central nucleus of primary fibres which thus becomes encased within them.   This process of gradual growth, whereby each fibre and each successive layer of fibres cover the surface of those just previously formed, goes on until adult life with the

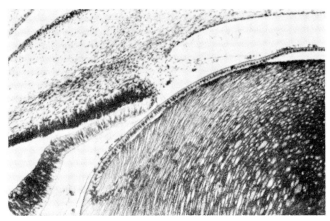

FIG. 180.—In a 41 mm. fœtus, to show the nuclear bow at the equator of the lens. Note the peripheral portion of the pupillary membrane running from the angle of the anterior chamber over the anterior lens capsule (G. Leplat).

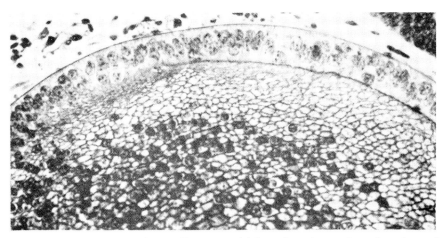

FIG. 181.—In a 41 mm. fœtus. Pre-equatorial frontal section to show the subcapsular epithelium and the lens fibres (F. Vrabec).

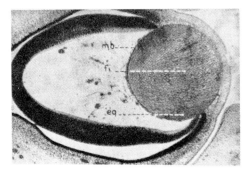

FIG. 182.—In a 50 mm. fœtus. Section cutting the lens obliquely. *eq*, equatorial zone producing new fibres ; *fi*, central fibres ; *mb*, basal membrane of the lens (C. Dejean).

result that the lens is continuously growing in size by the laying down of zones of fibres in the periphery. The process of accretion, indeed, continues up to old age. Until the stage of active proliferation of the equatorial epithelial cells the lens has remained spherical in shape; but the continued division and growth in this region increase the equatorial diameter in comparison with the axial and the structure gradually takes on the lentoid shape characteristic of the adult (Figs. 180 to 182).

The Zones of the Lens. Apart from the primary fibres which retain their embryonic transparency, as time goes on the successively formed secondary fibres become more sclerosed than the more recently formed superficial

Figs. 183 and 184.—The Structure of the Lens as shown in the Optical Beam of the Slit-lamp.

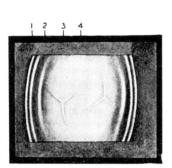

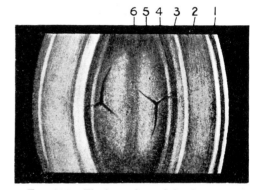

Fig. 183.—The lens of a 3-year-old infant.

1. Anterior capsule.
2. Infantile nucleus.
3. Fœtal nucleus.
4. Embryonic nucleus.

Fig. 184.—The lens of an adult of 40 years.

1. Anterior capsule.   4. Infantile nucleus.
2. Cortex.   5. Fœtal nucleus.
3. Adult nucleus.   6. Embryonic nucleus.

ones; consequently as growth proceeds a definite stratification into zones appears which can best be made out optically, as by the slit-lamp (Vogt, 1921), a differentiation particularly obvious with polarized light (Babel and Baud, 1953). In the adult the following zones of discontinuity are seen[1] (Figs. 183 and 184).

A. NUCLEI. 1. *The embryonic nucleus,* an optically clear central area, formed in embryonic life (months 1 to 3) representing the primary lens fibres which retain their embryonic transparency.

2. *The fœtal nucleus,* formed from secondary fibres from the 3rd to 8th month of fœtal life.

3. *The infantile nucleus,* laid down during the last weeks of fœtal life and continuing to be formed up to puberty.

4. *The adult nucleus,* formed after puberty in adult life.

[1] For terminology, see Vol. II, p. 321.

B. CORTEX. The soft and young superficial fibres formed after puberty, lying between the nuclei and the subcapsular epithelium.

A further refinement was made by Goldmann (1937), using an elegant optical method, who found that the layers laid down in adolescence could be further divided into zones of discontinuity, each stratum taking about 4 years to form.

It is obvious that the localization of pathological changes in one or other of these layers allows an accurate reconstruction to be made of their ontogenetic history, the zones acting, as it were, like the rings in the sawn-off trunk of a tree.

The Sutures of the Lens. We have seen that the primary fibres reach uninterruptedly from the posterior to the anterior extremity of the lens, but none of the secondary fibres is sufficiently long to extend in a curved

FIGS. 185 to 187.—THE FORMATION OF THE SUTURES OF THE LENS.

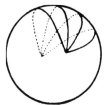 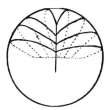 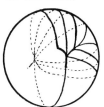

FIG. 185.   FIG. 186.   FIG. 187.

course all the way from one pole to the other. Their lines of junction must therefore be linear ; sutures are thus formed and since a fibre starting at a suture line nearest one pole must terminate at a point furthest from the other pole, the pattern of sutures must be reversed on the anterior and posterior aspects of the lens. The ends of the fibres are slightly tapered and flattened, fitting in snugly with those they meet so that the region of union is flat and optically undisturbed—less so, in fact, than would result if all the fibres met at a point at either pole (Fig. 185).

The earliest suture lines are seen in the fœtal nucleus throughout which they run. During a transient stage in development these form the simplest pattern of two lines running in a vertical direction anteriorly and a horizontal direction posteriorly (Fig. 186) (an arrangement which remains permanently in lower vertebrates) ; according to Yamasaki (1957) the posterior suture is evident as a horizontal line towards the end of the 2nd month to be fully formed in the 3rd month, in the middle of which the anterior suture begins to form. After a short period, towards the end of the 3rd month, these lines branch into a triradiate form resembling the letter Y, orientated in the erect position anteriorly and the inverted position posteriorly (Figs. 187, 188, 189). As the path of the fibres increases in length with age, the suture

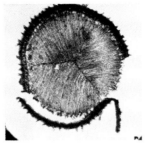

FIG. 188.—THE LENS OF A HUMAN EMBRYO OF 30 MM.

Frontal section of the lens showing the fibres inserted along the line of the Y-suture (G. Leplat).

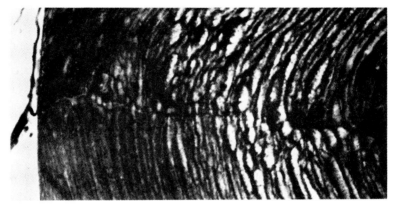

FIG. 189.—THE POSTERIOR SUTURE OF THE LENS IN A 4-MONTH FŒTUS (F. Vrabec).

lines of successive zones must become more complex. In the infantile
nucleus the simple Y becomes a star ; in the adult nucleus the suturing is
variable but usually is based upon a vertical line which bifurcates above and

FIGS. 190 and 191.—THE SUTURES OF THE ADULT LENS AS SEEN BY THE SLIT-LAMP.

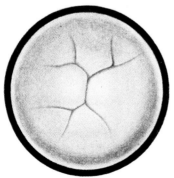
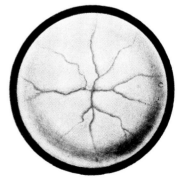

FIG. 190.—The adult nucleus.   FIG. 191.—The adult cortex.

below (Fig. 190) ; and in the cortex this arrangement becomes still more complex, the vertical line sending out 9 to 12 branches to form the *lens star* (Fig. 191).

THE LENS CAPSULE

Around the vesicle a structureless hyaline capsule is evident as a well-formed layer at about the 8 mm. stage (Fig. 181). It was said by the older authors to be secreted by the underlying ectodermal cells (Kessler, 1877 ; von Kölliker, 1887 ; Rabl, 1898 ; and others). On the other hand, the suggestion has been made that the vascular elements which eventually surround the developing lens take a share in its formation (Truc and Vialleton, 1903) ; but this (mesodermal) tunica vasculosa lentis[1] is probably a quite separate structure. The capsule would seem to be of ectodermal origin, and is developed as a thickening of the fine basement membrane lining the inner aspect of that portion of the surface ectoderm which is destined to form the lens vesicle and is necessarily carried in with it as it becomes invaginated (O'Rahilly and Meyer, 1960). According to Dejean (1958) all the ecto-dermal surfaces of the eye are similarly clothed with membranes which tend to grow by accretion ; indeed, in his view, the same material in a less condensed form constitutes the greater part of the vitreous body and the zonule.[2]

At a later stage of development we shall see presently[3] that the " tertiary vitreous " which forms the suspensory mechanism of the lens associates itself with the lens capsule. Commencing at the 5th month the fibres of the zonule, at this stage fine and delicate, are seen to run from the ciliary epithelium to the equatorial region of the lens where they establish themselves as a fine continuous membrane superficial to the capsule (the ZONULAR LAMELLA). While adequate developmental studies are lacking, the adult capsule is thus composed of two layers, an inner, the capsule proper which is PAS-positive and orthochromatic, and a thin outer layer which is metachromatic and contains much reticulin (Wislocki, 1952).

THE CORNEAL EPITHELIUM

After the separation of the lens vesicle, the surface epithelium fuses to form a single layer of cubical cells from which is developed the corneal epithelium, provided with its basement membrane. During the 6th week (14 mm. stage) a double layer of cells is formed, the surface layer being composed of flattened cells with large nuclei (Fig. 192). No change occurs until the 8th week when a layer of polyhedral cells appears between the first two layers ; after the 7th month a fourth layer develops and a fifth and sixth after birth (Figs. 217 to 221). The epithelium covering the eye is transparent and fails to develop the glandular structures characteristic of other epidermis, but is structurally continuous with the surface epithelium covering the conjunctiva and the lids and shares a common basement membrane with the former (O'Rahilly and Meyer, 1960).

[1] p. 192.   [2] p. 142.   [3] p. 150.

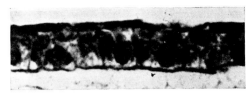

FIG. 192.—THE CORNEAL EPITHELIUM.

In a 20 mm. embryo, showing the main (basal) layer of epithelium, a second layer of flat cells is seen superficially. The beginning of the third layer is occasionally visible (F. Vrabec).

As takes place in the skin, renewal of the epithelium is constantly occurring, the cells in the basal layer dividing by mitosis at intervals of approximately a week (Friedenwald and Buschke, 1944). Few cells remain in the basal layer more than 2 days after division and by tagging the nuclei with tritium-labelled thymidine injected into the anterior chamber and thus following the fate of the cell by radio-autographs, Hanna and O'Brien (1960) demonstrated that most cells had reached the superficial layer and desquamated into the tear film a few days after they had left the basal layer (4 days in the rat ; 6 days in the mouse).

Babel and Baud. *Atti Cong. Soc. oftal. ital.*, **14,** 153 (1953).

von Baer. *Ueber Entwicklungsges. d. Thiere*, Königsberg, **2** (1837).

Cirincione. *Arch. Anat. Entwickl.*, Beil., 171 (1897).

Dejean. Dejean, Hervouët and Leplat's *L'embryologie de l'œil et sa tératologie*, Paris, 309 (1958).

Friedenwald and Buschke. *Arch. Ophthal.* (Chicago), **32,** 410 (1944).

Goldmann. *Arch. Augenheilk.*, **110,** 405 (1937).

Hanna and O'Brien. *Arch. Ophthal.* (Chicago), **64,** 536 (1960).

His. *Anatomie menschlicher Embryonen*, Leipzig (1880–85).

Huschke. *Arch. Anat. Physiol.*, **6,** 1 (1832).

Kessler. *Zur Entwicklung d. Auges d. Wirbelthiere*, Leipzig (1877).

von Kölliker. *Zur Entwicklung d. Auges*, Würzburg (1887).

Koniukhov and Lishtvan. *Arkh. Anat.* (Moskva), **37,** 32 (1959).

Langman. *J. Embryol. exp. Morph.*, **7,** 193, 264 (1959).

Mann. *Development of the Human Eye*, Camb. (1928) ; 2nd ed. (1949).

Meyer, H. *Arch. Anat. Physiol.*, 202 (1851).

O'Rahilly and Meyer, D. B. *Z. Anat. Entwickl. Gesch.*, **121,** 351 (1960).

Rabl. *Z. wiss. Zool.*, **63,** 496 ; **65,** 257 (1898) ; **67,** 1 (1899).

Ueber d. Bau u. Entwicklung d. Linse, Leipzig (1900).

Schwann. *Mikr. Untersuch. ü. d. Ueberein-stimmung in d. Struktur u. d. Wachsthum d. Thiere u. Pflanzen*, Berlin (1839).

Stroeva. *Dokl. Akad. Nauk.*, **125,** 461 (1959).

Truc and Vialleton. *Encycl. franç. Ophtal.*, Paris, **1,** 499 (1903).

Valentin. *Hb. d. Entwickelungsges. d. Menschen*, Berlin (1835).

Vogt. *Lhb. u. Atlas d. Spaltlampenmikros-kopie*, Berlin (1921).

Wislocki. *Amer. J. Anat.*, **91,** 233 (1952).

Yamasaki. *Yokohama med. Bull.*, **8,** 251 (1957).

CHAPTER VI

THE SECONDARY ECTODERMAL STRUCTURES

No book dealing with the embryology of the eye would be complete without a tribute to AUREL VON SZILY [1880–1945] who contributed so richly to our knowledge of this subject (Fig. 193). A Hungarian by birth who became professor of ophthalmology at Münster and eventually returned to occupy the chair in his native Budapest just before his death, his interests in ophthalmology were spread over an unusually wide range ; and with his enthusiasm, thoroughness in his researches and his comprehensive grasp of the essentials of a problem, to each subject in which he interested himself he made a noteworthy contribution. His work on anaphylactic reactions in the eye, on sympathetic ophthalmitis, on the pathology of the lens and on war injuries will survive as long as our specialty excites interest ; but one of his greatest contributions which occupied his earlier days was his painstaking histological studies on all aspects of ocular development. In no phase of this complex subject did he interest himself more than in the debatable questions of the origin of the vitreous body and the scaffolding of the anterior chamber.

There is still a considerable amount of controversy regarding the origin of two structures which are intimately associated with ectoderm : the vitreous body and the groundwork of the cornea. The problem centres round the interpretation of the histological appearance of the material which separates the surface ectoderm and the neural ectoderm. It will be seen from Fig. 193 that in histological preparations, between the two layers there stretches a network of fibrillæ which appears to demonstrate some degree of protoplasmic continuity (van Pée, 1902; v. Lenhossek, 1903); and it was postulated that after the lens vesicle had formed, that portion bridging over the gap between the lens vesicle and the optic vesicle took part in the formation of the vitreous body, while that between the lens vesicle and the surface epithelium (the " anterior vitreous ") gave rise to the ectodermal basis of the cornea (Fig. 195).

von Szily (1908) pointed out that this appearance was the rule between all surfaces in the early embryo, and concluded that the fibrillæ established direct continuity between the ectodermal layers and mesodermal cells, thus forming a tissue containing both components. Bach and Seefelder (1911), however, showed that these fibrils could be demonstrated within the " anterior vitreous " at a stage before the mesoderm has encroached upon this region ; a mesodermal component is therefore not essential to their formation. When the early vitreous is examined histologically a similar appearance is seen—a network of fibrillæ, interconnected with each other and connected with every tissue-element in their vicinity, the surrounding ectoderm and the ingrowing mesoderm. From its appearance in such sections it is quite impossible to postulate of any one fibril how much of it is

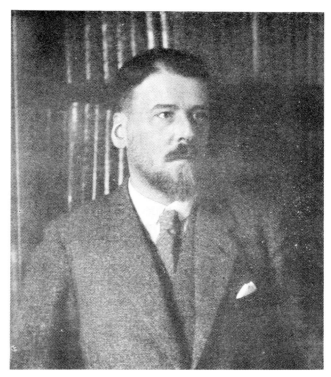

Fig. 193.—Aurel von Szily
[1880–1945].

ectodermal and how much mesodermal, and, consequently, a theory of a mixed origin of the vitreous received much support.

It was pointed out, however, in discussing the anatomy of the vitreous body,[1] that the fibrillæ seen in histological preparations are merely coagulative artefacts produced by fixation whereby the hydrated micellæ of an amorphous gel are condensed and aggregated to form the pseudo-framework of a coagel, a transformation which can be exactly simulated in any dilute colloid solution ; consequently it seems obvious that embryological arguments based merely on this artificial picture cannot be reasonably accepted without further confirmation. Unfortunately, up to the present time there is no technique available which is capable of providing an answer to these questions, which in the present state of our knowledge must therefore remain, to some extent at any rate, unsolved. Many of the appearances seen in sections could well be interpreted as the coagula of a protein-rich fluid formed by the action of histological fixatives.

THE VITREOUS BODY AND ZONULE

Inasmuch as the vitreous body is not a tissue but a cell-product, the problem of its origin resolves itself into a determination of the cells which form it, and every possible tissue has at one time or another been implicated. In accordance with the earliest views on its anatomical structure whereby it was considered a specialized form of areolar connective tissue, the theory was advanced by Schöler (1848) that the vitreous body was *mesodermal*, and for a long time this theory received universal agreement (Virchow, 1852 ; von Kölliker, 1879 ; Angelucci, 1881 ; and others). Some controversy existed whether the mesoderm penetrated at a very early stage between the neural and surface ectoderm, whether it entered by the embryonic fissure, whether it was associated with the hyaloid vessels (Kessler, 1877 ; Spampani, 1901), or whether it was merely derived from wandering cells (Bertacchini, 1901) ; but the theory remained unchallenged until Tornatola (1897–1904) of Palermo pointed out that the vitreous body continued to be formed after the mesoderm had all been extruded and the hyaloid system had atrophied.

Tornatola therefore concluded that the vitreous body was *ectodermal* in origin and because of the convincing histological pictures he obtained in sections of mammalian embryos showing fibres running from the border of the retina into the vitreous (the " fibres of Tornatola "), he suggested that it was secreted by the *retina*, a view which was accepted by Rabl (1899) in fishes and amphibians and Fischel (1900) who stressed the importance of the ciliary region in its formation.

Variations in this theory were suggested. Addario (1901) considered that the ciliary epithelium was the sole origin of the fibres ; Haemers (1903) postulated a derivation from retinal neuroglial cells which van Duyse (1905) and Wolfrum (1906–7) pin-pointed as the cells of Müller, while Magitot and Mawas (1912–13) ascribed its growth to wandering glial cells migrating from the retinal tissue as well as to the cone of glial cells originally forming Bergmeister's papilla at the optic disc[2] and subsequently becoming associated with the hyaloid vessels forming their sheaths.

An alternative ectodermal origin from the *lens* was initially suggested by von Lenhossek (1903), a view which seemed to receive confirmation at a later date by Beckwith (1927) who showed that the vitreous failed to develop if the lens vesicle were removed at an early stage. We have seen, however, that this failure could be

[1] Vol. II, p. 294.   [2] p. 198.

due to a lack of the inductive effect of the lens on the normal development of the retina.[1] Immediately after von Lenhossek's suggestion was published, both views were compounded by Cirincione (1903–4) who advocated a *dual origin* partly from the retinal and partly from the lenticular ectoderm, a concept which has had many subsequent advocates particularly as applied to the earlier stages of development (Howard, 1920 ; Jokl, 1928 ; Seefelder, 1930 ; and others).

Meantime a third school of thought had sprung up which attempted to reconcile the two opposing views by assigning to the vitreous body a *mixed origin*, both ectodermal and mesodermal (van Pée, 1902 ; von Szily, 1903–8 ; and others). Most adherents of this view considered that the mesoderm made an unimportant contribution. Cirincione (1903) and Froriep (1906) considered that it took part in the formation of the late-formed " secondary vitreous " ; Druault (1904–13) thought that it was responsible for the " primary vitreous " originally in association with the hyaloid artery, and remained throughout life as the hyaloid canal ; Howard (1920) suggested a transitory contribution in association with the hyaloid artery ; and Mann (1927) a small share in the primary vitreous. Fracassi (1923–25) and Monesi (1926) attributed to the mesoderm a more important role (see Carrère, 1925).

A fourth theory, which may be termed the *humoral hypothesis*, defined the vitreous body as a transudate or a secretion. Kessler (1877) and Spampani (1901) considered it a simple transudate from the blood vessels with sufficient protein to form a coagulum on chemical fixation, while Cirincione (1897) viewed it as the fluid filling the optic vesicle.

Finally, that the vitreous body was developed from the *basement membranes* of the retina and lens surrounding the posterior segment was suggested initially by Lieberkühn (1871–72) and supported by Franz (1913), Dejean (1923–32) and Redslob (1932). Franz, indeed, defined the vitreous embryologically as " the basement membrane of the retina ". In Dejean's interpretation its formation dates from the time when the limiting membrane of the optic vesicle approximated that of the lens plate ; when these two membranes separate they secrete a homogeneous substance which maintains continuity between them, the greater part of which is supplied by the limiting membrane of the retina. Dejean (1958) described a hypertrophy and thickening of the internal limiting membrane of the retina at the 7 mm. stage, whereafter the primary vitreous filled the cavity of the optic cup as a clear homogeneous substance merging with and emanating from the membrane which gradually tended to lose its definition.

It is to be remembered, however, that most of these polemics are based on fallacious arguments, depending essentially on histological artefacts, and that in the present state of our knowledge no pragmatic answer can be supplied to a problem that must in the meantime remain a riddle. On the whole it seems most probable that *the vitreous body is essentially ectodermal, being formed originally from the neural and surface epithelium and at a later stage from the retina*, perhaps through the medium of the basal membrane ; any contribution from mesoderm is problematical. The zonule is generally considered to be developed in a similar way from the ciliary epithelium (Stuart, 1891 ; Schön, 1895 ; Baldwin, 1912 ; Carlini, 1912 ; Druault, 1914 ; Carrère, 1925 ; Mann, 1927–49; Dejean, 1928–58 ; and others). In the meantime, the most practicable approach is to recount objectively the facts as we know them, laying as little stress upon theory as possible.

The development of the vitreous body and zonule may be conveniently divided into three stages as they concern the primary (or hyaloidean) vitreous, the secondary (or definitive) vitreous, and the tertiary vitreous (or zonule).

---

[1] p. 65.

THE PRIMARY (OR HYALOIDEAN) VITREOUS

It will be recalled that when the lens vesicle becomes separated from the primary optic vesicle on the invagination of the latter, some sort of continuity is maintained between them by a protein-rich PAS-positive material which on coagulation by fixatives appears histologically as a series of " protoplasmic

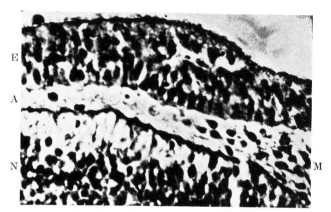

FIG. 194.—THE ANTERIOR VITREOUS.

In a 5 mm. embryo. Between the surface epithelium (E), thickened in this locality to form the lens plate, and the neural epithelium of the optic vesicle (N), there is a fibrillar meshwork as seen in a histological section, the anterior vitreous (A), which is being invaded by mesodermal cells (M) from the periphery (F. Vrabec).

bridges " connecting the two epidermal layers (Fig. 194). This apparent continuity of tissue is not confined to the region of the optic cup but is present to some degree wherever the neural ectoderm is contiguous with that of the surface and appears to be formed from the basement membranes

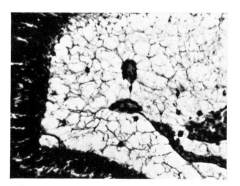

FIG. 195.—THE " VITREOUS FIBRILS ".

In an embryo of 18 mm., to show the continuity of the " vitreous fibrils " with the mesoderm and the ectoderm (W. A. Manschot).

bounding the surface, lenticular and neural ectodermal layers (O'Rahilly and Meyer, 1960). As the optic cup deepens, therefore, its cavity is occupied by these threads apparently derived from both retinal and lenticular epithelium. By the 10 mm. stage, however, vascularized mesoderm enters the embryonic fissure and invades the developing vitreous space, whereafter histological preparations show similar threads from the mesodermal cells

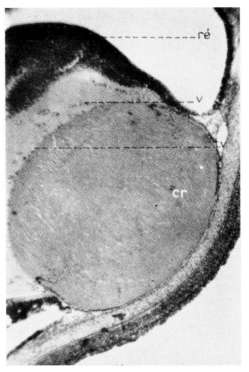

Fig. 196.—The Primary Vitreous.

In an embryo of 22 mm., showing the primary vitreous, v, containing mesodermal elements of the hyaloid system, separated from the lens, cr, by the tunica vasculosa lentis, tv ; ré, retina (C. Dejean).

merging with the ectodermal processes to form a syncytium in which no separate constituent can be analysed (Fig. 195). At the 8 to 13 mm. stage the hyaline capsule of the lens is formed, and as the cavity of the optic cup becomes increasingly permeated by a network of fine capillaries with the ingrowth of the hyaloid artery, the lens becomes progressively more isolated from the primary vitreous by the layer of vascular tissue which becomes interposed between them (Fig. 196). So far as conclusions drawn from histological specimens thus lead us, the primary vitreous could be formed from the lens initially, the retina all the time, and (problematically) elements

THE DIFFERENTIATION OF THE EYE

(Hamilton, Boyd and Mossman, *Human Embryology*, Heffer and Sons, Cambridge).

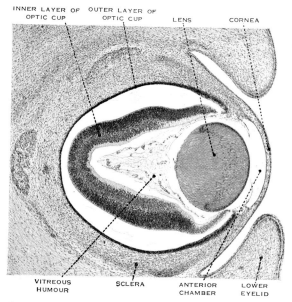

FIG. 1.—Sagittal section through the eye and orbit of a 25 mm. human embryo. The vitreous humour is the highly vascularized primary vitreous ($\times$ *ca.* 36).

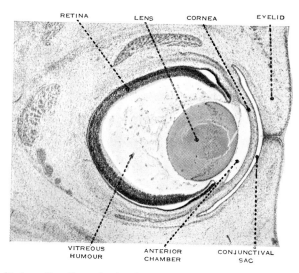

FIG. 2.—Sagittal section through the developing eye and orbital region of a 40 mm. human embryo. The secondary vitreous has become established; in the lens the embryonic nucleus is seen ($\times$ *ca.* 25).

of the mesoderm either derived from invaginating cells or from the hyaloid system. Its origin from the retina, however, seems clear and in specimens which have undergone shrinkage the internal limiting membrane adheres to the vitreous more readily than to the retina, cleavage taking place along the same plane as occurs in later life in a subhyaloid hæmorrhage (Fig. 197).

At first homogeneous, the primary vitreous soon takes on a fibrillar appearance in histological preparations, the bundles of coagulated fibres being arranged parallel to the surface of the retina and enmeshing the

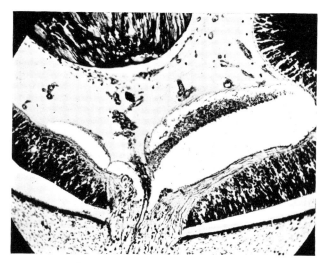

FIG. 197.—THE PRIMARY VITREOUS.

In an embryo of 21 mm. The hyaloid artery is well developed and the primary vitreous is rich in vasa hyaloidea propria. Note that in the region where the vitreous has been torn away from the retina the internal limiting membrane separates from the latter and associates itself with the vitreous (Henry Haden).

invading capillaries of the hyaloid system (Plate II, Fig. 1). Towards the equator of the lens these lamellæ become more condensed as they converge to form a fan-like formation intervening between the lens and the anterior lip of the optic cup (Fig. 199). As the vitreous space enlarges, however, the configuration of the fibrils becomes increasingly irregular so that the fan-like arrangement remains only in the anterior region (30 mm. stage). Radial fibres also extend perpendicularly from the internal limiting membrane of the retina running towards the lens (the fibres of Tornatola), the orientation of which is presumably due to traction between the epithelia of the lens vesicle and the optic cup as they become increasingly separated during the growth of the latter.

THE SECONDARY (OR DEFINITIVE) VITREOUS

The second period of vitreous formation lasts from the 13 to the 70 mm. stage and is initiated by the appearance in contact with the inner surface of the retina of a layer of vitreous which is finer but denser than that of the

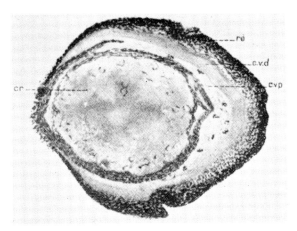

FIG. 198.—THE DEVELOPMENT OF THE VITREOUS.

Section of a human fœtus of 36 mm., showing the large lens (cr), the primary vitreous (c.v.p.), with the hyaloid vessels and the emergence of the secondary (definitive) vitreous (c.v.d.), surrounding the retina (ré) (C. Dejean).

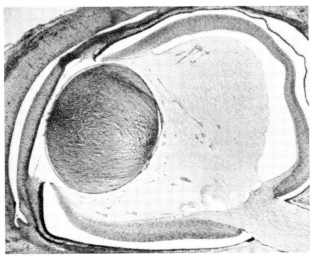

FIG. 199.—THE SECONDARY VITREOUS.

In a fœtus of 45 mm. The vascularized primary vitreous is surrounded by the non-vascularized secondary vitreous. It will be seen that when torn from its attachment in the process of preparation it adheres to the anterior rim of the optic cup (the vitreous base) in the region where the pars plana of the ciliary body will be situated when the rim of the cup has grown forward. A similar attachment is seen in the region of the optic disc (Henry Haden).

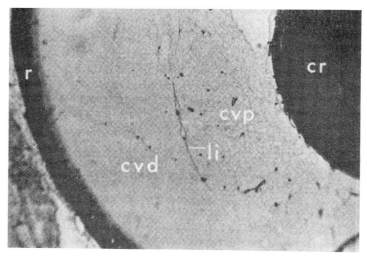

FIG. 200.—THE DEVELOPMENT OF THE VITREOUS.

In a 70 mm. fœtus. The secondary vitreous, cvd, has become more consolidated and the intravitreal membrane, li, between it and the primary vitreous, c.v.p., is less marked. cr, lens; r, retina (C. Dejean).

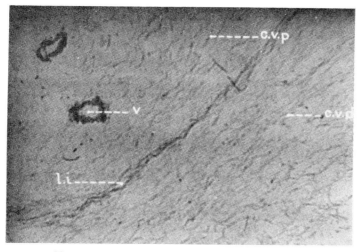

FIG. 201.—THE DEVELOPMENT OF THE VITREOUS.

In a 110 mm. fœtus. The intravitreal membrane, li, is seen between the primary, c.v.p., and the secondary vitreous, c.v.d. ; in the former are large hyaloid vessels, v (C. Dejean).

primary vitreous. This secondary vitreous as seen in histological sections is composed of fine undulating fibres initially orientated parallel to the retina, and its structure is sharply differentiated from the vascularized primary vitreous (Figs. 198–9 ; Plate II, Fig. 2). Its fibres are thicker at the anterior peripheral region at the rim of the optic cup, and most anteriorly those which abut against the mesoderm insinuating itself between the lens and the rim of the cup form a definite *marginal bundle* (the " faisceau isthmique " of Druault, 1914), which radiates inwards and backwards towards the equatorial region (Fig. 199). Here the vitreous is securely attached to the internal limiting membrane of the retina and embryologically this constitutes the main " zone of origin " of the secondary vitreous (Wolfrum, 1906–7) (the *vitreous base* of Salzmann, 1912) (Fig. 199). Tenuous connections with the internal limiting membrane of the retina throughout its extent, however, persist into adult life (Grignolo, 1952 ; Schepens, 1954), while a slight attachment also remains to the posterior

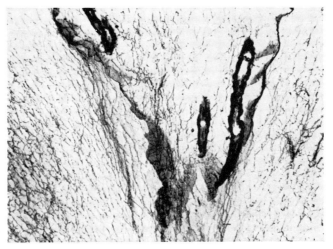

FIG. 202.—THE DEVELOPMENT OF THE VITREOUS.

In a fœtus of 5 months. The V-shaped mass in the centre is the primary vitreous, the structure of which is becoming attenuated but which still contains hyaloid vessels. It is surrounded by a secondary vitreous (F. Vrabec).

surface of the lens capsule in the form of a ring 8 to 9 mm. in diameter (the hyaloideo-capsular ligament of Wieger, 1883, or Egger's line, 1924) as well as to the region of the optic disc (Fig. 199).

The progressive growth of the secondary vitreous together with the cessation of growth of the primary vitreous, the atrophy of the branches of the hyaloid artery and the increase in size of the eye as a whole, eventually result in the relegation of the primary vitreous together with the remnants of the hyaloid vascular system to a narrowly constricted zone in the centre of the vitreous cavity, the undulant line of demarcation between them being clearly visible in histological preparations as a condensation of vitreous fibrillæ (the *intra-vitreal limiting membrane*) (36 mm. stage) (Figs. 200–1). As the zone becomes increasingly smaller and the vessels fewer in number, it is eventually reduced to a poor remnant of its former self, consisting of a

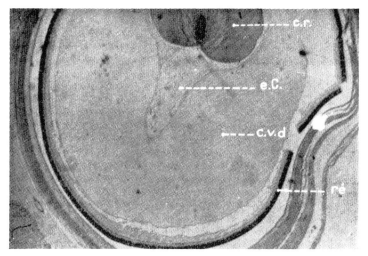

FIG. 203.—THE DEVELOPMENT OF THE VITREOUS.

In a 110 mm. fœtus. A general view showing the primary vitreous contracting, e.C., attached to the lens, c.r., and enveloped in the secondary vitreous, c.v.d. The retina, ré. (C. Dejean).

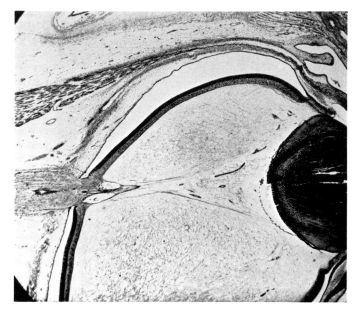

FIG. 204.—THE DEVELOPMENT OF THE VITREOUS.

In a 7-month fœtus. The primary vitreous now containing only atrophied hyaloid vessels has assumed the general configuration of the canal of Cloquet (hyaloidean vitreous) (C. Dejean).

central cone with its apex towards the disc and its base extending towards the posterior aspect of the lens (70 mm. stage) (Figs. 202 to 204). Eventually this " hyaloidean vitreous " shows little or no structural differentiation and is most clearly delineated by the intra-vitreal membrane surrounding it. It is attached posteriorly around the margin of the optic disc leaving a posterior expansion over this structure (the area of Martegiani, 1814) ; it runs through the vitreous anteriorly in a downward sagging course as the canal of Cloquet ; and it expands again anteriorly to form an optically empty space (the retrolental space of Erggelet, 1914). In any part of this portion of the vitreous persistent remnants of the hyaloid vascular system may be seen in adult life.[1]

THE TERTIARY VITREOUS OR ZONULE

During the 3rd month at the 70 mm. stage the secondary vitreous is almost completely developed and fills two-thirds of the optic cup, while the primary vitreous is restricted to the central region and its peripheral wings extend between the rim of the optic cup and the lens (Fig. 205). As the rim of the cup grows forward to form the ciliary region, the vitreous occupying the triangular area between the developing ciliary body and the lens becomes clearly demarcated by a curved intravitreal membrane from the secondary vitreous posteriorly. At the 170 mm. stage in histological preparations well-formed fibrils can be seen running from the ciliary processes towards the lens (Fig. 205), guided, according to Pau (1957), and their topographical arrangement determined, by the transient blood vessels of the vascular sheath. These fibres at first run anteriorly parallel to the ciliary epithelium for a short distance before passing inwards to traverse the triangular zone of vitreous ; here they run at right angles to the main mass of its fibres and eventually reach the lens where their terminations unite to form fine lamellæ on the surface of the capsule ; we shall see that the capsulo-pupillary portion of the vascular tunic of the lens[2] has almost disappeared in this region at this stage. As the eye grows in size and the developing ciliary body and the margin of the cup become increasingly withdrawn from the equator of the lens, these fibrillæ progressively become longer, stronger and more defined until eventually they become grouped in two bundles, an anterior group running behind the iris, and a posterior running parallel to the intravitreal membrane. It is from these compact and well-defined bands of fibres that the adult system of the zonule is derived (Fig. 205). In the meantime, the most anterior triangular zone of the secondary vitreous atrophies so that this tissue retains its connection with the retina only up to the level of the ora serrata ; here it remains anchored throughout life, forming the " base of the vitreous ", thus leaving the tertiary vitreous in front attached to the ciliary body. There is thus complete embryological continuity between the secondary vitreous and the zonule. It is to be

[1] p. 200.   [2] p. 201.

remembered, however, that in the adult eye, viewed during life or *in vitro* before fixation, the zonule (like the vitreous body) appears as continuous gel-like membranes ; it is only after fixation and coagulation of the protein basis of the gel that the artefact of " fibres " emerges. There is no reason to suspect that the embryonic condition is otherwise.[1]

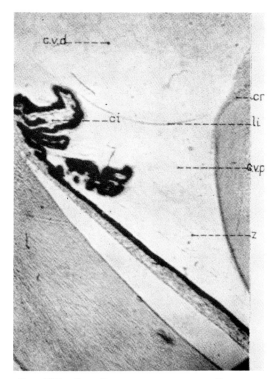

FIG. 205.—THE DEVELOPMENT OF THE ZONULE.

In a 6-month fœtus.   Between the lens, cr, and the ciliary processes, ci, lie the remains of the primary vitreous, c.v.p., through which run the fibres of the tertiary vitreous (zonule, z). Separating this from the secondary vitreous, c.v.d., is the intravitreal membrane, li (C. Dejean).

It is generally held that the *zonular lamella of the lens* is formed by the fusion of the termination of these zonular fibres over the lens capsule ; but the possibility that the entire lens capsule including this lamella is either a secretory product of the epithelial cells of the lens or is derived from their basement membrane cannot as yet be definitely excluded.

Owing to the difficulty of interpreting fixed microscopic preparations of the gel, the origin of the zonular fibres has been disputed. According to Dejean (1958) the first sign of their emergence is a thickening of the basement membrane of the ciliary epithelium which thereafter breaks up into minute

[1] Vol. II, p. 327.

fibrils at first parallel to the epithelium before running towards the lens. In the view of this author this basement membrane, like that of the retina, consists of a series of very fine lamellæ the innermost of which peel off (as it were) to form in the one case the zonule and in the other case the vitreous. Electron-microscopic studies have confirmed the view originally put forward by Salzmann (1900) and supported by Carlini (1912) that the zonular fibres do indeed arise from the internal limiting membrane lining the ciliary epithelium (Pappas and Smelser, 1958 ; and others). Alternative suggestions—that they arise from the epithelial cells themselves, from between the cells, from the cuticular portion of the forward prolongation of the membrane of Bruch, or from the outer (pigmented) layer of the ciliary epithelium—have been discussed in a previous volume[1] where the relevant bibliography is cited.

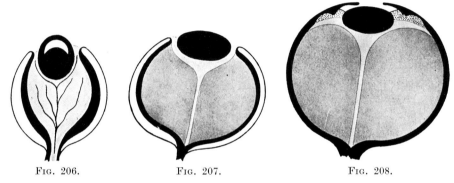

Fig. 206.   Fig. 207.   Fig. 208.

Fig. 206 to 208.—Stages in the Development of the Vitreous Body.

The primary vitreous is shown in light shading, the secondary in dark shading, and the tertiary is marked by dots. In Fig. 206 the primary vitreous alone is present, in Fig. 207 the secondary vitreous occupies the greater part of the picture, and in Fig. 208 the tertiary vitreous has appeared (after Ida Mann).

The relationship of the three stages of development of the vitreous is demonstrated in Figs. 206 to 208, where it will be seen that in the adult the primary vitreous fills up Cloquet's canal and the retrolental space, the secondary vitreous fills up the great mass of the cavity, and the tertiary vitreous comprises the zonule.

The Hyaloid and Intravitreal Membranes. Opinion has long been divided as to whether there is any evidence for the separate existence of a hyaloid membrane surrounding the vitreous body or intravitreal membranes separating its various parts. Everyone is agreed that no cellular membrane exists. It is true that histological sections give the appearance of the existence of such structures. There is, however, no evidence—embryological or otherwise—that any such membranes exist as separate and individualistic structures other than the condensation of the otherwise disorientated protein micellæ such as occurs on the surface of any colloid gel and is accentuated by coagulation in histological sections.[2]

[1] Vol. II, p. 333.   [2] For discussion, see Vol. II, p. 306.

THE ECTODERMAL BASIS OF THE ANTERIOR SEGMENT

We have seen that the " anterior vitreous " is the name applied to the filaments joining the lenticular and surface epithelia (van Pée, 1902 ; von Lenhossek, 1903) (Fig. 194). At an early stage in development this ectodermal matrix becomes invaded by mesodermal cells, and soon afterwards (12 to 13 mm. stage) it can no longer be recognized ; evidence has been brought forward, however, which points to the possibility that it may play a part in the formation of the basis of the cornea and anterior chamber.

The classical theory describing the development of the anterior chamber is due to von Kölliker (1861), who suggested that it developed as a chink in the mesoderm between the lens vesicle and the surface epithelium, a view which is still held by many authorities. Inasmuch as it appeared difficult to say how far the anterior vitreous was ectodermal and how far mesodermal, it was considered probable by some that ectoderm also entered into the structures of the walls of the chamber (Seefelder and Wolfrum, 1906 ; von Szily, 1908). Thus Descemet's endothelium was interpreted as a differentiated product of the anterior vitreous, the corneal membranes (of Bowman and of Descemet) were said to be ectodermal, and the substantia propria was considered to contain both ectodermal and mesodermal elements, just as (in von Szily's opinion) did the vitreous body itself.

A third view attributed to the ectoderm the primary function of moulding the structure of the anterior segment of the eye, while the mesoderm played the subsidiary role of travelling along already formed paths : a mutual relationship of this kind is of very general application in embryology. Kessler (1877) described (in birds) a fine structureless membrane developing at an early stage in the anterior vitreous which seemed to lay a basis for the developing cornea ; his observation was verified by Knape (1910), who considered it an ectodermal directing membrane (" Richtungshäutchen "), and was confirmed by Lindahl (1915), Laguesse (1923), Giesbrecht (1925), and others. Further, from a wide study of comparative embryology, Hagedoorn (1928) concluded that such a transient *ectodermal primitive cornea* was laid down in the primary vitreous in all vertebrates, posterior to which mesodermal elements grew in as the endothelium (which secreted Descemet's membrane at a later stage), and anterior to which mesoderm grew in wedgewise between the primitive cornea and the surface epithelium to form the substantia propria.

In a somewhat similar manner, Seefelder (1926) considered that the pupillary membrane was also initially laid down as a thin ectodermal lamella, a view which received support from the observations of Hagedoorn (1928). This author considered that such a cell-free membrane was first laid down in the anterior vitreous, which, in mammals, was invaded by mesoderm secondarily and thus became cellular and vascularized.

The whole question, however, is in need of further investigation, for it seems possible that " directional membranes " of this nature may be coagulative artefacts of fixation in a gel in which, presumably, lines of stress exist.[1] While the " fibrils " seen between the lens and the surface epithelium have been ascribed to artefacts due to shrinkage and cleft-formation during the process of fixation, there is no doubt that they are visible in histological preparations. Their origin is not clear, whether from the ectoderm of the

[1] Vol. II, p. 300.

lens or of the surface epithelium or both ; quite probably, as was suggested by Redslob (1935), they merely represent a coagulate of the albuminous fluid which fills the cavity of the embryo.

Whatever the derivation of this ground substance may be, there is no universal agreement regarding the part played (if any) by the anterior vitreous in the early development of the cornea. According to Mann (1928) the interconnecting filaments lose their connection with the lens at the 13 to 14 mm. stage and soon thereafter, as the cells of the mesoderm surrounding the rim of the optic cup invade the area, they can no longer be recognized. They therefore disappear so long before either Descemet's or Bowman's membrane becomes visible that it is impossible to ascribe to them any part in the formation of these structures. It is possible, however, that in the early stages of development this acellular substance may act as a basis upon which the mesodermal elements of the cornea are built up (Redslob, 1935 ; Thomas, 1955 ; Dejean, 1958).

Addario. *Ann. Ottal.*, **30**, 721 (1901).
Angelucci. *Arch. mikr. Anat.*, **19**, 152 (1881).
Bach and Seefelder. *Atlas z. Entwicklungs-geschichte d. mensch. Auges*, Leipzig (1911–14).
Baldwin. *Arch. mikr. Anat.*, **80**, 274 (1912).
Beckwith. *J. exp. Zool.*, **49**, 217 (1927).
Bertacchini. *Soc. Chir. Modena*, **3**, 1 (1901).
Carlini. *v. Graefes Arch. Ophthal.*, **82**, 75 (1912).
Carrère. *C.R. Soc. Biol.* (Paris), **92**, 769 (1925).
Cirincione. *Arch. Anat. Entwickl.*, Beil., 171 (1897).
   Zbl. prakt. Augenheilk., **27**, 161 (1903).
   Anat. Anz., **23**, Erg., 51 (1903).
   Arch. Augenheilk., **50**, 201 (1904).
Dejean. *C.R. Acad. Sci.* (Paris), **177**, 220, 360 (1923).
   Arch. Ophtal. (Paris), **41**, 659 (1924) ; **43**, 257 (1926) ; **45**, 65, 145 (1928).
   C.R. Soc. Biol. (Paris), **92**, 1051 (1925).
Dejean, Hervouët and Leplat's *L'embryo-logie de l'œil et sa tératologie*, Paris, 220 (1958).
Druault. Poirier's *Anatomie*, Paris, **5**, 1005 (1904).
   Arch. Ophtal. (Paris), **33**, 645 (1913) ; **34**, 1 (1914).
van Duyse. *Encycl. franç. Ophtal.*, Paris, **2**, 189 (1905).
Egger. *v. Graefes Arch. Ophthal.*, **113**, 1 (1924).
Erggelet. *Klin. Mbl. Augenheilk.*, **53**, 449 (1914).
Fischel. *Anat. Hefte*, **14**, 1 (1900).
Fracassi. *v. Graefes Arch. Ophthal.*, **111**, 219 (1923) ; **115**, 215 (1925).
Franz. Oppel's *Lhb. vergl. mikr. Anat. d. Wirbeltiere*, Jena, **8**, 153 (1913).
Froriep. *Hb. d. vergl. u. exper. Entwickl-ungslehre d. Wirbeltiere*, Jena, **2**, 139 (1906).
Giesbrecht. *Z. wiss. Zool.*, **124**, 305 (1925).

Grignolo. *Arch. Ophthal.* (Chicago), **47**, 760 (1952).
Haemers. *Arch. Ophtal.* (Paris), **23**, 103 (1903).
Hagedoorn. *Brit. J. Ophthal.*, **12**, 479 (1928).
Howard. *Amer. J. Ophthal.*, **3**, 589 (1920).
Jokl. *Vergleichende Untersuch. ü. d. Bau u. d. Entwicklung d. Glaskörpers*, Uppsala (1928).
Kessler. *Dorpat med. Z.*, 589 (1874).
   Zur Entwicklung d. Auges d. Wirbelthiere, Leipzig (1877).
Knape. *Mitt. Augenkl. Carol. Inst. Stockholm*, **11**, 107 (1910).
von Kölliker. *Entwicklungsgeschichte d. Menschen*, Leipzig (1861).
Laguesse. *C.R. Soc. Biol.* (Paris), **89** 543, 871 (1923).
von Lenhossek. *Die Entwickl. d. Glaskörpers*, Leipzig (1903).
Lieberkühn. *Schrift. d. Ges. z. Beforderung d. gesammten Naturwiss. z. Marburg*, No. 3 (1871) ; **10** (1872).
Lindahl. *Anat. Hefte*, **52**, 195 (1915).
Magitot and Mawas. *Arch. Anat. micr.*, **14**, 41 (1912).
   Ann. Oculist. (Paris), **147**, 475 (1912) ; **150**, 323, 390 (1913).
Mann. *Trans. ophthal. Soc. U.K.*, **47**, 172 (1927).
   Development of the Human Eye, Camb. (1928) ; 2nd ed., London (1949).
Martegiani. *Novae observationes de oculo humano*, Napoli, 19 (1814).
Monesi. *Ann. Ottal.*, **54**, 220 (1926).
O'Rahilly and Meyer. *Z. Anat. Entwickl. Gesch.*, **121**, 351 (1960).
Pappas and Smelser. *Amer. J. Ophthal.*, **46** (2), 299 (1958).
Pau. *Ophthalmologica*, **134**, 320 (1957).
van Pée. *Arch. Biol.* (Liège), **19**, 317 (1902).
Rabl. *Z. wiss. Zool.*, **67**, 1 (1899).

Redslob. *Ann. Oculist.* (Paris), **168,** 29 (1931).

Le corps vitré, Paris (1932).

Arch. Anat. (Strasbourg), **19,** 135 (1935).

Salzmann. *Die zonula ciliaris*, Wien (1900).

Anat. u. Histol d. mensch. Augapfels, Leipzig (1912).

Schepens. *Amer. J. Ophthal.*, **38** (2), 8 (1954).

Schöler. *De oculi evolutione in embryonibus gallinaceis* (Diss.), Dorpat (1848).

Schön. *Arch. Anat. Entwickl.*, 417 (1895).

Seefelder. *Arch. Augenheilk.*, **97,** 156 (1926).

Kurzes Hb. d. Ophthal., Berlin, **1,** 476 (1930).

Seefelder and Wolfrum. *v. Graefes Arch. Ophthal.*, **63,** 430 (1906).

Spampani. *Monit. zool. ital.*, **12,** 145 (1901).

Stuart. *Proc. roy. Soc. B*, **49,** 137 (1891).

von Szily. *Anat. Anz.*, **24,** 417 (1903).

Anat. Hefte, **35,** 649 (1908).

Thomas. *The Cornea*, Springfield (1955).

Tornatola. *Rev. gén. Ophtal.*, **16,** 543 (1897).

Ann. Ottal., **31,** 711 (1902).

Anat. Anz., **24,** 536 (1904).

Virchow. *Virchows Arch. path. Anat.*, **4,** 468 (1852).

Wieger. *Ueber Canalis Petiti u. ein Ligamentum hyaloideo-capsulare*, Strasburg (1883).

Wolfrum. *Ber. dtsch. ophthal. Ges.*, **33,** 341 (1906).

v. Graefes Arch. Ophthal., **65,** 220 (1907).

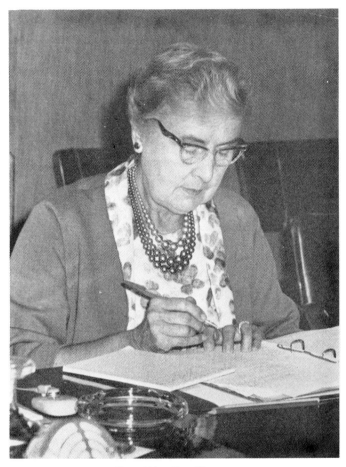

FIG. 209.—IDA MANN
[1893——].

CHAPTER VII

THE BULBAR MESODERM

SOMEWHERE in this book must go the portrait of IDA CAROLINE MANN [1893———]
(Fig. 209) who in the English-speaking world has contributed most to our knowledge
of embryology ; and the present chapter seems most suitable in view of the extent and
excellence of her work on the evolution of the vascular system of the eye. Moreover,
in an otherwise male gallery, it is good on one occasion to have a woman who is good
to look upon. Graduating at St. Mary's Hospital, London, she was stimulated by
J. E. Frazer to undertake an elaborate and sustained research on the embryology of the
eye at the Institute of Pathology at that hospital, the results of which, fully annotated
and richly illustrated with her own delightful drawings, appeared in her two classical
publications, *The Development of the Human Eye* (1928, 1949) and its logical sequel,
Developmental Abnormalities of the Eye (1937, 1957). Her interests have not been confined
to embryology. The extent of her researches into the comparative anatomy of the eye
is indicated by the magnificent series of coloured illustrations of the vascular arrangements and the form of the iris in the lower vertebrates seen in the first volume of this
System. An able pathologist, she became an equally good clinician. The only woman
to be a surgeon to Moorfields Eye Hospital in its history of a century and a half (in
which capacity she more than held her own !), she became the first professor of ophthalmology at the University of Oxford ; during her tenure of this office the work she did
on chemical injuries on the outer eye is classical.[1] Migrating to Australia at the end of
the Second World War, she extended her interests to a study of the incidence of
ophthalmic diseases, particularly of trachoma, in the aborigines of that continent and
the neighbouring islands of the Pacific, realizing in so doing her passion for uncharted
and adventurous travel[2] ; her survey of the comparatively new and fascinating
subject of geographical ophthalmology—the variation of the incidence and characteristics
of diseases in different races, climates and social conditions—is to be found in her Bowman
Lecture to the Ophthalmological Society of the United Kingdom in 1961.

As the optic vesicle expands outwards from the cerebral vesicle it
grows into the paraxial mesoderm and is entirely surrounded by it except
when it is temporarily associated with the surface ectoderm ; and when,
on the invagination of the vesicle to form the optic cup, this structure
dissociates itself from the surface and retreats before the developing and
advancing lens vesicle, mesodermal cells insinuate themselves between the
surface and neural ectodermal layers so that the developing eye is entirely
surrounded by mesenchymal tissue. From this tissue the stromal basis of
the globe is developed and since it is highly vasoformative, in it the vascular
system develops. Even although the latter to a considerable extent precedes
and determines the configuration of the former, it will be convenient to
describe the two elements separately.

[1] See *Textbook*, Vol. VI, p. 6702.
[2] See her delightful book, *The Cockney and the Crocodile*, Faber & Faber, London, 1962,
written under her married name, Caroline Gye.

The Ocular Stroma

THE UVEAL TRACT

THE CHOROID. At first the mesoderm surrounding the optic vesicle shows no differentiation, and it is in this type of tissue that the endothelial spaces which eventually develop into the choriocapillaris appear at the 5 to 6 mm. stage (Fig. 210). The vascular tissue is abundant but the stromal elements are tenuous and always remain so in the choroid. This meso-

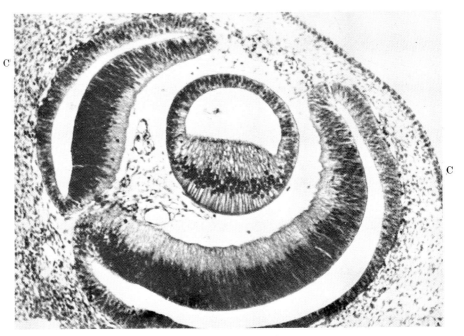

FIG. 210.—THE BEGINNING OF THE CHORIOCAPILLARIS.

In a 14 mm. embryo. The endothelial spaces developing into the choriocapillaris are well seen on the external aspect of the outer layer of the optic cup opposite C and C (F. Vrabec).

dermal layer is sharply differentiated from the ectoderm of the optic vesicle by the limiting membrane which lines the outer aspect of the pigment epithelium and becomes conspicuous as the cuticular layer of the membrane of Bruch at the 14 to 18 mm. stage ; it is not until the 70 mm. stage that the elastic elements of the choroidal stroma have condensed sufficiently to allow the outer (elastic) lamina of Bruch's membrane to become histologically visible. This membrane is therefore of bipartite origin, being composed of an inner ectodermal (cuticular) lamina and an outer mesodermal lamina. On its outer aspect the choroid is less definitely delimited ; but during the 3rd month when the large venous channels which form its most prominent feature are making their appearance, a condensation of the surrounding tissue demarcates the denser scleral tissue from the loose uveal stroma ; the differentiation, however, remains incomplete, a feature which survives in the merging of the lamina fusca of the sclera with the epichoroidal tissue in the adult. By the 5th month chromatophores are beginning to make their appearance, first in the posterior region and spreading forwards, and always initially in the outermost layers and gradually spreading towards the inner layers which remain permanently less densely pigmented than the former (Igo, 1957) (Fig. 211). At this period the choroid is well differentiated and resembles the adult tissue except that it is more richly nucleated ; even at birth it is more cellular than in the adult.

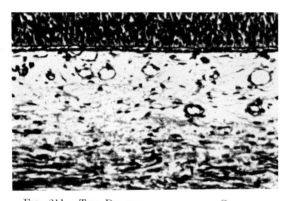

Fig. 211.—The Development of the Choroid.
In a 5 month fœtus. The vascular basis of the choroid is well developed and chromatophores are beginning to make their appearance (F. Vrabec).

THE CILIARY BODY AND IRIS. When the anterior rim of the optic cup commences its rapid phase of growth during the 3rd month (65–70 mm. stage) the paraxial mesoderm immediately outside it shows the same tendency to condensation as did the corresponding mesodermal tissue round the more posterior parts of the optic cup. As the epithelial layers become deformed into radial folds and ridges in the region just behind the growing edge, the mesoderm external to it fills the spaces of the folds to form the stroma of the corona ciliaris, each of the 70 to 75 convolutions differentiating into a ciliary process which eventually becomes richly vascularized (Fig. 267).[1] As the continued peripheral growth of the vesicle extends anteriorly and inwards over the lens, the reservoir of mesoderm at the rim of the optic cup, which has already supplied the basis of the cornea, grows inwards, following the forward and axial extension of the neural ectoderm and maintains its process of consolidation to form the posterior leaf of the meso-dermal portion of the iris (Fig. 212). We shall see at a later stage[2] that the

[1] p. 202.   [2] p. 196.

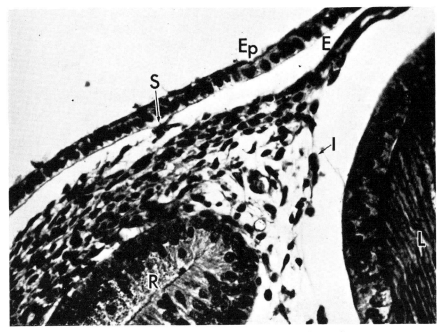

FIG. 212.—MESODERM AT THE RIM OF THE OPTIC CUP.

To show the three waves of mesoderm which grow out from the mass on the rim of the optic cup. (1), the endothelium of the cornea, E ; (2), mesodermal cells migrating into the mesostroma between the endothelium and the surface epithelium to form the cells of the corneal stroma, S ; (3), mesodermal cells destined to form the stroma of the iris, I. L, lens; R, rim of optic cup ; Ep, epithelium (F. Vrabec).

anterior leaf is so intimately connected with the development of the vascular system in the formation of the pupillary membrane that its consideration is best omitted in the meantime (Fig. 213).

In fœtal life a fine diaphanous layer of endothelium is seen on the anterior surface of the iris which seems to be a continuation of the corneal endothelium. In post-natal life this tends to atrophy particularly in the region of the crypts (Fuchs, 1885) ; Vrabec (1951–52) considered that the layer disappeared in man between the 1st and 2nd year of post-natal life, whereafter the cells assume the characteristics of immature fibroblasts. The extent of this disappearance has given rise to controversy and several authors deny its persistence into adult life (Krückmann, 1908 ; Wolfrum, 1926 ; Tousimis and Fine, 1959). Magari (1957), however, demonstrated its existence although the interstices between the flat endothelial cells are usually filled by the processes of cells in the immediately subjacent layers.

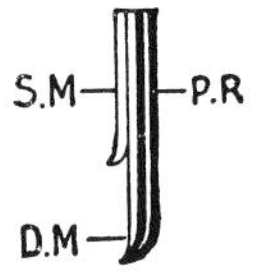

FIG. 213.—STRUCTURE OF THE IRIS OF PLACENTALS.

SM, DM, superficial and deep mesodermal layers. PR, the two posterior retinal layers containing between them the potential cavity of the optic vesicle.

THE CILIARY MUSCLE. The ciliary muscle plays an important role in the development of the anterior segment of the globe (Sondermann, 1932 ;

Abraitis, 1939 ; Badtke, 1942 ; Allen *et al.*, 1955 ; and others). It is developed as a specialized aspect of the general mesodermal condensation that envelops the optic cup ; in contrast to the musculature of the iris it is therefore of mesodermal origin. The earliest condensation appears in the area of mesoderm which lies between the outer surface of the optic cup at its margin and the inner surface of the scleral condensation. In meridional section the area involved is triangular in shape, the base of the triangle being directed towards the angle of the anterior chamber and the apex posteriorly. During the 3rd month the cells here become regularly arranged in longitudinal formations until by the 5th month the meridional portion of the muscle is evident, its fibres running antero-posteriorly in the outer part of the mesodermal triangle. They are directly continuous with a dense condensation of scleral fibres which at about the 5th month grow obliquely

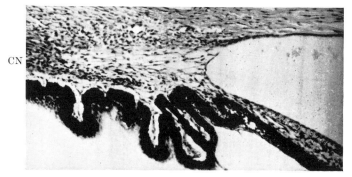

CN

FIG. 214.—THE DEVELOPMENT OF THE CILIARY MUSCLE, CN, IN A 6 MONTH FŒTUS
(F. Vrabec).

inwards across the base of the triangle to form the scleral spur from which the meridional fibres of the muscle therefore take origin (Fig. 214). Not only is this portion of the muscle ontogenetically the older but it is interesting that it is also phylogenetically the first to appear among mammals since oblique fibres are found only in carnivores and primates.[1] It is not until the 6th month in the human fœtus that these latter fibres are recognizable ; by the 7th month they are still represented only by a small group at the inner side of the meridional portion of the muscle near its anterior end ; and, while development of the meridional fibres is more or less complete at birth, the oblique fibres continue to increase for a variable time thereafter, the degree of their development possibly depending to some extent upon the refractive power of the eye and the amount of work the muscle is therefore called upon to perform (Lange, 1901).

Although the ciliary muscle remains in its original position anchored, as it were, to the scleral spur, it would appear during the rapid development of the anterior seg-

[1] Vol. I, p. 460.

ment of the eye to change its relative position. At the 6th month its anterior border lies on a level with the ora serrata ; by the 8th month the mid-portion of the muscle is related to this landmark. During the 9th month the posterior border of the muscle occupies this position, and after birth the posterior extremity of the main mass of muscle lies anterior to the ora although many of its meridional fibres run posteriorly to the equator and beyond.

The development of the pigment of the uveal tract and the embryological nature of the chromatophores and the clump cells of the iris will be dealt with separately in a later chapter (Chapter VIII).

THE SCLERA

Shortly after the 18 to 20 mm. stage of development, in the hitherto undifferentiated paraxial mesoderm immediately surrounding the vascularized layer which ultimately forms the uveal tract, there begins a process of consolidation and condensation wherein the mesodermal cells arrange

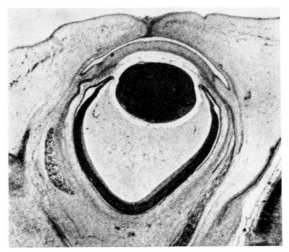

FIG. 215.—THE DEVELOPMENT OF THE SCLERA.

In a 41 mm. foetus. The scleral condensation is seen as a definite layer of consolidation running posteriorly from the limbus in the anterior part of the globe ; posterior to the equator it is not well defined (C. Dejean).

themselves concentrically with the contour of the optic vesicle. Prior to this time there is nothing to distinguish the future sclera from the other orbital tissues. This process starts at the limbus where the consolidating fibres are continuous with those of the already-formed cornea, near the region of the future insertions of the rectus muscles (Fig. 215). Thereafter it extends posteriorly to reach the equator at the end of the 2nd month ; at this time, posterior to the equator there is no distinction between the sclera and the tissues of the orbit. Only at a considerably later stage, towards the end of the 5th month, does the condensation reach the posterior pole.

Meantime, during the 3rd month, the mesodermal cells become differentiated into collagenous and elastic fibres, a process which also starts anteriorly and extends posteriorly ; while during the 5th month and thereafter the scleral envelope becomes progressively thicker by the gradual accretion of new fibres in its periphery. During the same month chromatophores begin to appear in the deeper layers which eventually form the lamina fusca. At the 45 mm. stage, during the 3rd month, a further and still more peripheral condensation indicates the beginning of the capsule of Tenon near the equatorial region (Casari, 1953).[1]

It is important to remember, as was pointed out by Badtke (1952), that the sclera plays little or no part in determining the shape and configuration of the eye. These are regulated essentially by the growth of the retina, and the sclera, with its late development, acquires an effective density of its tissues only after the period of rapid ocular development has passed. It, as well as the choroid and pigment epithelium, is essentially shaped by the development of the inner layer of the optic cup ; but it is possible that the late development of the posterior part of the sclera may be associated with its weakness in myopia.

In the earlier stages of development it is interesting that the scleral tissues show a slight degree of metachromatic staining, a process which gradually accentuates to attain its maximum between the 150 and 200 mm. stage. During the last 3 months of fœtal life, however, the intensity of the staining gradually diminishes until at birth little is evident. In the cornea, on the other hand, metachromatism increases progressively up to term and remains permanently (Aurell and Holmgren, 1953 ; François and Rabaey, 1952).

THE OPTIC NERVE

THE LAMINA CRIBROSA. We have already noted that the ectodermal basis of the lamina cribrosa is laid down at an early stage, during the 3rd month, by a condensation of glial cells which become orientated at right angles to the fibres of the optic nerve. Towards the end of the 5th month mesodermal elements from the developing sclera begin to invade this region and reinforce its glial basis (Maggiore, 1923 ; Redslob, 1956). Initially collagenous fibres become arranged in palisade-like formations along the edge of the scleral canal and invade the interior of the nerve, sending in two types of septum, the one short and penetrating only a small distance into the substance of the nerve anchoring it to the edge of the canal, the other, on a level with the anterior third of the sclera, penetrating deeply into the network of glial cells which form the primitive lamina to constitute its scleral component. These are much in evidence by the 7th month, during which they are reinforced by elastic fibres, the whole being supplemented during the 8th month by similar elements from the choroid, the nerve sheaths and the central core of connective tissue associated with the hyaloid vessels. Even at the end of the 9th month, however, the lamina is quite supple and is not fully consolidated until some time after birth (Fig. 162).

THE DURAL SHEATH OF THE OPTIC NERVE is similarly formed by a

[1] p. 230.

condensation of the mesodermal tissue around the optic stalk, a process which is said by Barber (1955) to be apparent as early as the 10 mm. stage when the cells begin to arrange themselves longitudinally in regular formation. It is usually accepted that by the beginning of the 5th month the dural sheath is thus well differentiated with its collagenous and elastic fibres continuous with the sclera anteriorly and with the corresponding cerebral sheath posteriorly ; it is during this period that the optic nerve becomes rapidly elongated. We have already seen that the pial and arachnoid sheaths are essentially ectodermal in nature.[1]

THE CORNEA

The different views held as to the origin of the cornea have already been noted.[2] The classical theory of von Kölliker (1861) was that the anterior layers of the mesoderm which insinuates itself between the surface epithelium and the lens vesicle became differentiated to form the cornea. Of these the innermost cells rearranged themselves *in situ* to form the endothelium of Descemet's membrane, which itself was a cuticular formation elaborated by these cells, while Bowman's membrane was formed as a condensation of the superficial layers of the substantia propria. The cornea was thus assumed to be entirely mesodermal ; and being continuous with the mesodermal condensations on either side, could be considered of tripartite origin, containing a subcutaneous (subconjunctival), a scleral, and a uveal component (von Kölliker, 1861 ; Kessler, 1877). Some doubt remained, however, as to how much of the substantia propria should be apportioned to the subconjunctival and choroidal mesoderm, and how much of the central layers was derived from the sclera.

We have already seen, however, that on the separation of the surface ectoderm and the lens vesicle the intervening space is filled by an indeterminate material which has been variously interpreted as representing, on the one hand, protoplasmic continuity between the two surfaces and, on the other, tissue-fluid from which the richly protein matrix has been precipitated in the process of fixation (the " anterior vitreous ").[3] In one view this material forms an ectodermal basis for the cornea (Seefelder and Wolfrum, 1906; von Szily, 1908; Laguesse, 1923), into the composition of which many authors have admitted a mesodermal element derived from the cells of the paraxial mesoderm which insinuate themselves between the surface layer and the anterior rim of the optic cup (the " mesostroma ").[4] We have also seen that the evidence of comparative embryology might suggest that a fine structureless ectodermal membrane develops at an early stage immediately behind the surface ectoderm, a view enthusiastically supported by Hagedoorn (1928) (the *ectodermal primitive cornea*). Sondermann (1932–49) carried this suggestion a stage further. According to him the corneal endothelium

[1] p. 117.   [2] p. 153.
[3] p. 153.   [4] p. 139.

represented the remnants of the adhesions between the surface ectoblast and the lens vesicle and was in reality an epithelium. In this view the cornea was essentially mesodermal but was built upon a scaffolding of ectoderm.

However this may be, it is certain that mesodermal cells invade the space between the surface ectoderm and the lens vesicle as the latter is formed from the former (from the 6 to 9 mm. stage), and that when the

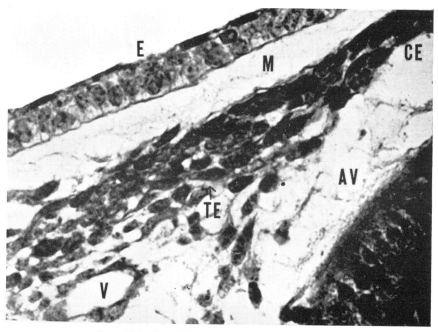

FIG. 216.—THE DEVELOPMENT OF THE CORNEA.

In a 20 mm. embryo. The cornea is seen in the region of the limbus. E, corneal epithelium ; M, indeterminate matrix in which the corneal stroma is eventually formed (mesostroma) ; CE, mesodermal cells destined to form the corneal endothelium ; AV, indeterminate tissue between the mesoderm and the lens in which the anterior chamber develops (anterior vitreous) ; TE, the initial cellular basis of the trabecular endothelium ; V, circular vessel surrounding the anterior rim of the optic cup (F. Vrabec).

vesicle detaches itself the mesoderm grows across, almost immediately forming a thin layer between the two (12 mm. stage). Initially this is loosely organized and as the globe enlarges it is drawn out to form a single lamina of flattened cells immediately behind the surface epithelium ; this lamina represents the future posterior endothelium of the cornea (Fig. 216). Subsequently, at about the 13·5 mm. stage, the surface ectoderm has begun to differentiate into two layers when it may be said to take on the characteristics of corneal epithelium.[1]

[1] p. 137.

In the endothelial cells of very young animals mitosis is seen over the entire extent of the layer, but as maturity is reached, cell-division is restricted more and more to the periphery (Mills and Donn, 1961 ; von Sallmann et al., 1961), while the cells themselves grow wider and flatter (Stocker, 1953). Since corneal swelling can be induced by anoxia shortly before birth in the rabbit, Smelser (1960) concluded that it began at this early stage to transport fluid actively out of the cornea. This function, however, is not fully effective until some days after birth.

Intervening between the ectodermal and endothelial layer there remains a fine stratum of acellular fibrillar material. Whether or not this forms an ectodermal basis determining the future architecture of the cornea seems

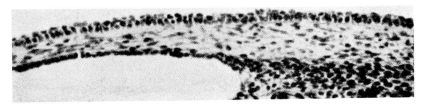

FIG. 217.—THE DEVELOPMENT OF THE CORNEAL STROMA.

In an embryo of 23 mm. The cellular corneal stroma begins to become evident made up of mesodermal cells migrating from the region of the rim of the optic cup (G. Leplat).

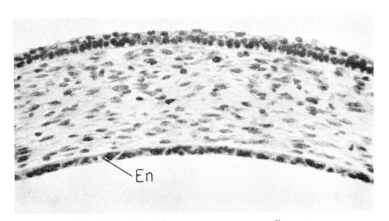

FIG. 218.—THE DEVELOPMENT OF THE CORNEA.

At the 30 mm. stage. Note that the epithelium consists of two layers and the endothelium, En, of a single layer (A. N. Barber).

relatively immaterial ; it is established that, insinuating itself into this space between the surface ectoderm and the endothelium, a second wave of mesodermal cells grows inwards from the proliferating tissue at the margin of the optic cup and gradually becomes more and more compact until, at the 22 mm. stage, the entire space is filled with regularly arranged mesodermal cells of a fibroblastic nature having their long axes parallel to the surface of the cornea, the whole gradually increasing in thickness ; the arrangement is continuous peripherally with that of the scleral condensation of mesoderm. At the earliest stages of differentiation it has been demonstrated that radio-active sulphate is incorporated into sulphated mucopolysaccharides (Smelser, 1960) ; from these cells collagen fibres are formed which immediately acquire their orientation and are of a remarkable uniformity of diameter (Schwarz, 1961). By the 20 mm. stage a relatively thick cornea is evident and the presence of collagen can be detected, and at the 25 mm. stage collagenous fibres make the picture of the substantia propria recognizable (Figs. 217–8).

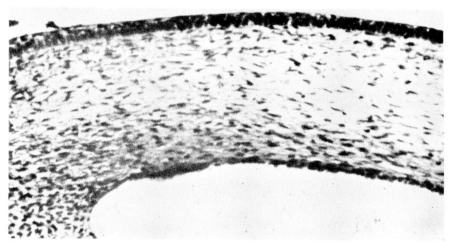

FIG. 219.—THE DEVELOPMENT OF THE CORNEA.

In a 90 mm. fœtus. Showing the beginnings of differentiation of the deeper layers of the corneal stroma (F. Vrabec).

By the 30 mm. stage the lamellar structure of the substantia propria becomes apparent first in the deeper layers and gradually progressing superficially, a process associated with an increase in collagen fibres and mucopolysaccharide and a reduction in the number of nuclei (A. and J. Coulombre, 1961) (Fig. 219). As occurs in other collagenous tissue the proportion of mucopolysaccharide drops in the early stages of development but rises again in the more mature fœtus (Smits, 1957)[1] ; but after the framework is completed collagen synthesis continues, a process for which the presence of the epithelium appears to be essential (Herrmann, 1961). As the stroma continuously consolidates, first in its posterior third, it gradually becomes more uniform in appearance and about the 7th month this structure

[1] During the development of the mammalian stroma an intense metachromasia occurs first in the inner lamellæ and then throughout the tissue (man, Gemolotto and Patrone, 1955 ; rat, Alagna, 1954, Seo, 1955 ; rabbit, Smelser and Ozanics, 1957–59). The significance of this is not clear ; it may represent an increase in the rate of synthesis of mucopolysaccharide, the appearance of new compounds of the same type. or an increase of concentration of pre-existing mucopolysaccharides associated with the dehydration and thinning of the stroma.

approaches that seen at birth (Fig. 220).   All the time the fibrous elements
increase proportionately to the cellular, a process which continues even
after birth for the number of corneal corpuscles gradually decreases through
the first 2 or 3 years of post-natal life.   At first the cornea is translucent and
it remains so until it acquires its normal hydration, an event which occurs
in the chick on hatching (A. and J. Coulombre, 1961), and in the rabbit
after the eyes open (Smelser, 1960).

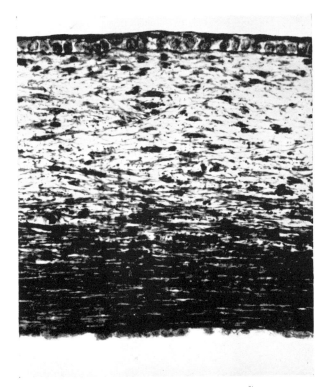

FIG. 220.—THE DEVELOPMENT OF THE CORNEA.

At the end of the 4th month. The basal membrane of the epithelium is well seen
and the consolidation of the deeper layers of the stroma is obvious (F. Vrabec).

The two *corneal membranes* are of relatively late formation.   Up to the
4th month the epithelium is separated from the underlying substantia
propria only by a basement membrane (which remains permanently) ; but
from this stage onwards a thin acellular lamina appears, formed by a feltwork of fine fibres derived from the substantia propria. This lamina gradually
thickens to form BOWMAN'S MEMBRANE which is easily recognizable by the
5th month (103 mm., Seefelder, 1930) and resembles the adult form by
the 7th ; while it remains sharply demarcated from the overlying epithelium,

FIGS. 221 and 222.—THE DEVELOPMENT OF THE CORNEAL MEMBRANES (George Smelser).

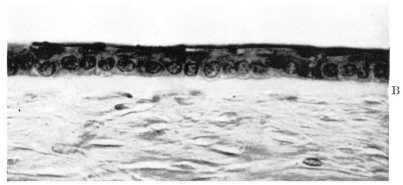

FIG. 221.—The superficial layers of the cornea. From a 6 months' human fœtus, showing the 3-layered epithelium and the presence of Bowman's membrane (B).

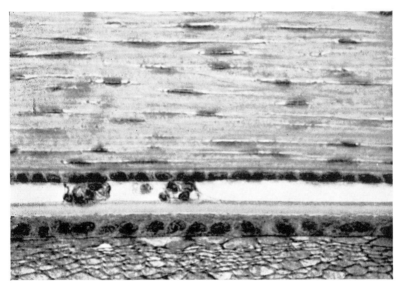

FIG. 222.—The deep layers of the cornea. From a 6 months' human fœtus, showing the endothelium and Descemet's membrane. Below is the subcapsular epithelium of the lens with the well-developed capsule ; note the shallowness of the anterior chamber.

it is firmly adherent to the underlying fibres of the substantia propria from which it is derived and with which it remains in continuity (Fig. 221).

DESCEMET'S MEMBRANE is universally accepted as formed from the corneal endothelium, but there is a considerable difference of opinion as to the stage at which it first becomes apparent. Thus Barber (1955) described its first appearance as a thin refractile line at the 30 mm. stage ; Mann (1928) noted that it could first be recognized at 49 mm. ; Seefelder

(1930) recognized it with certainty at the 76 mm. stage, Redslob (1935) and Thomas (1955) during the 6th month (160 mm. stage), and Fischer (1933) not until the 320 mm. stage (Fig. 222). This diversity of opinion has most probably arisen owing to confusion in the interpretation when the basal membrane of the endothelium should be called Descemet's membrane.

The *nerve fibres* enter the fœtal cornea at 3 months and reach the corneal epithelium by the 5th month. Between the 6th and 9th months they multiply and increase their ramifications until eventually a diffuse nerve-net is formed throughout the substantia propria (Kitano, 1955–57). It is interesting that when the lids separate and the palpebral aperture opens the cornea is provided with a well-developed innervation (Vasilieva, 1959).

From the early stages of development the cornea and sclera have the same radii of curvature. During the 3rd month, however, at the 48 mm. stage at the time when the anterior chamber is rapidly developing, the corneal curvature begins to become greater than that of the main part of the globe.

It has been shown by Smelser and Ozanics (1957) in the rabbit that the mucopolysaccharide ground substance (as indicated by metachromatic staining and the incorporation of radio-active sulphate) precedes the formation of collagenous fibres ; but whereas scleral metachromasia decreases with development, that of the cornea increases in degree and in resistance to the action of hyaluronidase. In this respect the line of demarcation between the two at the limbus is sharp after birth.

Up to the 85 mm. stage both cornea and sclera are transparent but while the cornea maintains its embryonic optical character, the sclera thereafter becomes progressively opaque. This persistent transparency of the cornea is in part due to the uniform arrangement of its fibres and to the retention of the thick mucoid ground substance which progressively disappears in the sclera after this stage. In a sense, therefore, the transparency of the cornea may be considered as a case of " arrested development ".

THE LIMBUS

Between the 25 and 30 mm. stages the anlage of the corneo-scleral junction appears (Fig. 224). Its emergence is marked by a change in the appearance of the corneal stroma at the periphery, characterized by a transition from the uniform type of stromal cells to those of a more polymorphic shape and the loss of a regular orientation. By the 40 to 45 mm. stage the relatively acute corneal curvature is differentiated in this region from that of the sclera ; at the 50 mm. stage the limbal condensation has become more pronounced ; and at 65 mm. the corneo-scleral junction is well demarcated (Fig. 223).

At about the same time, during the latter part of the 3rd month (65 mm.), the CANAL OF SCHLEMM first makes its appearance as a small plexus of venous channels[1] within the fibres of the corneo-scleral condensation, at this period level with the deepest part of the angle of the anterior chamber,

[1] p. 173.

not in front of it as in the full-term fœtus (Kawai, 1955). Sometime thereafter, about the 5th month, a triangular wedge of dense scleral condensation
appears immediately behind the canal of Schlemm continuous with the
meridional fibres of the ciliary muscle and gradually consolidates to form
the SCLERAL SPUR ; like the ciliary muscle, however, it is slow to reach its
full development which is not achieved until shortly before birth (Fig. 223).
By the 8th month of gestation an outflow path exists connecting Schlemm's
canal with the scleral veins (Araki, 1957).

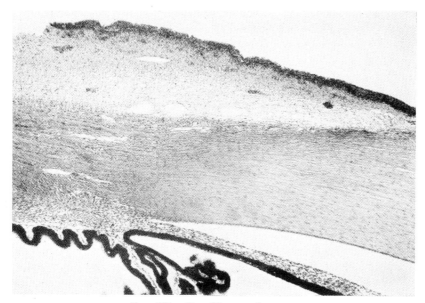

FIG. 223.—THE MATURE LIMBUS.

In a human fœtus of 7 months, showing the structure of the limbus and also the
late fœtal configuration of the angle of the anterior chamber (George Smelser).

THE ANTERIOR CHAMBER

The anterior chamber begins to form at a relatively early stage as a
space surrounded by mesoderm, long before the rim of the optic cup grows
forwards and inwards to form the ectodermal basis of the ciliary body and
iris. There are, however, considerable differences of opinion as to when and
how it first becomes apparent.[1]

The original view of von Kölliker (1861) was that it was formed early
in embryonic life as a narrow chink in the mesoderm which had insinuated

---

[1] The literature on the development of the anterior chamber is quite extensive. The early
classical work of von Kölliker (1861) has been followed by papers—among others—by Gabriélidès (1895), Jeannulatos (1896), Fritz (1906), Seefelder and Wolfrum (1906), Speciale-Cirincione
(1917), Hagedoorn (1928), Glücksmann (1929–34), Sondermann (1931–32), Seefelder (1930),
Fischer (1931–33), Allen and his co-workers (1955).

itself between the surface ectoderm and the anterior surface of the lens vesicle. Its early appearance has been corroborated by later writers such as Mann (1928), Grosser (1934) and Barber (1955), who described it as being present at the end of the 6th week (about 18 mm.). Everyone is agreed, however, that by the 5th month it is present as a well-marked cleft between the corneal endothelium anteriorly and the mesodermal portion of the iris posteriorly (Seefelder and Wolfrum, 1906 ; Speciale-Cirincione, 1917) ; Hagedoorn, 1928 ; and others). The doubt regarding its initial appearance is due to the difficulty of interpreting fixed histological specimens of a delicate tissue such as an embryo the content of which is filled with an albuminous fluid ; the appearance of clefts and spaces between its various more solid constituents and layers depends largely on the degree of shrinkage that has occurred ; the fresher the specimen and the better the fixation, the fewer and the smaller are the spaces that appear histologically, and it is difficult to say how far these are related to the configuration during life (see Nussbaum, 1908 ; Lindahl, 1915).

The mode of the formation of the anterior chamber is also a matter of controversy. von Kölliker's view that it developed as a chink in pre-existing mesoderm is now generally discounted, and it is usually conceived as resulting from the ingrowth in stages of mesoderm from the proliferative mass of this tissue which lies between the rim of the optic cup and the surface ectoderm. The first ingrowth forms the corneal endothelium just before the 12 mm. stage ; then, a considerable time later, a second ingrowth determines the corneal stroma ; at the 18 mm. stage a third wave of mesoderm forms the iris stroma extending axially posterior to the endothelium and anterior to the lens. The cleft between the first and third mesodermal ingrowths is the anlage of the anterior chamber which only develops into a large space as a result of the rapid growth of the anterior segment of the globe after the 5th month (Dejean, 1958) (Fig. 212).

A third hypothesis ascribes the determination of the topography of this region to ectodermal elements surviving from the surface and neural ecto-dermal layers as the " anterior vitreous ".[1] This, and the validity of the evidence on which the argument is based, have already been discussed. In this view the " primitive ectodermal cornea " determines the configuration of the corneal endothelium and stroma (Seefelder and Wolfrum, 1906 ; von Szily, 1908 ; Knape, 1909 ; Giesbrecht, 1925), a similar ectodermal lamina determines that of the pupillary membrane posteriorly, both of these laminæ being subsequently permeated with mesoderm (Hagedoorn, 1928). Apart from the determining influence of the ectodermal laminæ acting as a scaffolding, the sequence of events is the same as in the preceding description.

It is interesting that Mawas and Magitot (1912) considered that the primitive aqueous is also an ectodermal secretion, being derived from the glial cells forming the sheaths of the vessels of the anterior parts of the hyaloid system.

[1] p. 153.

THE ANGLE OF THE ANTERIOR CHAMBER. At the stage when the anterior chamber is relatively small its periphery is occupied by the mesodermal tissue lying between the rim of the optic cup and the surface ectoderm, which contributed to the formation of its walls. At this period the angle of the anterior chamber does not exist, and, indeed, it cannot be said to become evident before the 6th month—2 months after the canal of Schlemm[1] has become visible (Figs. 224–5). During development of the eye from the 120

FIGS. 224 and 225.—THE DEVELOPMENT OF THE ANTERIOR CHAMBER.

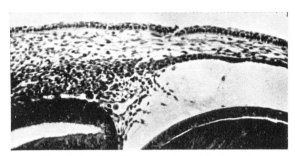

FIG. 224.—In a 23 mm. embryo (G. Leplat).

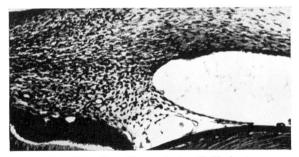

FIG. 225.—In a 90 mm. fœtus (F. Vrabec).

The angle of the anterior chamber is filled with mesodermal tissue, continuous with the deeper layer of the corneal stroma and with the pupillary membrane.

mm. stage to its adult size, the cross-sectional area of the angle increases over six times while the volume-increase between the two stages is 35 times (Burian *et al.*, 1954–56 ; Allen *et al.*, 1955). During this time as the angle deepens the loose mesodermal tissue lying between the canal of Schlemm and the root of the iris differentiates as a fan-like bundle of widely-spaced anastomosing strands which ultimately constitutes the scleral and uveal portions of the trabeculæ (Figs. 226–7).

It should be noted, however, that following the examination of an anencephalic eighth-month fœtus, Sondermann (1951) found the uveo-scleral meshwork to consist of

[1] p. 170.

FIGS. 226 and 227.—THE DEVELOPMENT OF THE ANTERIOR CHAMBER.

(L. Allen, H. M. Burian and A. E. Braley.)

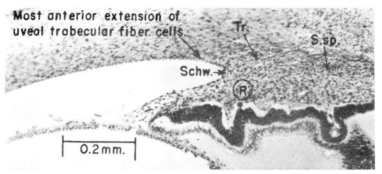

FIG. 226.—At the 120 mm. stage. Schw., rudimentary anterior border ring of Schwalbe ; **Tr,** trabecular cells ; S.sp., scleral spur ; R, the region to be occupied later by the oblique **fibres** of the ciliary muscle.

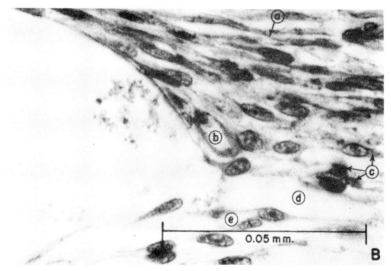

FIG. 227.—In a fœtus of 5 months. Detail of the trabecular region showing corneo-scleral trabecular fibres (a) ; b, spiral fibres destined to form the anterior border ring of Schwalbe ; c, uveal trabeculæ ; d, cleft formation starting between the trabecular tissue and the tissue of the iris and ciliary body (e).

a mass of blood-filled capillaries, a finding which led him to suggest that the trabecular fibres are normally formed from vascular tissue.

As the angle of the anterior chamber becomes gradually deeper, insinuating itself progressively into the mesodermal tissue between the corneo-scleral condensation and the mesoderm forming the iris, considerable alterations in topographical relationships necessarily occur (Rytkölä, 1952). The mutual relationship between the canal of Schlemm, the uveo-scleral

Figs. 228 and 229.—The Angle of the Anterior Chamber (A. N. Barber).

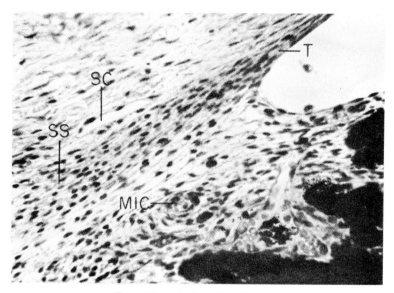

Fig. 228.—At about the 6th month.

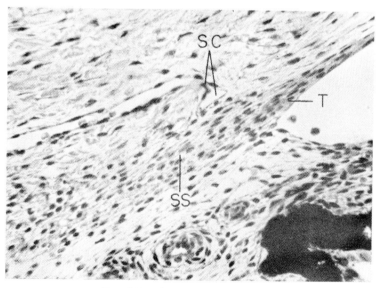

Fig. 229.—At about the 7th month.

The relative topography of the region at these stages is seen. The atrophy of the mesoderm filling the angle has progressed so that it now lies about the middle of the trabecular meshwork, T. SS, scleral spur ; SC, Schlemm's canal ; MIC, major circle of the iris.

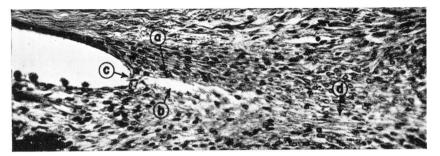

FIG. 230.—THE ANGLE OF THE ANTERIOR CHAMBER.

In a fœtus of 220 mm. To show the process of cleavage (c) between the uveal trabecular tissue (a) and the anterior aspect of the mesoderm of the ciliary body and iris (b). The cleft will shortly open into the angle and will eventually extend as far as the level marked d (Allen, Burian and Braley).

trabeculæ and the scleral spur, of course, remains fairly constant, but their positions with regard to the angle of the anterior chamber change continually as the position of the developing angle progressively shifts posteriorly (Figs. 228–9). Thus at the 6th month the angle is level with the anterior border of the trabeculæ ; by the 7th month it lies about the middle of the trabecular fibres, and the canal of Schlemm and the scleral spur are

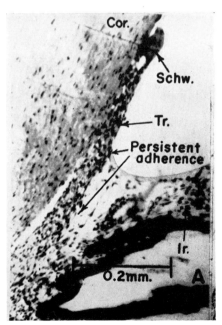

FIG. 231.—THE ANGLE OF THE ANTERIOR CHAMBER.

In a fœtus of 8½ months. Atrophy of the mesodermal trabeculæ has increased considerably leaving persisting adherences between the trabecular tissue, Tr., and the iris, Ir. Schw., indicates the border ring of Schwalbe ; Cor., cornea (Allen, Burian and Braley).

behind it ; and at birth it has reached the posterior or basal portion of the meshwork, with the scleral spur and the canal of Schlemm well in front of it.

During these changes there is in addition. a marked inequality of growth in this region, well demonstrated by the fact that the major circle of

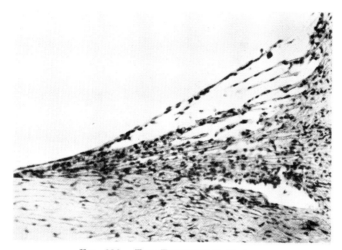

FIG. 232.—THE TRABECULAR REGION.

In the 2nd year after birth. Many of the trabeculæ are still showing regressive changes (F. Vrabec).

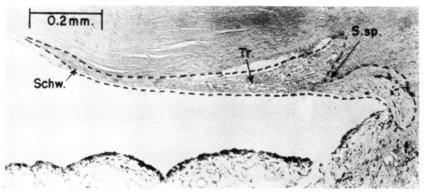

FIG. 233.—THE ANGLE OF THE ANTERIOR CHAMBER.

Orientation of the structures round the angle in the adult. Tr, trabecular fibres ; Schw., ring of Schwalbe ; S.sp., scleral spur. The dotted line indicates the outline of the trabecular region in the adult (Allen, Burian and Braley).

the iris is anterior to the level of Schlemm's canal when the latter is first developed while in the adult eye it arrives at a point behind the scleral spur. Probably the greatest contribution to this change in topographical relationship in this area and a factor contributing largely to the formation of the angular cleft is provided by the development of the ciliary muscle, the increasing mass of which has the effect of forcing the ciliary processes and the root of the iris progressively further from the trabecular region in an axial direction. The result is that the ciliary tissues, formerly resting against the uveal trabeculæ, are pulled away thus helping to extend the periphery of the anterior chamber outwards and backwards (Figs. 228 to 233).

The process by which the angle is thus excavated has always been classically considered to be one of atrophy. This is a feature of much of the mesodermal tissues in this region of the eye, seen most markedly, as we shall see presently,[1] in the disappearance of the pupillary membrane. The excavation of the neighbouring mesoderm which initially fills the angle has been taken to be an extension of this process and so also has the looseness of the tissues of the trabecular area. Allen and his co-workers (1955), however, have brought forward evidence that the essential process is not mesodermal absorption but rather a simple separation of two dissimilar layers of mesodermal tissue which suffer unequal growth (Figs. 227, 230), the cleavage occurring along the line of the inner layer of the uveal trabeculæ ; the displacement caused by the growth of the ciliary muscle probably aids the process. To some extent this element may play a part in determining the ultimate configuration of the tissues.

In the classical view congenital glaucoma may be due to a failure of the mesodermal tissue in the angle to undergo atrophy ; in the second view to a failure in separation.

THE CAPSULA PERILENTICULARIS FIBROSA

An indefinite condensation around the lens which is transient in nature has been described by this somewhat inappropriate term. At an early stage (6–7 mm.) the mesoderm which invaginates between the margin of the optic cup and the surface ectoderm and insinuates itself between the rim of the cup and the lens in association with the primitive vitreous, gradually surrounds the lens as it is formed by the separation of the lens vesicle. Initially the condensation contains only a few stellate mesodermal cells. We shall see at a later stage that this tissue becomes invaded by the hyaloid artery advancing from behind so that by the 10 mm. stage this condensation connects the mesoderm outside the optic cup with that forming the hyaloid artery ; it thus becomes vascularized to be replaced by the tunica vasculosa lentis.[2]

Abraitis. *Anat. Anz.*, **87**, 375 (1939).
Alagna. *Arch. Ottal.*, **58**, 259 (1954).
Allen, Burian and Braley. *Arch. Ophthal.* (Chicago), **53**, 783, 799 (1955).
Araki. *Acta Soc. ophthal. jap.*, **61**, 1485 (1957).
Aurell and Holmgren. *Acta ophthal.* (Kbh.), **31**, 1 (1953).
Badtke. *v. Graefes Arch. Ophthal.*, **145**, 321 (1942) ; **152**, 671 (1952).
Barber. *Embryology of the Human Eye*, St. Louis (1955).
Burian, Braley and Allen. *Trans. Amer. ophthal. Soc.*, **52**, 389 (1954). *Arch. Ophthal.* (Chicago), **55**, 439 (1956).
Casari. *Arch. Anat.* (Strasbourg), **35**, 203 (1952–3).
Coulombre, A. J. and J. L. Smelser's *The Structure of the Eye*, N.Y., 405 (1961).

Dejean. Dejean, Hervouët and Leplat's *L'embryologie de l'œil et sa tératologie*, Paris, 392 (1958).
Fischer. *v. Graefes Arch. Ophthal.*, **126**, 504 (1931) ; **131**, 318 (1933).
François and Rabaey. *Bull. Soc. belge Ophtal.*, No. 102, 568 (1952).
Fritz. *S.B. Akad. Wiss. Wien*, **115**, 485 (1906).
Fuchs. *v. Graefes Arch. Ophthal.*, **21** (3), 39 (1885).
Gabriélidès. *Arch. Ophtal.* (Paris), **15**, 176 (1895).
Gemolotto and Patrone. *G. ital. Oftal.*, **8**, 42 (1955).
Giesbrecht. *Z. wiss. Zool.*, **124**, 305 (1925).
Glücksmann. *Z. Anat. Entwickl. Gesch.*, **88**, 529 (1929). *v. Graefes Arch. Ophthal.*, **132**, 51 (1934).

[1] p. 201.   [2] p. 192.

Grosser. *Med. Klin.*, **29**, 837 (1933).
  Z. mikr.-Anat. Forsch., **36**, 516 (1934).
Hagedoorn. *Brit. J. Ophthal.*, **12**, 479 (1928).
Herrmann. Smelser's *The Structure of the Eye*, N.Y., 421 (1961).
Igo. *Jap. J. Ophthal.*, **1**, 124 (1957).
Jeannulatos. *Arch. Ophtal.* (Paris), **16**, 529 (1896).
Kawai. *Acta Soc. ophthal. jap.*, **59**, 1834 (1955).
Kessler. *Zur Entwicklung d. Auges d. Wirbelthiere*, Leipzig (1877).
Kitano. *Acta Soc. ophthal. jap.*, **59**, 1094 (1955).
  Jap. J. Ophthal., **1**, 48 (1957).
Knape. *Anat. Anz.*, **34**, 117 (1909).
von Kölliker. *Entwicklungsgeschichte d. Menschen*, Leipzig (1861 ; 1879).
Krückmann. *Graefe-Saemisch Hb. d. ges. Augenheilk.*, 2nd ed., Leipzig, **5**, 514 (1908).
Laguesse. *C.R. Soc. Biol.* (Paris), **89**, 543 (1923).
Lange. *Klin. Mbl. Augenheilk.*, **39** (1), 202 (1901).
Lindahl. *Anat. Hefte*, **52**, 195 (1915).
Magari. *v. Graefes Arch. Ophthal.*, **159**, 257 (1957).
Maggiore. *Ann. Ottal.*, **51**, 727 (1923).
Mann. *The Development of the Human Eye*, Camb. (1928) ; 2nd ed., London (1949).
Mawas and Magitot. *Arch. Anat. micr.*, **14**, 41 (1912).
Mills and Donn. Smelser's *The Structure of the Eye*, N.Y., 435 (1961).
Nussbaum. *Graefe-Saemisch. Hb. d. ges. Augenheilk.*, 2nd ed., Leipzig, **2**, 1 (1908).
Redslob. *Arch. Anat.* (Strasbourg), **19**, 135 (1935).
  Ann. Oculist. (Paris), **189**, 749 (1956).

Rytkölä. *Ann. Acad. Sci. fenn.*, Ser. *A*, No. 33, 3 (1952).
von Sallmann, Caravaggio and Grimes. *Amer. J. Ophthal.*, **51** (2), 83 (1961).
Schwarz. Smelser's *The Structure of the Eye*, N.Y., 393 (1961).
Seefelder. *Kurzes Hb. d. Ophthal.*, Berlin, **1**, 476 (1930).
Seefelder and Wolfrum. *v. Graefes Arch. Ophthal.*, **63**, 430 (1906).
Seo. *Kyushu Mem. Med. Sci.*, **5**, 169 (1955).
Smelser. Duke-Elder and Perkins's *The Transparency of the Cornea*, Oxon., 23, 125 (1960).
Smelser and Ozanics. *Amer. J. Ophthal.*, **44** (2), 102 (1957) ; **47**, 100 (1959).
Smits. *Biochim. biophys. Acta*, **25**, 542 (1957).
Sondermann. *Zbl. ges. Ophthal.*, **24**, 193 (1931).
  v. Graefes Arch. Ophthal., **128**, 119 (1932) ; **129**, 238 (1932) ; **149**, 690 (1949).
  Ber. dtsch. ophthal. Ges., **57**, 282 (1951).
Speciale-Cirincione. *Ann. Ottal.*, **45**, 161, 249 (1917).
Stocker. *Trans. Amer. ophthal. Soc.*, **51**, 669 (1953).
von Szily. *Anat. Hefte*, **35**, 649 (1908).
Thomas. *The Cornea*, Springfield (1955).
Tousimis and Fine. *Amer. J. Ophthal.*, **48** (2), 397 (1959).
  Arch. Ophthal. (Chicago), **62**, 974 (1959).
Vasilieva. *Arkh. Anat.* (Moskva), **36** (6), 20 (1959).
Vrabec. *Biol. Listy, Suppl.* 2, 118 (1951).
  Ophthalmologica, **123**, 20 (1952),
Wolfrum. *v. Graefes Arch. Ophthal.*, **67**, 307 (1908).
  Graefe-Saemisch Hb. d. ges. Augenheilk. 2nd ed,, Leipzig, **1** (2) (1926).

The Vascular System

The ocular vascular system which develops from the paraxial mesoderm surrounding and at a later stage invaginating into the optic vesicle, plays a prominent part in the development of the eye ; indeed, few aspects of embryology are more interesting than the story of its evolution and the subsequent devolution of a great part of it after it has fulfilled its role of providing nutriment for the ocular tissues at the time when they are undergoing rapid differentiation.

THE PRIMITIVE VASCULAR SYSTEM

In the embryo the germ of the vascular system appears in the wall of the yolk sac as islands of cells which constitute the ANGIOBLAST, the outer cells of which differentiate into vascular endothelium and the inner into free blood cells, at first undifferentiated hæmocytoblasts which later develop either into erythroblasts or promyelocytes (Hughes, 1943 ; Weiss, 1953).

Within this tissue a plexiform system of tubes appears which rapidly become connected with one another to form a continuous capillary network, at first running diffusely throughout the mesenchyme and then becoming localized into separate plexuses elaborated in relation to differentiating tissues and organs. From this retiform arrangement the enlargement of definite channels in some places leads to the evolution of the primitive stem-vessels of the embryo through which blood, also formed from the angioblastic tissue, circulates from one locality to another, large vessels being formed by the fusion and confluence of adjacent channels, while portions where the flow is no longer required undergo retrogression and atrophy.

Blood vessels are initially formed in the embryonic mesoderm as simple endothelial tubes without other mesodermal tissue in their walls. Initially

FIGS. 234 and 235.—THE DEVELOPMENT OF BLOOD VESSELS (Ida Mann).

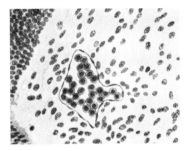 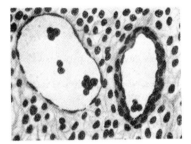

FIG. 234.—Transverse section across the internal carotid artery of a 4·5 mm. embryo ; the vessel wall is a single layer of endothelium.

FIG. 235.—Transverse section through an artery (right) and a vein (left) in a 16 mm. embryo. The wall of the artery has several rows of cells ; the vein is lined by a single layer of endothelium.

Note that the erythrocytes are nucleated.

there is no differentiation between arteries and veins and the channels appear merely as a plexus within which the direction of blood-flow is in many cases problematical (Fig. 234). This state of affairs remains for a considerable time. The annular vessel at the rim of the optic cup, for example, was originally called an artery by Fuchs (1905) in the light of histological researches, whereas Versari (1923), using an injection method, concluded that it was a vein ; probably it partakes of the nature of both and the term *annular vessel* is the best (Mann, 1928). Similarly, the loop-formation of the " arterial " circles of the iris might be more correctly termed " vascular " circles.[1] At the early stages, in fact, the nature of any vessel can be inferred only from its position and a knowledge of its future fate. It is only at the 16–18 mm. stage that the walls of the arteries can be differentiated as such in transverse section ; thereafter the arteries appear as small and discrete

[1] p. 201.

FIGS. 236 and 237.—HÆMATOPOIESIS (A. B. Reese and F. C. Blodi).

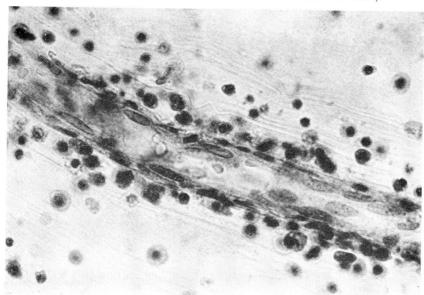

FIG. 236.—Immature blood-cells round the hyaloid artery in the primary vitreous in a premature infant of birth-weight 850 G., who lived for 62 hr. and 10 minutes.

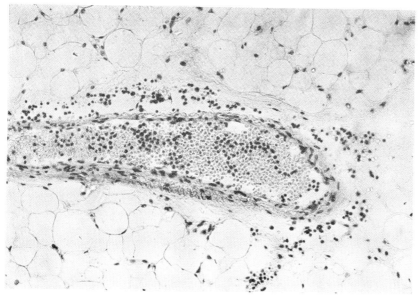

FIG. 237.—Immature blood-cells round a ciliary vessel in the orbit in a premature infant of birth-weight 1,021 G. who died after 67 days.

tubes with well-formed walls consisting of several rows of cells, while the
veins are still somewhat irregular channels made up of the coalescence of
loose blood-spaces lined by a single layer of endothelium (Fig. 235). It is to
be remembered, also, that the primitive blood-cells in the embryo and the
fœtus differ from those of the adult : the red cells are nucleated until the
end of the 2nd month whereafter the nuclei gradually disappear, while there
is a considerable leucocytosis with a preponderance of polymorphs over
leucocytes which persists until about the time of birth.

We have already seen that hæmatopoiesis first occurs in angioblastic islands in the
wall of the yolk sac and then throughout the mesenchyme generally. Finally, however,
the process is taken over by the bone marrow, extramedullary foci diminishing and

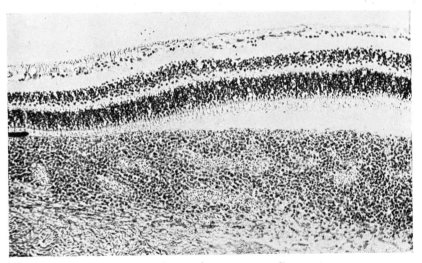

FIG. 238.—HÆMATOPOIESIS IN THE CHOROID.

The choroid of the same child as in Fig. 237, showing considerable thickening of this
tissue with foci of hæmatopoiesis containing eosinophilic myelocytes and leucocytes (A. B. Reese
and F. C. Blodi).

disappearing at or after birth. There is, however, evidence that such foci may persist
both in the eye and in the connective tissues of the orbit. Gilmour (1941) observed
such a focus in the connective tissue of the orbit in an 18 mm. embryo, while Reese
and Blodi (1954) noted its occurrence in this region around the ciliary vessels in premature or stillborn infants. In such cases the latter authors also described a series of
such foci within the eye, with some frequency in the choroid, occasionally in the iris,
and also in the primary vitreous around the hyaloid artery (Figs. 236 to 238). It may be
that these hæmatopoietic cells account in some degree at any rate for the haziness sometimes seen in the vitreous of premature infants, and the uveal foci have been confused
in the literature with inflammatory cells.

The early development of the arteries and veins of the head is an
extremely complicated process involving the appearance and disappearance
of some vessels, the formation of new vascular junctions and the abolition of

older channels to suit the needs of areas where active differentiation is occurring and to divert the excess of blood when the phase of activity has passed ; this process we shall discuss subsequently when we are describing the development of the vascular supply to the orbit.[1] In the meantime it is sufficient to say that in the early embryo (at about the 20-somite stage, Padget, 1948–54) the primitive internal carotid artery terminates in a plexus of fine endothelial tubes at the caudal aspect of the emerging optic vesicle (Fig. 239). In the 4 mm. embryo this plexus is replaced by several

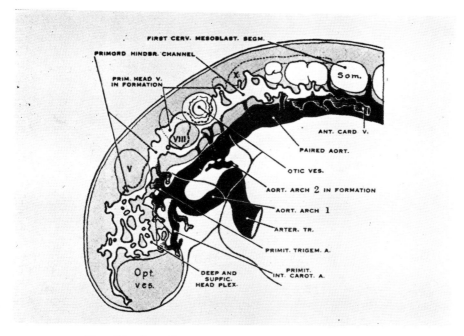

FIG. 239.—THE EARLY VASCULAR SYSTEM OF THE HEAD.

A human embryo of 20 somites. The first aortic arch gives off the primitive internal carotid and the primitive trigeminal arteries.

Veins in white, arteries in black. Som., somite in first cervical mesoblastic segment. V, VIII, X, cranial nerves. The primary head vein is seen in formation (D. H. Padget).

definitive branches, and by the time the embryo has attained 9 mm. the largest of these (termed by Padget the primitive DORSAL OPHTHALMIC ARTERY) ends in a capillary plexus over the dorsal aspect of the optic cup. At the 12 mm. stage the internal carotid artery gives off a second smaller branch (the VENTRAL OPHTHALMIC ARTERY) which becomes associated with the more medial part of the plexus now entirely investing the optic cup. By the 13 mm. stage these plexuses have extended anteriorly to the margin of the cup where their branches anastomose to form an ANNULAR VESSEL (Figs.

[1] p. 246.

240–1). Meanwhile, the primitive dorsal ophthalmic artery sends a branch (the HYALOID ARTERY) through the embryonic fissure into the interior of the optic cup, and the dilated end of the parent artery is recognizable as the COMMON TEMPORAL CILIARY ARTERY (Fig. 242).

At this stage the parent internal carotid artery passes upwards behind the optic stalk (Fig. 240) ; but as the stalk increases in length the VENTRAL OPHTHALMIC ARTERY develops from it, running along the lower border of the stalk and lengthening as the latter elongates, and to it the vascular channels surrounding and entering the optic cup are transferred (16–18 mm. stage). Up to the 18 mm. stage the ophthalmic artery supplies only the developing

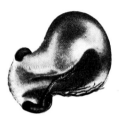

FIG. 240.—THE OPTIC CUP OF A 5 MM. HUMAN EMBRYO.

From the internal carotid artery, which passes up behind the optic stalk, two vessels are given off, the hyaloid penetrating into the optic cup, and a vessel vascularizing its margin.

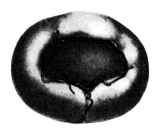

FIG. 241.—THE ANNULAR VESSEL.

The optic vesicle of a 10 mm. human embryo seen from in front. The embryonic fissure is seen below. Vessels are seen passing from the annular vessel at the margin of the cup behind the lens to join the hyaloid system (after von Szily).

eye, and all its ocular branches have been established by the time the embryo reaches 20 mm. ; the surrounding orbital tissues are initially supplied by the STAPEDIAL ARTERY, a branch of the internal carotid artery which initially assumes a transient importance (Figs. 242–3). Its complicated life-history will be described at a later stage[1] ; suffice it to say at present that in embryos of 20 mm. its supra-orbital division forms an anastomosis with the ophthalmic artery and, as its stem becomes progressively reduced in size, the latter vessel takes over the orbital vascular supply (Fig. 243).

Meantime the venous system is simultaneously developing, initially as two large venous plexuses to which the capillary plexus surrounding the optic vesicle is connected by loose irregular channels—the SUPRA-ORBITAL and INFRA-ORBITAL PLEXUSES (Fig. 246). The complex development of the vessels draining them will be discussed at a later stage.[2]

THE CHOROIDAL VASCULAR SYSTEM

The development of the posterior uveal vascular system may be conveniently described in three stages : (1) the early formation of a plexus of

[1] p. 253.   [2] p. 188.

FIGS. 242 and 243.—THE EARLY VASCULAR SYSTEM TO THE HEAD (D. H. Padget).

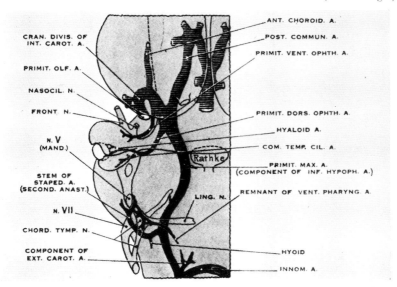

FIG. 242.—In a human embryo of approximately 14 mm. Both dorsal and ventral ophthalmic arteries are elongated and from the dorsal has developed the hyaloid artery.

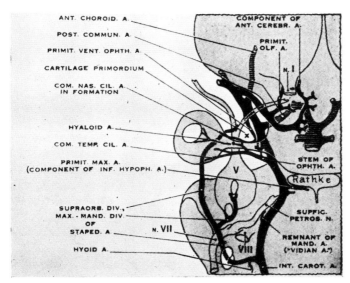

FIG. 243.—In a human embryo of approximately 18 mm. The primitive stem of the ophthalmic artery has appeared. A secondary anastomosis joins its hyaloid branch to the primitive ventral ophthalmic artery which is subsequently interrupted. The stapedial artery has formed its two primary divisions—the supra-orbital and maxillo-mandibular arteries.

small vascular channels lying next to the outer surface, first of the optic vesicle and then of the optic cup, the anlage of the future choriocapillaris, (2) the formation of venous spaces and channels more externally, the anlage of the future layer of large vessels (Haller's layer), and (3) the subsequent intrusion of arterial elements between the capillary and venous layers, the forerunner of the intermediate layer of small vessels in the choroid (Sattler's layer).

The first evidence of the uveal vascular system is the development of a rich plexus of endothelial blood-spaces in the undifferentiated paraxial mesoderm encircling the optic vesicle (Fig. 244). This commences as early

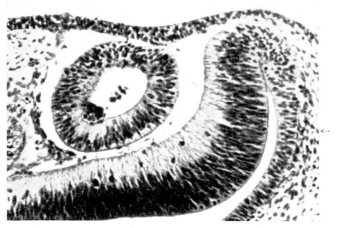

FIG. 244.—THE ENDOTHELIAL VASCULAR PLEXUS.
In an 8 mm. embryo. An endothelial plexus (arrowed) is forming around the outer aspect of the optic vesicle (F. Vrabec).

as the 3 to 4 mm. stage and can be regarded as an extension of the general surface vascularization of the neural tube which throughout its length is closely invested by minute vessels. This vascular layer is most pronounced over the lower and distal parts of the vesicle (which invaginate), and its formation is delayed over the upper part (which does not) ; it follows that when, at the 4·5 mm. stage, invagination commences, the outer layer of the cup is at first unclothed by capillaries and so it remains until pigment begins to appear within its cells at the 5 to 6 mm. stage. It is interesting that the development of the two processes, vascularization and pigmentation, are related in time as if the latter depended on the former. Thereafter, the development of the vascular spaces proceeds rapidly ; at 8 to 10 mm. the outer layer of the optic cup is covered by small vessels, and by 13 mm. the investing system of the choriocapillaris is complete.

The vessels surrounding the central nervous system (and the optic stalk) penetrate into its substance ; those investing the optic cup, however, do not do so but merely lie superficially upon it ; here the ectodermal and mesodermal elements remain separate, a relation further intensified when continuity between the two layers is rendered impossible by the development of the cuticular lamina of Bruch from the cells of the pigment epithelium.

As development proceeds, the plexus becomes denser and richer and its component vessels more conspicuous, and at the anterior rim of the cup they coalesce to form the ANNULAR VESSEL forming a circle, sometimes incomplete, around the margin (Fig. 245). The hyaloid artery (as we shall see presently) anastomoses with this vessel at the margin of the cup and also for a short time with the investing plexus at the margin of the embryonic fissure ; the closure of this fissure necessarily cuts off these latter anastomotic channels, the process occurring from behind forwards until it is complete at the 12 mm.

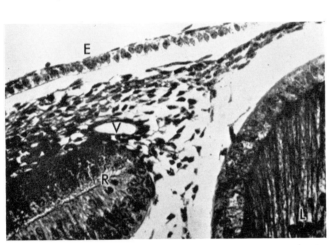

FIG. 245—THE ANNULAR VESSEL.
In a 20 mm. embryo. The annular vessel, V, is seen at the anterior border of the optic cup, R. L, lens ; E, surface epithelium (F. Vrabec).

stage. Initially the plexus is quite irregular but during the 2nd month a certain amount of pattern in the arrangement of the vessels appears whereby those investing the more anterior parts of the optic cup become orientated in parallel lines running in a postero-anterior direction except at the margin itself close to the annular vessel where they break up again into an irregular network (Fig. 246).

The second stage of development commences in the 3rd month. The loose venous channels which initially drained the choriocapillaris into the supra- and infra-orbital venous plexuses become aggregated into a wide-meshed network between the capillary layer and the mesodermal condensation now developing around the optic cup to form the sclera. This second plexus is made up of relatively large channels which form the basis of the future choroidal layer of large vessels and from it a few large trunks emerge,

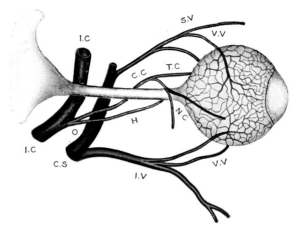

FIG. 246.—THE DEVELOPMENT OF THE VASCULAR SYSTEM.

Reconstruction of an 18 mm. embryo.

C.C. Common ciliary artery.　　　　　　O. Ophthalmic artery.
C.S. Cavernous sinus.　　　　　　　　　S.V., I.V. Superior and inferior ophthalmic
H. Hyaloid artery.　　　　　　　　　　　veins.
I.C. Internal carotid artery.　　　　　　T.C., N.C. Temporal and nasal ciliary arteries.
　　　　　　　　　　V.V. Vortex veins.

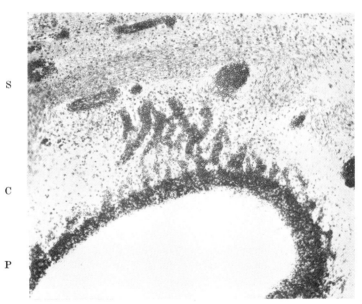

FIG. 247.—THE DEVELOPMENT OF THE CHOROIDAL VESSELS.

Tangential section in a fœtus of $3\frac{1}{2}$ months. S, the scleral condensation ; C, the beginnings of the choroidal layer of large vessels and vortex veins ; P, pigment epithelium (G. Renard).

perforating the sclera to form the vortex veins (Fig. 247) ; between the plexus and the sclera lies a layer of loose mesodermal tissue, the future suprachoroidal laminæ. It will be seen that at this period the vascular system of the choroid is entirely capillary-venous in nature.

The third and final stage of development is the interposition of a layer of vessels of arterial nature between the first two plexuses to form the future intermediate layer of small vessels, a process recognizable during the 4th month and gradually spreading from behind forwards. Some time previously (18 mm.), the primitive dorsal ophthalmic artery as it runs under the optic stalk has given off a considerable branch, the COMMON TEMPORAL CILIARY ARTERY which passes upwards on the temporal side of the optic stalk, while,

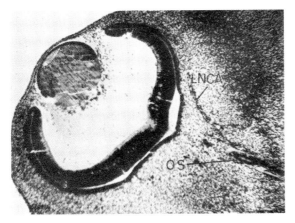

FIG. 248.—THE CILIARY ARTERIES.

In an 18 mm. embryo. A portion of the nasal long posterior ciliary artery, LNCA, is seen running forwards alongside the optic stalk, OS, towards the eye, extending through the chorio-scleral condensation (A. N. Barber).

on the lower and nasal side of the eye, the primitive ventral ophthalmic artery terminates in the COMMON NASAL CILIARY ARTERY. Soon after their origin these two common ciliary arteries give off anastomotic branches forming a ring around the optic stalk (Fig. 243) ; and shortly thereafter the portion of the nasal vessel between the anastomotic connections disappears, and the common nasal ciliary artery is annexed by the (dorsal) ophthalmic. It follows that both these ciliary arteries now take origin directly from the stem of the ophthalmic. These two ciliary arteries (the precursors of the nasal and temporal long posterior ciliary arteries) run forwards on either side of the optic nerve to the eye (Fig. 248) ; reaching it they traverse the scleral condensation and continue between it and the choroid to form a terminal anastomosis at the margin of the optic cup (the GREATER CIRCLE OF THE IRIS) ; the subsequent evolution of this vessel will be described presently.[1]   By the 60 mm. stage the short posterior ciliary arteries develop from the ophthalmic artery close to the origin of the long posterior arteries ; they first appear as 5 or 6 small branches running forwards around the optic nerve but soon break up into 12 or 15 small twigs which perforate the sclera to reach the choroid and supply the choriocapillaris encircling the outer wall of the optic cup.

By 5 months all the layers of the choroid are visible and by 7 months they are fully differentiated.

THE HYALOID SYSTEM AND THE TUNICA VASCULOSA LENTIS

The hyaloid vessels in association with the vascular tunic of the lens constitute an imposing and complex vascular system invading the developing eye posteriorly and anteriorly and forming an extensive ramification within it.   But, as occurs so often in the embryonic vascular system, it is transitory ; nourishing the structures within the eye during the period of their active growth, it begins to atrophy practically as soon as it has reached full maturity and almost completely disappears before birth.   It resembles a scaffolding erected at a crucial stage of building, to be dismantled when its function is completed.

A system so dramatic in its evolution and devolution naturally excited much interest among early writers by whom its embryology was well understood.   Henle (1832), Arnold (1832), and Valentin (1833) noted the complex vascular formations round the lens and their origin from a central artery running through the vitreous ; the system was more intimately described by von Ammon (1858), Richiardi (1869), Arnold (1874), von Kölliker (1879–1904), Schultze (1892), Kollmann (1898), Corrado (1901), and in great detail in the rabbit by Fuchs (1905).   There followed the observations of Dedekind (1908), Cosmettatos (1910), Seefelder (1909), and Bach and Seefelder (1911).   Most of this work was done by serial sectioning and construction therefrom, but owing to the difficulty of tracing complicated and minute structures from section to section, several points remained in doubt.   Versari, whose results were summarized in a valuable monograph (1923), adopted the more satisfactory method of studying injected specimens either whole or after free-hand sectioning, and in this way was able to settle the few debatable points left over from the earlier work.   Subsequent observations, more especially on the vessels of the iris (Wolfrum, 1922 ; Mann, 1925), while amplifying details, have been largely confirmatory in nature.

The HYALOID ARTERY, originally a major branch of the primitive dorsal ophthalmic artery,[2] enters the proximal part of the groove in the optic vesicle which marks the beginning of the embryonic fissure (5 mm. stage) (Fig. 240), and, running forwards in its depths, rapidly (6 to 7 mm.) reaches the posterior pole of the lens vesicle.   While the fissure is open the artery communicates freely with the capillary plexus forming the vascular network of the developing choroid ; but as the lips of the fissure fuse, this anastomosis is progressively obliterated from behind forwards, the connections at the distal end remaining the longest.   At this stage the main trunk enters the

----

[1] p. 203.   [2] p. 251.

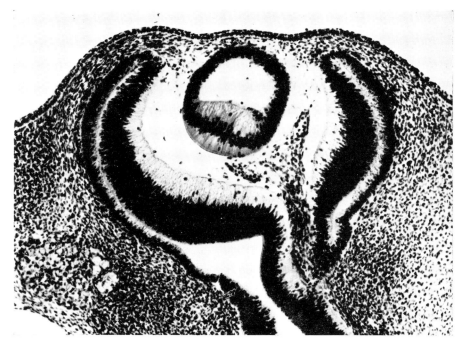

FIG. 249.—THE HYALOID ARTERY.

In a 12 mm. embryo. The hyaloid vessels and their associated mesoderm are seen entering the proximal part of the open embryonic fissure (G. Renard).

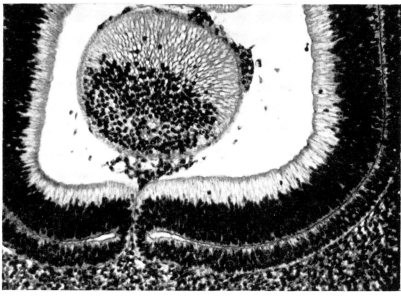

FIG. 250.—THE HYALOID SYSTEM.

In an 11·7 mm. embryo showing the closure of the embryonic fissure at the junction between a notch on the rim of the optic cup and an already closed portion of the fissure. The hyaloid artery and the tunica vasculosa lentis are well seen (R. O'Rahilly, Carnegie Institute of Washington).

optic stalk and emerges into the optic cup in the region of the future optic
disc ; as in the case of other developing vessels, its walls consist of a single
layer of endothelium and the calibre of the channel is markedly irregular
(Fig. 249).

Growing forwards through the primary vitreous, the hyaloid artery
arrives in the neighbourhood of the posterior pole of the lens where it meets
the capsula perilenticularis fibrosa, the mixture of vasoformative mesodermal cells associated with ectodermal elements which we have already
seen to have invaginated between the anterior rim of the optic cup and the

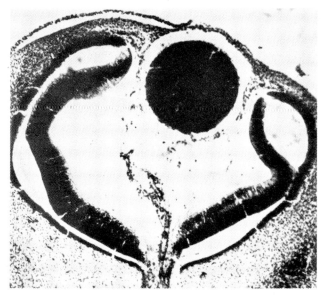

Fig. 251.—The Hyaloid System.

In an embryo of 20 mm. The hyaloid artery has reached the posterior aspect of the lens;
its branches, the vasa hyaloidea propria, are seen in the primary vitreous, and it has anastomosed with the vasoformative mesoderm invaginating from the anterior rim of the optic
cup to form the tunica vasculosa lentis (Henry Haden).

surface ectoderm to surround the lens vesicle.[1] In the meshes of this tissue
the hyaloid vessels spread by budding over the posterior surface of the lens
to form a wide-meshed capillary net—the POSTERIOR PART OF THE TUNICA
VASCULOSA LENTIS—a process which occurs at the 8 to 9 mm. stage. At
first this network makes communication with the extra-ocular (choroidal)
vessels inferiorly in the region of the embryonic fissure, but in a short time
two other systems of channels can be recognized, a temporal and a nasal,
on either side of the lens vesicle, passing between this structure and the rim
of the optic cup to establish connection with the annular vessel (10 mm.
stage). Three sets of capillaries (inferior, nasal and temporal) are thus

[1] p. 178.

formed, establishing connection between the hyaloid system within the eye and the choroidal vessels outside it, and as they do so they usually indent the margin of the optic cup below and on either side (Figs. 251 and 252).

Soon after the 10 mm. stage the posterior network of vessels sends out a large number of straight channels running anteriorly in a palisade arrangement which connects the hyaloid system with the annular vessel so that the mesodermal tissue around the equator of the lens becomes richly vascularized —the LATERAL OR CAPSULO-PUPILLARY PORTION OF THE TUNICA VASCULOSA LENTIS (Plate III, Fig. 1). Somewhat later (17 mm.) small buds appear in the annular vessel itself from which vascular loops run along the anterior surface of the lens, until eventually (25 mm.) an elaborate ANTERIOR PORTION

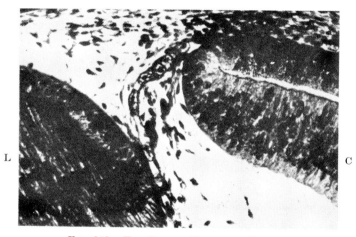

L   C

FIG. 252.—THE TUNICA VASCULOSA LENTIS.

In a 19 mm. embryo. Capillary vessels are seen running between the anterior border of the optic cup (C) and the lens (L) to form the lateral part of the tunica vasculosa lentis (F. Vrabec).

OF THE TUNICA VASCULOSA LENTIS becomes evident (Plate III, Fig. 2). It will be remembered that at this stage no anterior chamber has yet been formed so that the vascular loops run in the deepest cells of the mesodermal layer intervening between surface ectoderm and lens ; they run in one plane in close apposition to the lens and without ramifications within the mass of mesoderm.

During the time the embryo is growing from 40 to 60 mm. the hyaloid system reaches its greatest degree of development, providing an elaborate and rich vascularization for the interior of the rapidly developing eye. The single hyaloid trunk now entering the optic cup through the optic disc has ramified into a large number of branches, the VASA HYALOIDEA PROPRIA, which anastomose freely amongst each other and with the posterior part of the vascular tunic of the lens, filling the entire cavity of the optic cup, at this stage relatively small and occupied by the primary vitreous (Plate III, Fig. 2). At the disc the vessels are provided with a glial sheath derived from the ectodermal elements of Bergmeister's papilla[1] ; this is usually considered to accompany the hyaloid artery along the first third of its course (Seefelder,

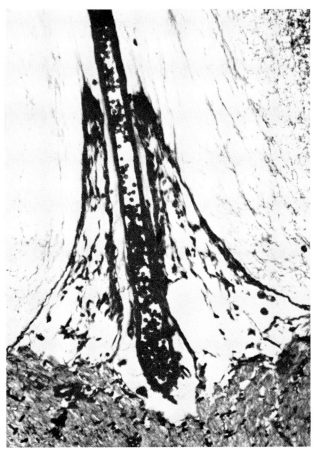

FIG. 253.—THE HYALOID ARTERY.

At the end of the 3rd month. The artery, now well formed, is seen emerging from the optic disc surrounded by glial tissue (F. Vrabec).

1910 ; Mann, 1928), but Mawas and Magitot (1912) claimed that glial elements are continued up to its terminal ramifications at the anterior part of the lens. At the optic nerve-head, however, the sheath is particularly conspicuous and reaches its greatest development at the 180 mm. stage (Figs. 253 and 254).

[1] p. 109.

The function of the hyaloid system presumably is the supply of nutriment to the rapidly developing lens and indirectly to the retina. In human embryos the vessels never appear to come into direct contact with the retina which, at this stage, has no vascular supply of its own. In certain lower vertebrates such as some fishes, amphibians and snakes[1] a MEMBRANA VASCULOSA RETINÆ develops from the peripheral vessels of the vasa hyaloidea propria from which the definitive retinal blood supply is ultimately formed ; in man, however, as the hyaloid system atrophies, the retina develops its own direct vascular system to supply its nutritive needs.

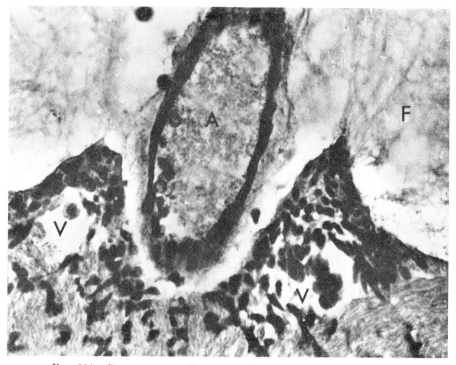

FIG. 254.—DETAIL OF THE PROXIMAL PART OF THE HYALOID ARTERY.

As seen in Fig. 253. A, hyaloid artery, surrounded by its sheath ; V, venous vessels of the optic nerve-head ; F, fibres of the secondary vitreous attached to the glial tissue of the optic nerve-head (F. Vrabec).

While the hyaloid system is developing, the vascular tunic of the lens is rapidly consolidating (Figs. 255–7), both the close network of the posterior portion and the palisade arrangement of the lateral portion; the latter runs forwards between the equator of the lens and the margin of the optic cup to drain initially into the annular vessel and subsequently into the loops of the network which replaces it. Meantime, the vascular buds growing axially from the annular vessel and carrying mesodermal tissues with them, are covering the anterior surface of the lens with vascularized tissue (Plate III,

[1] Vol. I, p. 482.

Fig. 2). Whether this grows along a preformed ectodermal lamina is unproven[1] (Seefelder, 1926 ; Hagedoorn, 1928) ; but in any event, at the 22 mm. stage the anterior chamber can be recognized and its posterior wall is seen to be made up of mesodermal cells richly vascularized from the annular vessel at the periphery and clinging closely to the anterior surface of the lens—the LAMINA IRIDO-PUPILLARIS (Jeannulatos, 1896). The peripheral portion is thick and cellular and remains permanently to form the superficial mesodermal layer of the iris ; but the central portion is almost acellular and extremely diaphanous and ultimately disappears (the PUPILLARY MEMBRANE) (Plate IV; Figs. 257–8). While this vascular proliferation is taking place, the anterior margin of the optic vesicle from which the ectodermal portion of

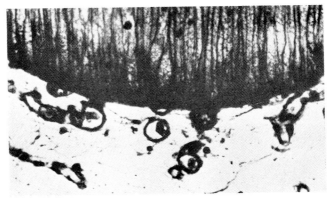

FIG. 255.—THE TUNICA VASCULOSA LENTIS.
In a 22 mm. embryo. Numerous vessels are seen forming the vascular tunic around the posterior surface of the lens (F. Vrabec).

the iris is formed, is growing forwards behind the thick layer of peripheral mesoderm towards the axis of the globe, and as the margin of the vesicle advances, the terminal branches of the long ciliary arteries, as we shall see,[2] grow into the base of the iris to reinforce the circulation and form the major circle of the iris. Thence the vessels grow axially as a series of loops arranged in three and occasionally four tiers of arcades, a process which reaches its height at 5 months at which stage the whole or practically the whole of the mesoderm covering the anterior part of the lens is vascularized (Plate IV, Fig. 2).

Having thus reached a remarkably high stage of differentiation, the hyaloid system then commences to atrophy. This process is first seen at the 60 mm. stage when the smallest peripheral branches of the vasa hyaloidea propria begin to shrink at their proximal ends and eventually, losing connection altogether with their parent artery, they hang from their distal ends

[1] p. 153.   [2] p. 203.

Figs. 256 and 257.—The Hyaloid System.

In a 34 mm. embryo ; injected with Indian ink (F. Vrabec).

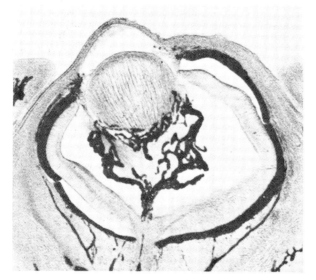

Fig. 256.—Injected embryo to show the hyaloid artery, its branches within the vitreous, and the posterior part of the tunica vasculosa lentis.

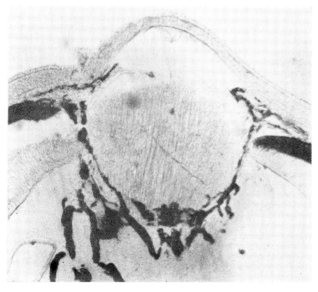

Fig. 257.—Showing the anastomosis between the anterior uveal system and the hyaloid system to form the tunica vasculosa lentis.

suspended in spiral form from the vessels on the posterior surface of the lens (Fig. 262) ; their peculiar and characteristic corkscrew-like shape is presumably determined by the inherent elasticity of their walls.   By $8\frac{1}{2}$ months the atrophy of these vessels is almost complete, and only a few remnants are left which may persist throughout life when they may be subjectively evident as muscæ volitantes.   Meantime, the vessels of the posterior tunic fail to keep pace with the rapid growth of the lens, and become stretched,

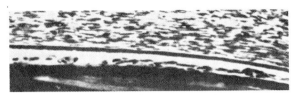

FIG. 258.—THE PUPILLARY MEMBRANE.

In a 4 months' fœtus. Mesodermal tissue is seen clothing the anterior surface of the lens below ; the cornea is above. Note the extreme shallowness of the anterior chamber owing to celloidin embedding by Gros-Schultze's method (× 180) (F. Vrabec).

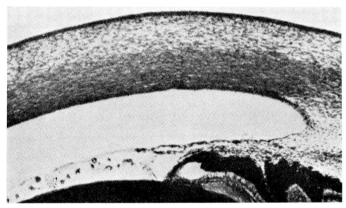

FIG. 259.—THE FORMATION OF THE PUPILLARY MEMBRANE.

In a fœtus of $4\frac{1}{2}$ months. Vasoformative mesodermal tissue spreads over the anterior surface of the lens from the mesoderm at the anterior rim of the optic cup (G. Leplat).

reduced in calibre and finally atrophy.   During the 7th month the main trunk of the hyaloid itself also narrows and becomes impervious, first in its central part, a process which proceeds proximally so that by the end of the 7th month the ectodermal elements which constitute Bergmeister's papilla also begin to atrophy, ultimately leaving a physiological cup on the disc (Figs. 260–1).   Finally, during the 8th month the central artery has lost all connection with the disc and, curling up into a spiral form, extends backwards from the posterior pole of the lens, a withered remnant of its former self.   Meantime, as the hyaloid system degenerates, the primary vitreous in which the

FIGS. 260 and 261.—THE ATROPHY OF THE HYALOID SYSTEM.
(F. Vrabec)

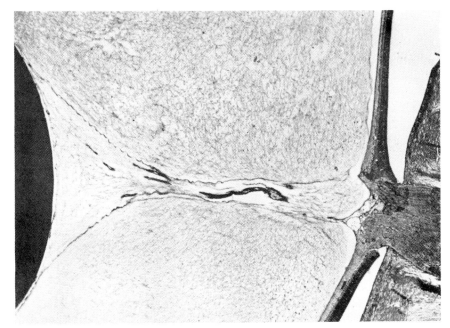

FIG. 260.—In an early 5 month fœtus. The hyaloid vessels are degenerating but are well seen in the primary vitreous running from the optic disc to the posterior aspect of the lens ; at this stage the canal of Cloquet is rich in mesodermal tissue. It is surrounded by the avascular secondary vitreous.

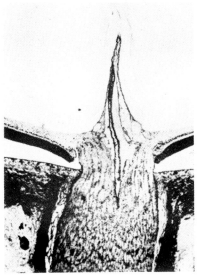

FIG. 261.—In a late 5 month fœtus. Showing the remnants of the hyaloid vessels surrounded by glial tissue emerging from the optic disc.

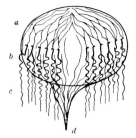

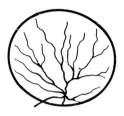

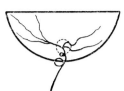

FIG. 262.—THE VESSELS ON THE LENS AT THE BEGINNING OF ATROPHY OF THE VASA HYALOIDEA PROPRIA.

a. Anterior vascular capsule (pupillary membrane).
b. Capsulo-pupillary vessels.
c. Vasa hyaloidea propria.
d. Main trunk of hyaloid (after Versari).

FIG. 263.—THE RETROGRESSION OF THE POSTERIOR VASCULAR CAPSULE OF THE LENS IN A FŒTUS OF 280 MM. (Versari).

FIG. 264.—THE LENTAL END OF THE HYALOID ARTERY AT BIRTH (Versari).

vessels ramify is becoming progressively concentrated into the central axis of the optic vesicle by the development of the secondary vitreous, so that at birth the coiled artery floats freely in the narrow confines of Cloquet's canal. After the 4th or 5th year of life, under the influence of gravity, it is frequently visible hanging vertically downwards corkscrew-like from the posterior

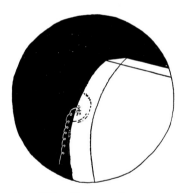

FIG. 265.—HYALOID REMNANTS.

Diagrammatic representation of the hyaloid remnant in the adult seen with the slit-lamp. The arc line is seen on the posterior surface of the lens and the cork-screw-like remnant of the hyaloid artery hangs downwards from it in the hyaloidean space (after Ida Mann).

pole of the lens. In this form it can be observed throughout life with great frequency (Vogt, 1919), although atrophy often proceeds further so that practically no trace of the artery or any of its branches remains (Figs. 262 to 265).

Meantime, the process of atrophy has spread to the lateral part of the tunica vasculosa lentis. We have seen that this portion of the embryonic

PLATE III

THE HYALOID SYSTEM

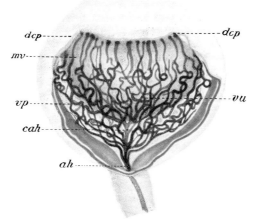

FIG. 1.—In human embryo of 40 mm. (second week of third month).

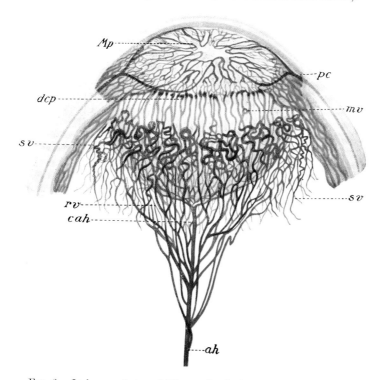

FIG. 2.—In human fœtus of 85 mm. (beginning of fourth month).

ah. Hyaloid artery.
cah. Central branch of hyaloid artery.
dcp. Distal extremity of capsulo-pupillary system forming the annular vessel.
Mp. Pupillary membrane.
mv. Capsulo-pupillary portion of the tunica vasculosa.

pc. Long posterior ciliary artery.
sv. Superficial vessel of vitreous in stage of involution.
vp. Vasa hyaloidea propria (superficial).
vu. Vasa hyaloidea propria (deep).

(After Versari.)

PLATE IV

The Pupillary Membrane

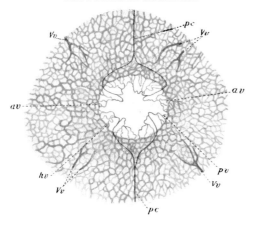

Fig. 1.—In a human embryo of 32 mm.

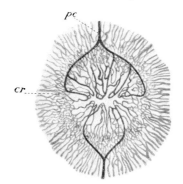

Fig. 2.—In a human embryo of 60 mm.

pc. Long posterior ciliary artery.
Vv. Collecting branches of vortex veins.
av. Annular vessel.

hv., pv., Vessels of pupillary membrane.
cr. Capillary network of the ciliary processes.

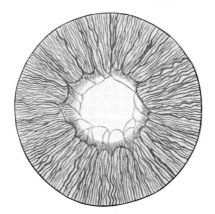

Fig. 3.—In a human embryo of 7 months.

Figures 1 and 2 after Versari; Figure 3 after Ida Mann.

vascular system constitutes a series of parallel vessels running round the equator of the lens, draining the hyaloid system and the posterior part of the tunic into the most anterior loops of the choroidal net. As the lens grows in dimensions the vessels of this portion of its tunic also do not seem to be able to compete and they become progressively stretched, a process accentuated as they bend over the ectodermal margin of the optic cup now rapidly growing forwards to form the ciliary body and iris ; moreover, as the posterior part of the hyaloid system gradually atrophies, their function of draining the blood anteriorly into the choroid progressively diminishes. These vessels therefore shrink and begin to disappear where they are constricted at the growing margin of the optic cup (50 mm.) until finally, during the 4th month, they cease to be visible here, a retrogression which, incidentally, makes room for the development of the ciliary processes and the suspensory ligament of the lens.

The first change in the vascular system comprising the anterior or pupillary portion of the tunica vasculosa lentis occurs at about the 48 mm. stage when its peripheral portion begins to lose its original connections with the capsulo-lenticular vessels as these suffer atrophy. At the 7th month, however, the process of atrophy which has long before been marked in the posterior part of the vascular tunic, becomes evident in the central attenuated part of the pupillary membrane (Plate IV, Fig. 3). The most central tier of arcades begins to shrink, and as the second tier atrophies it tends to recede away from the growing border of the deeper stromal layer which now forms the pupillary margin, leaving a slight cleft of variable extent between itself (the pupillary membrane) and the latter (the angle of Fuchs). By 8½ months most of the central loops have disappeared, occasionally leaving a few persistent remnants attached to the superficial leaf of the iris[1] ; only the first arcade persists to form a series of arterio-venous anastomoses which remains permanently as the LESSER CIRCLE OF THE IRIS. Since the persistence of this vascular circle provides a circulatory channel for the blood in the peripheral portion of the pupillary membrane, this superficial sheet of mesoderm persists and its vessels form the radial superficial vessels of the fully developed iris. The tendency to atrophy is, however, usually present occurring in isolated patches, a process which may continue during the first year of life and gives rise to the formation of crypts and establishes the delicate architecture of the final pattern of the iris. The same process of atrophy, as we have seen,[2] affects the superficial layer of endothelium.

THE CILIO-IRIDIC CIRCULATION

It will be remembered that in the formation of the choroid the capillary-venous system was the first to develop ; the same sequence occurs in the ciliary body. We have seen[3] that in the anterior parts of the choroid the vessels of the primitive capillary network assume a parallel arrangement,

---

[1] See Part 2, p. 775.   [2] p. 160.   [3] p. 187.

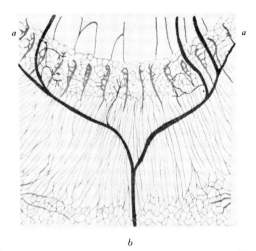

FIG. 266.—THE VASCULARIZATION OF THE CILIARY REGION.
In a 110 mm. fœtus. *a*, commencing ciliary veins ; *b*, long ciliary artery.
The veins are in grey ; the arteries in black (after Versari).

and that still more anteriorly in the region of the future ciliary processes an irregular network is again formed (Fig. 266). This occurs during the 4th month. This network is essentially capillary-venous in nature, and as the ciliary folds develop the vessels under a fold mount up to the summit and dip down again to the general level of the net, presenting anteriorly a prominent rounded curve and anastomosing to form an arcade-like arrangement within each process (Fig. 267).

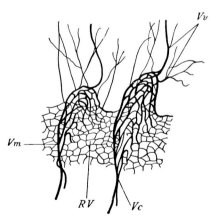

FIG. 267.—THE VESSELS OF THE CILIARY PROCESSES.
From a 210 mm. fœtus (Versari).

Vm. Marginal vessel of a ciliary process.   *Vc.* Vessels leaving the process posteriorly.
RV. Vascular network in the valley between   *Vv.* Vessels entering the process anteriorly.
    two processes.

While the capillary-venous foundation of the ciliary circulation is thus being laid, the arterial elements are growing forwards to participate in the definitive blood supply of the anterior segment of the eye. We have seen that at a relatively early stage of development (18 mm.) the ophthalmic artery gives off, on the one hand, the common ciliary artery which passes upwards on the temporal side of the optic stalk, and, on the other, several anastomosing channels which pass towards the nasal side of the eye and eventually fuse to form the nasal ciliary artery. From the former there develops the temporal ciliary artery ; and the subsequent atrophy of the portion of the common ciliary artery between the nasal and temporal ciliary arteries determines a configuration in which the two ciliary arteries (now the NASAL and TEMPORAL LONG POSTERIOR CILIARY ARTERIES) take origin directly from the ophthalmic. These two arteries run forwards on either side of the optic nerve, traverse the scleral condensation and continue between it and the choroid towards the margin of the optic cup. Here each divides into two terminal branches which, traversing the mesoderm in this region, anastomose with the peripheral vessels of the anterior portion of the vascular tunic of the lens to form eventually an anastomotic circle, the GREATER CIRCLE OF THE IRIS, in the deeper layer of the mesoderm, a process which is completed during the 6th month (Plate IV, Figs. 1 and 2). The anastomosis is further reinforced by small tributaries from the muscular and lacrimal branches of the ophthalmic artery in the anterior part of the orbit, some of which, appearing about the 90 mm. stage, pierce the sclera as the ANTERIOR CILIARY ARTERIES and eventually anastomose with branches of the long posterior ciliary arteries to take part in the formation of the greater circle of the iris. From this vascular circle three sets of vessels are given off :

(1) *Superficial branches* to the iris, combining with those of the pupillary membrane to supply its vascular arcades.

(2) *Intermediate branches* running deeply into the peripheral portion of the mesoderm to form a network in the deeper layer of the iris stroma. Taking mesodermal tissue with them, these vessels grow from the periphery running in an axial direction underneath the superficial layer of stroma (the pupillary membrane), keeping in step with the axial growth of the rim of the optic cup. When the sphincter muscle of the pupil is formed from the ectodermal layer of the iris and migrates forwards into the stroma, these vessels participate in its activity by forming two associated plexuses. Branches invade the muscle itself carrying with them mesodermal elements so that it is divided into bundles by vascularized connective tissue septa by an INTER-SPHINCTERIC PLEXUS, while a SUB-SPHINCTERIC PLEXUS insinuates itself between the bulk of the muscle and its parent epithelium. At this time, therefore, during the 7th month, four layers of vessels are present in the iris near the pupillary margin : (a) the arcades of the pupillary membrane lying superficially ; (b) the radial vessels of the iris stroma; (c) the inter-sphincteric plexus in the substance of the sphincter muscle; and (d) the sub-sphincteric

plexus lying most deeply between the muscle and the pigment epithelium of the iris (Fig. 147).

(3) *Recurrent ciliary branches* running backwards to the ciliary body. These are the last to be formed and by the 8th month one branch has reached each ciliary process and vascularized it and is extending backwards to anastomose with the vessels of the middle (arterial) layer of the choroid.

THE RETINAL CIRCULATION

The retina of the human embryo is entirely avascular for when the hyaloid artery enters the proximal end of the embryonic fissure in the earlier stages of development, it gives off no branches until it reaches the cavity of the optic vesicle. It would appear that at a very early stage a venous tributary of the primitive maxillary vein ramifies at the base of the optic vesicle and that it receives vessels from the fissure (5–8 mm. stage) (Padget, 1957). This is presumably the anlage of the future central retinal vein. Mann (1949), however, could find no vein accompanying the central retinal artery until the 3rd month when two venous channels could be traced running on either side of the artery in the optic nerve ; these finally anastomose and unite at a variable distance behind the optic disc, leaving the nerve as a single trunk. At a later stage, during the 4th month (100 mm.), a bulbous swelling, which marks the posterior point to which the atrophy of the hyaloid artery will extend, appears in its trunk in the region of the pre-papillary cone

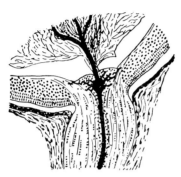

FIG. 268.—THE DEVELOPMENT OF THE CENTRAL ARTERY OF THE RETINA.

Diagram in a 4-month fœtus. The bulb of the hyaloid artery is seen at the disc and from it the branches of the central retinal artery are budding out into the retina (after Ida Mann).

of Bergmeister, and from it grow two small solid buds which represent the primordia of the upper and lower branches of the central retinal artery (Fig. 268). It is generally accepted that from these further buds ramify, at first within the cone itself, and later more widely in the nerve-fibre layer of the immediately adjacent retina, which soon become canalized ; Nilausen (1958), however, failed to confirm the presence of such buds and suggested that the vascular net expands peripherally by a continuous differentiation of mesenchymal cells into endothelium. Whatever the mechanism may be, a well-marked zone of vascularization appears around the disc, the temporal vessels being always in advance of the nasal (Fig. 269). As occurs with the hyaloid artery, these vessels are clothed with a glial sheath derived from the cone itself. Thereafter vascularization spreads progressively out towards the periphery (Fig. 270), until during the 8th month the vessels reach the neighbourhood of the ora serrata. Collateral

FIGS. 269 and 270.—THE DEVELOPMENT OF THE RETINAL VESSELS.
(I. C. Michaelson).

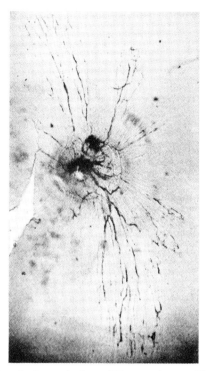

FIG. 269.—Injected retinal vessels in a 110 mm. fœtus. Four vessel-complexes can be distinguished, upper and lower temporal, upper and lower nasal. These measure in extent 2·28 mm., 1·92 mm., 1·39 mm., and 1·39 mm. respectively (× 17).

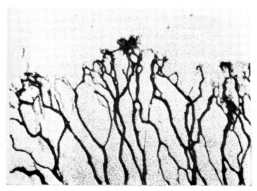

FIG. 270.—The formation of capillary loops in the periphery of the retina of a 230 mm. fœtus (× 23).

venous channels appear coincidentally with the tributaries of the retinal arteries and drain into the two venous channels which accompany the central retinal artery within the distal end of the optic nerve.

The retinal capillary networks are formed by a process of budding from

FIGS. 271 and 272.—THE DEVELOPMENT OF THE RETINAL CAPILLARIES.
(I. C. Michaelson).

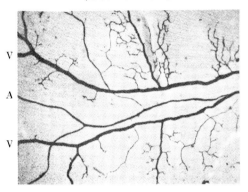

FIG. 271.—The injected retina showing capillary budding from the sides of two veins (V) (above and below) remote from the intervening artery (A), in a 190 mm. fœtus (× 20).

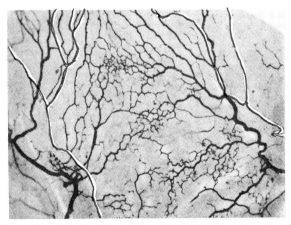

FIG. 272.—Capillary formation in the retina. Injected fœtus showing the capillary formation taking place entirely from the veins. Arteries in red, veins in black (× 20).

pre-existing vessels ; this is a function of the veins only, and where a vein and artery are close to each other, budding takes place initially from the side of the vein remote from the artery (Michaelson, 1948). Capillaries are first present only in the nerve-fibre layer, the deep capillary network being formed subsequently from the superficial (Figs. 270 to 272).

THE VESSELS OF THE OPTIC NERVE

As occurs throughout the remainder of the central nervous system, the optic nerve is vascularized essentially by vessels which penetrate its substance from the primitive vascular plexus which is formed around it at an early stage of development ; in this it differs from the optic vesicle for the corresponding plexus which forms the choriocapillaris sends in no penetrating branches, a process which seems to be easy only when the superficial nervous layer consists of nerve fibres. These vessels, ultimately derived from the pial sheath, carry with them into the substance of the nerve the ectodermal

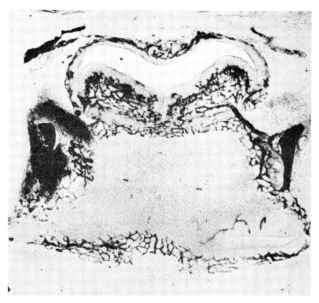

FIG. 273.—THE EMBRYONIC VASCULAR SYSTEM OF THE CHIASMA.

An injected specimen in a 2nd month embryo of 34 mm., showing the rich pial vascular plexus around the chiasma, anastomosing with the vascular system of the infundibulum (× 28) (F. Vrabec).

and mesodermal elements which form their glial sheaths and the system of septa ; they are the sole supply of the proximal part of the optic nerve, the chiasma and the lower visual pathways (Fig. 273). Distal to the point of entry of the hyaloid artery, however, a second source of vascularization is added, for here small capillary offshoots from the central artery penetrate between the bundles of nerve fibres, forming the essential blood supply for the axial portion of the distal part of the nerve.

In the region of the optic disc anastomoses occur between the ciliary and retinal vessels for the ciliary arteries forming the circle of Zinn can also penetrate among the nerve fibres in the same way as do the pial vessels. It is interesting that in some carnivores these anastomotic channels enlarge to form the definitive retinal blood supply, taking the place of the central artery of the retina.[1] Occasionally an enlarged anastomosis may become established between one of the posterior ciliary arteries and a small branch derived from the bulb of the hyaloid artery at the disc to form a cilio-retinal artery.

Among vertebrates the degree of development of the hyaloid artery varies greatly, and upon the extent of its persistence depends in large measure the variations in the ultimate vascular arrangement of the eye. We have already studied the various arrangements met with.[2] In fishes the hyaloid system is represented merely by a ridge of vascularized mesoderm lying at the site of the embryonic fissure (the *processus falciformis*) ; this is the only vascularized tissue inside the optic cup, and it remains stationary without any tendency to atrophy. In Sauropsidæ a well-defined hyaloid vessel enters the upper end of the embryonic fissure and passes across the lower part of the eye leaving by a notch at the rim of the optic cup without coming into relation with the lens ; this lays the foundation of the *cone* of reptiles and the *pecten* of birds. In mammals, on the other hand, a complex system with numerous vessels in the vitreous and a vascular tunic of the lens is formed and the degree of subsequent atrophy determines the final varieties of retinal blood supply. Complete atrophy of the hyaloid vessel determines an avascular retina ; the persistence of vasa hyaloidea propria determines a *membrana vasculosa retinæ* ; invasion of the retina itself by vessels, which varies considerably in the extent to which it occurs, determines the vascularized retina of mammals. Finally, since a tunica vasculosa lentis is present only in mammals, no species lower than these possess a pupillary membrane, and their iridic vessels are represented only by the deeper system of the iris stroma which is associated with the greater circle of the iris and the sphincteric plexuses.

von Ammon. *v. Graefes Arch. Ophthal.*, **4**, 1 (1858).

Arnold. *Anat. u. phys. Untersuch. ü d. Auges d. Menschen*, Heidelberg (1832).
    Beitr. z. Entwickelungsges. d. Auges, Heidelberg (1874).

Bach and Seefelder. *Atlas zur Entwicklungsgeschichte d. mensch. Auges*, Leipzig (1911-14).

Corrado. *G. Ass. Napol. Med. Nat.*, **5**, 318 (1901).

Cosmettatos. *Arch. Ophtal.* (Paris), **30**, 480 (1910).

Dedekind. *Anat. Hefte*, **38**, 1 (1908).

Fuchs. *Anat. Hefte*, **28**, 1 (1905).

Gilmour. *J. Path. Bact.*, **52**, 25 (1941).

Hagedoorn. *Brit. J. Ophthal.*, **12**, 479 (1928).

Henle. *De membrana pupillari aliisque oculi membranis pellucentibus* (Diss.), Bonn (1832).

Hughes. *J. Anat.* (Lond.), **77**, 266 (1943).

Jeannulatos. *Arch. Ophtal.* (Paris), **16**, 529 (1896).

von Kölliker. *Entwicklungsgeschichte d. Mensch.*, Leipzig (1879).
    Z. wiss. Zool., **77**, 1 (1904).

Kollmann. *Lhb. d. Entwickelungsges. d. Mensch.*, Jena (1898).

Mann. *Brit. J. Ophthal.*, **9**, 495 (1925).
    Development of the Human Eye, Camb. (1928) ; 2nd ed., London (1949).

Mawas and Magitot. *Arch. Anat. micr.*, **14**, 41 (1912).

Michaelson. *Trans. ophthal. Soc. U.K.*, **68**, 137 (1948).

Nilausen. *Acta ophthal.* (Kbh.), **36**, 65 (1958).

Padget. *Contrib. Embryol. Carneg. Instn.*, **32**, 212 (1948) ; No. 247, 81 (1957).
    Anat. Rec., **119**, 349 (1954).

Reese and Blodi. *Amer. J. Ophthal.*, **38** (2), 214 (1954).

Richiardi. *Sopra il sistema vascolare sanguifero dell'occhio*, Bologna (1869).

Schultze. *Zur Entwickelungsges d. Gefässsystems im Säugertierauge* (*Festschr. v. Kölliker*), Würzburg (1892).

Seefelder. *v. Graefes Arch. Ophthal.*, **70**, 448 (1909) ; **73**, 419 (1910).
    Arch. Augenheilk., **97**, 156 (1926).

Valentin. *v. Ammons Z. Ophthal.*, **3**, 302 (1833).

Versari. *Ric. Morfol.*, **3**, 1 (1923).

Vogt. *v. Graefes Arch. Ophthal.*, **100**, 328 (1919).

Weiss. *J. Embryol. exp. Morph.*, **1**, 181 (1953).

Wolfrum. *v. Graefes Arch. Ophthal.*, **109**, 106 (1922).

[1] Vol. I, p. 479.   Vol. I, p. 482.

SECTION III

THE DEVELOPMENT OF THE OCULAR ADNEXA AND PIGMENT

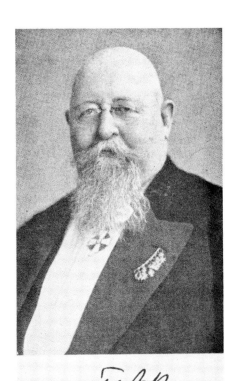

FIG. 274.—FRITZ ASK
[1876–1934].

CHAPTER VIII

THE OCULAR ADNEXA

WE are introducing this chapter with a portrait of FRITZ ASK [1876–1934] because of his fundamental work on the development of the lacrimal passages (Fig. 274). One of the best known Swedish ophthalmologists of his time, he was chief of the Ophthalmic Clinic at Lund, and apart from his contributions to our science he was a well-known international figure and a member of the International Council of Ophthalmology. Cast in a massive physical mould, he was an unusually delightful and kindly colleague with erudition sufficient to allow him to make international addresses in Latin for the sake of those who were not acquainted with the Scandinavian languages.

THE ORBIT

By the 4th week (3·5 to 4 mm. stage) the head-fold[1] is well developed and the visceral mesoderm bounding the stomatodæum (primitive mouth) together with the overlying ectoderm undergoes condensation and becomes raised up to form the localized mass of the MANDIBULAR PROCESSES (Figs. 275–6). At the 6 mm. stage an epithelial thickening (the *nasal* or *olfactory placode*) appears on either side of the front of the head above the stomatodæum ; initially forming ill-defined swellings on the surface, these gradually become transformed into depressions (the olfactory pits) owing to the proliferation of the surrounding mesoderm, a process particularly marked on either side of each olfactory pit leading to the formation of the medial and lateral nasal folds. The two medial nasal folds together with the intervening area above the stomatodæum form the central FRONTO-NASAL PROCESS while on each side the LATERAL NASAL PROCESS separates the olfactory pit from the developing optic vesicle (Figs. 275 to 282). While these changes are going on, a somewhat triangular process of visceral mesoderm grows ventrally on each side of the head from the cephalic side of the dorsal end of the mandibular arch as the MAXILLARY PROCESS, and as growth proceeds it eventually meets the lateral nasal fold. At this stage (8–12 mm.), therefore, the optic vesicle is encircled by the lateral nasal process and the maxillary process.

At the 12 mm. stage these two masses of mesoderm have met, the ectoderm along the line of fusion being buried under the surface to form a solid rod of cells, forming the anlage of the naso-lacrimal duct (Fig. 282). Thereafter the maxillary process extends forwards and upwards to fuse with its fellow on the opposite side of the developing face, so that by the 16 mm. stage it forms an uninterrupted shelf underneath the eye, while after the 20 mm. stage the depressions between these facial processes normally

---

[1] p. 25.

14—2

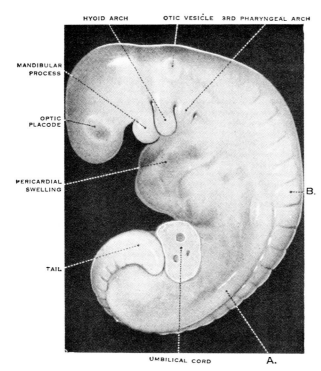

HYOID ARCH OTIC VESICLE 3RD PHARYNGEAL ARCH

MANDIBULAR PROCESS

OPTIC PLACODE

PERICARDIAL SWELLING

TAIL

UMBILICAL CORD A.

B.

FIGS. 275 and 276.— HUMAN EMBRYOS (G. L. Streeter; from Hamilton, Boyd and Mossman's *Human Embryology*, W. Heffer, Cambridge).

FIG. 275.—The left side of a 28-somite human embryo (4 mm. C.R. length; about 30 days). A, elevation caused by the mesonephros B, somites ($\times c. 20$).

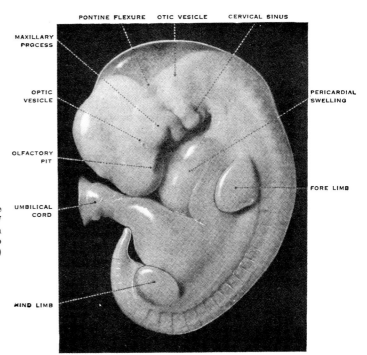

PONTINE FLEXURE OTIC VESICLE CERVICAL SINUS

MAXILLARY PROCESS

OPTIC VESICLE

OLFACTORY PIT

UMBILICAL CORD

PERICARDIAL SWELLING

FORE LIMB

HIND LIMB

FIG. 276.—The left side of a 6·7 mm. C.R. length human embryo (about 34 days) ($\times c. 12$).

Figs. 277 and 278.—
Human Embryos (G. L.
Streeter ; from Hamilton,
Boyd and Mossman's
Human Embryology, W.
Heffer, Cambridge).

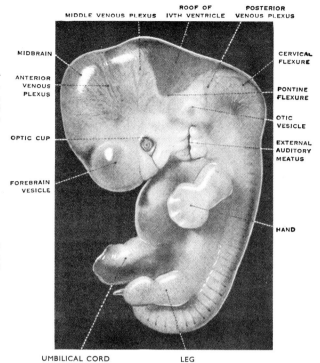

MIDDLE VENOUS PLEXUS — ROOF OF IVTH VENTRICLE — POSTERIOR VENOUS PLEXUS

MIDBRAIN

ANTERIOR VENOUS PLEXUS

OPTIC CUP

FOREBRAIN VESICLE

CERVICAL FLEXURE

PONTINE FLEXURE

OTIC VESICLE

EXTERNAL AUDITORY MEATUS

HAND

UMBILICAL CORD — LEG

Fig. 277.—The left side
of a 13·4 mm. C.R. length
human embryo (about 40
days) (× c. 6·5).

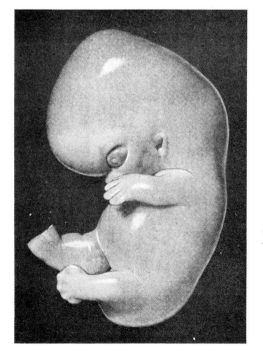

Fig. 278.—The left side of a 17 mm.
C.R. length human embryo (about 46
days) (× c. 4·7).

Figs 279 to 282.—The Development of the Face in the Human Embryo.

Drawings of the ventral aspect of the head region of a human embryo (Hamilton, Boyd and Mossman, based on Streeter ; *Human Embryology*, Heffer and Sons Ltd., Cambridge).

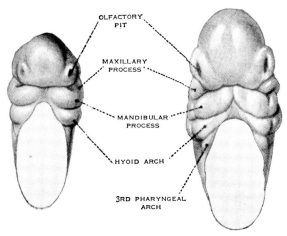

FIG. 279.—An embryo of 5·7 mm.   FIG. 280.—An embryo of 6·7 mm.

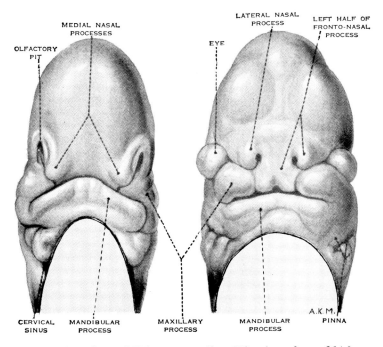

FIG. 281.—An embryo of 11·8 mm.   FIG. 282.—An embryo of 14·0 mm.

disappear (Fig. 278). The constitution of the face in the adult derived from these elements is seen in Fig. 283.

The swinging forwards of the axes of the orbits with a consequent swing of the visual axes is essentially due to the forward extension of the maxillary processes. As these increase in size they gradually move upwards and forwards, insinuating themselves on either side between the paraxial mesoderm and the surface ectoderm ; it is essentially this growth which is responsible for a swinging forwards of the axes of the orbits and the transference of the visual

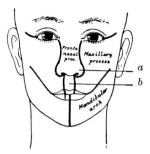

Fig. 283.—The Forerunners of the Face (Gray's *Anatomy*). Lateral nasal (*a*) and globular (*b*) processes.

axes from a lateral to a more frontal position (Figs. 284–5). Up to the 7 mm. stage the optic vesicles and stalks lie in the same coronal straight line ; there they remain in many mammals, but in man at the 7 to 9 mm. stage the angle

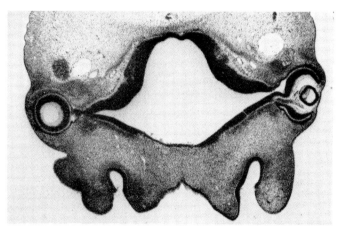

Fig. 284.—Section of the Head of an 11 mm. Embryo. To show the lateral position of the optic cups (F. Hervouët).

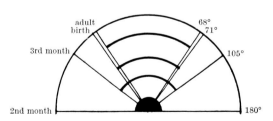

Fig. 285.—The Orbital Axis in Development.

The gradual swing forward in the orbital axis between the second lunar month in the embryo (180°) to an angle of 71° at birth and 68° in the adult (after Armstrong and Scammon).

between the optic axes is 160° ; at the 16 mm. stage it is reduced to 120°. By the 40 mm. stage, following the rapid increase in bulk of the maxillary process, the angle is further reduced to 72° ; and stabilization is eventually reached at 45°. Fink (1956) has pointed out that the development of the maxillary process and the anterior swinging of the eye in primates may be regarded as correlated with the increasing size and complexity of the brain ; the transference is, of course, necessary for the attainment of binocular vision.

THE ORBITAL WALLS

THE BONY WALLS OF THE ORBIT are formed from the mesoderm surrounding the developing eye (Spöndli, 1846 ; von Kölliker, 1861 ; Schultze, 1896 ; Fawcett, 1910). The floor and lateral wall of the orbit are derived from the visceral mesoderm of the maxillary process from which arise the zygomatic bone and maxilla (with the exception of its frontal process). The roof is developed in the paraxial mesoderm forming part of the capsule covering the forebrain ; while the medial wall of the orbit is developed from the lateral nasal process from which are derived the frontal process of the maxilla, the nasal bone, the lacrimal bone and lateral mass of the ethmoid bone. Between that part of the lateral nasal process which gives rise to the frontal process of the maxilla and the maxillary process a patent channel determines the naso-lacrimal canal. Posteriorly a portion of the sphenoid bone is derived from the base of the skull and completes the orbital wall ; while a gap between the primitive pre- and orbito-sphenoid portions of this bone allows the passage of the optic nerve. At the 5th week the sphenoid mesoderm sends out a wing-like process on each side to determine the future great wing of the sphenoid, while more anteriorly, processes extend laterally which eventually determine the lesser wings of the sphenoid.

At $3\frac{1}{2}$ months the bony boundaries of the orbit are apparent, although they are still incomplete, but during the 4th month the walls are well developed. Initially the orbital boundaries appear to be moulded by the growth of the optic cup so that up to the 6th month its margin is approximately circular (Whitnall, 1921) ; it is, however, outpaced by the growth of the globe so that between the 6th and 7th months its margin extends only to the equator of the globe and is closely applied to it instead of arching over it (Fig. 286). Thereafter the shape of the orbital cavity becomes modified by its contents among which the developing globe, the lacrimal apparatus and the oblique muscles seem all to play an important role in the moulding process.

At birth the margin of the orbit is sharp and strongly developed, circular in outline and fitting closely around the globe. The height and breadth are thus approximately equal, a proportion retained until puberty, and although it keeps much the same proportion to the cranium at all ages, it changes considerably relative to the height of the face : the marginal

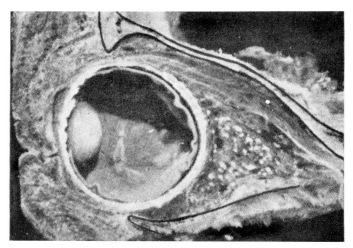

FIG. 286.—THE ORBIT OF A 6 TO 7 MONTH FŒTUS.
Sagittal section showing that the orbital walls (outlined) do not enclose the globe. Note
the thickness of the eyelids (× 4) (S. E. Whitnall).

height at birth is about half the height of the face while in the adult it is
about one-third (Fig. 287). At this time the fossa for the lacrimal gland is
deep and conical, that for the lacrimal sac is cylindrical and faces anteriorly
(instead of laterally), the supra-orbital notch is situated about the
middle of the supra-orbital margin, and the infra-orbital foramen is quite

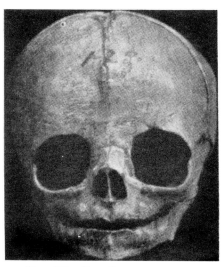

FIG. 287.—THE SKULL AT BIRTH.
Note the roundness of the orbital margin, the broad posterior wall of the fossa for the
lacrimal sac, and the accentuation of the posterior lacrimal crest (× 2/3) (S. E. Whitnall).

close to the infra-orbital margin. The subsequent changes occurring during childhood and adolescence will be discussed at a later stage.[1]

It should be noted that although the bones of the skull are formed from the mesoderm investing the cerebral vesicles, the developing skull passes through two stages, a blastemal followed by a cartilaginous stage, before the osseous stage is reached. The secondary stage of chondrification, however, is incomplete and most of the cranial vault, including the frontal bone and portions of the base of the skull, are ossified in membrane and are not preformed in cartilage. The number and approximate positions of the

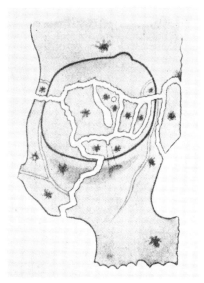

FIG. 288.—THE CENTRES OF OSSIFICATION OF THE BONES OF THE ORBIT.
As they appear between the 6th and 8th weeks of embryonic life (after S. E. Whitnall).

centres of ossification are shown in Fig. 288 ; they appear between the 6th and 7th weeks of embryonic life, and except for the sphenoid, have fused into the component bones during the 6th and 7th months of fœtal life (Whitnall, 1921). At birth the bones are still widely separated and the orbital walls are completed by membrane. In very rare cases one or more of the secondary centres of ossification may remain ununited so that supernumerary ossicles appear.[2]

In the *frontal bone* a primary centre of ossification appears in the central area of the frontal tuberosity about the 6th or 7th week, while three centres of ossification emerge on each side at a somewhat later stage, one for the frontal spine, one above each trochlear pit and one for each zygomatic process. At birth the two bones are separated in the midline by the metopic suture. The *nasal bone* is developed from a

[1] 308.   [2] Part 2, p. 942.

single centre appearing at the end of the 2nd month in the membrane covering the anterior part of the cartilaginous nasal capsule. On the same membranous basis the single centre for the *lacrimal bone* appears at the beginning of the 3rd month. Ossification of the *ethmoid* occurs initially in the cartilage of the nasal capsule, wherein a single centre appears on each side during the 4th or 5th month near the lamina papyracea ; from this centre the conchæ are also ossified about the 9th month. Some time after birth, about the end of the 1st year, a centre appears on either side of the crista galli, ossifying this part of the bone and the perpendicular plate, but the process is not complete until the 5th or 6th year. The *zygoma* ossifies in membrane, the process starting about the 10th week in a centre in the body of the bone and is continued by two secondary centres, one directed to the temporal fossa and the other on the medial extension below the orbital margin.

The ossification of the *maxilla* is complicated. It commences in membrane from a centre in the region of the canine tooth ; somewhat later an orbito-nasal element is formed, the infra-orbital canal and foramen indicating the junction between the two in the adult ; while the premaxillary element (an independent bone supporting the superior incisor teeth) is developed from two centres, a facial and a palatine, the line of fusion with the main bone being readily seen in young skulls and sometimes giving rise to a type of cleft palate.

The *sphenoid bone* is formed by the fusion of two parts (Levi, 1900 ; Fawcett, 1909–10) : the pre-sphenoid and the post-sphenoid, both of which (with the exception of the medial pterygoid lamina which develops in membrane from a single nucleus appearing about the 9th or 10th week) are formed in cartilage. The post-sphenoid ossifies first. About the end of the 2nd month a centre appears in the root of the great wing (alisphenoid) between the foramina ovale and rotundum from which ossification spreads to the wing and the lateral pterygoid lamina. About the same time two centres appear in the basi-sphenoid in relation to the floor of the hypophysial fossa on either side of the cranio-pharyngeal canal which they obliterate. Somewhat later two centres appear in the lateral aspect of the body of the bone. The last four centres fuse completely by the 6th month. A short time previously, in the middle of the 3rd month, a pair of centres appears lateral to the optic foramina from which the small wings (orbito-sphenoids) develop ; and almost simultaneously a pair appears medial to the optic foramina to form the body of the pre-sphenoid. At birth the bone consists of three parts—the body of the pre-sphenoid fused with the basi-sphenoid and the orbito-sphenoids centrally, and the alisphenoids on either side. Fusion occurs towards the end of the 1st year, but the dorsum sellæ remains as a cartilaginous plate separating the sphenoid from the basi-occipital bone which does not become completely ossified until the age of 25.

In general the skull grows secondarily to the brain, adapting itself to the latter in its development by growth during childhood and adolescence at right angles to the main sutures ; growth at the coronal suture determines the length of the front of the head, at the lambdoid suture the length of the back of the head, and at the sagittal suture its breadth. Although growth of the brain may be said to cease after puberty, these sutures do not normally fuse until after the 20th year, a gradual process which takes some time (Todd and Lyon, 1924).

THE ORBITAL CONTENTS

At first the paraxial mesoderm into which the optic vesicle evaginates is entirely undifferentiated forming a loose network of stellate cells apparently (in histological specimens) connected with each other by interlacing processes. This mesodermal mass is continuous with the paraxial mesoderm in which the central nervous system is embedded ; and as we have seen[1] it is invaded from below the optic vesicle by the visceral mesoderm derived from the maxillary process. Between the two masses of mesoderm there is little differentiation excepting slight differences in texture and a faint line where vascularization occurs between them. From the visceral mesoderm are developed the lower and outer walls of the orbit ; from the paraxial mesoderm surrounding the vesicle are developed all the orbital contents, its muscles, fascia and vessels as well as the mesodermal stroma of the globe.

The first sign of differentiation occurs at the 3 to 4 mm. stage when hæmatopoietic formation commences ; spaces containing blood cells surrounded by a single layer of flattened mesodermal (endothelial) cells are then evident, differentiating the mesodermal tissue into vascular and stromal elements. Within the latter tissue a condensation appears which indicates the commencement of the differentiation of the extrinsic ocular muscles.

THE EXTRINSIC OCULAR MUSCLES

The voluntary musculature throughout the body is derived mainly from the paraxial mesoderm as a development of the myomeres in the segmentally arranged somites lying on either side of the notochord. We have already noted[2] that such a segmentation is not seen in the head of the human embryo, but it has been suggested that in the human species the initial stages in the differentiation of the mesoderm of the head are so abbreviated that the development of cephalic mesoblastic somites has escaped observation. It follows that an understanding of the segmentation of the head is an extremely difficult problem ; nevertheless, it is of considerable ophthalmological importance since it affects our ideas of the phylogenetic and ontogenetic value of the ocular muscles. All that can be said at the present time is that metameric organization of the head has never been demonstrated in mammals.

Since conclusive evidence is lacking in man, and, indeed, in mammals, the metameric significance of the cephalic region in these higher forms must be analysed in the light of indirect evidence derived from the study of more simply constituted species in which the arrangement is more primitive ; but even among fishes and amphibians the morphology is so obscure that the theories put forward have been numerous and conflicting.[3] It has been commonly suggested that the vertebrate head is evolved from nine segments, four at least being occipital, but there is no general agreement on the final fate of these segments. Analysing the voluminous literature that has now accumulated on this subject, Wedin (1955) concluded that the morphogenesis of the head structures—the neuromeres, neural crest, head cavities, extrinsic eye muscles and pharyngeal gut—lends no support to the theory that the vertebrate head has any

---

[1] p. 42. [2] p. 47.
[3] Marshall (1881), von Wijhe (1883), Edgeworth (1902–11), Froriep (1906), von Schumacher (1907), Gaskell (1908), Neal (1914–18), Kingsbury (1926), and others.

metameric organization. At the present time this would seem to be the only safe conclusion.

The head-cavities, however, are in a different category, for from their walls the extrinsic ocular muscles are developed. The classical view is that in elasmobranchs there are four head-cavities lying on either side of the notochord evidently in series with the metameric somites behind them ; these have been assumed to represent a confluence of the myomeres taken into the head during evolution (Fig. 289). They are usually referred to as *A*, 1, 2 and 3 ; the reason for the somewhat curious notation is that *A* was discovered after the other three were known and designated. In any case the most anterior (*A*) is small and lies cephalad to the optic vesicle, but is transient and atrophies and disappears. The second (1), the *premandibular cavity* lies immediately behind the first on a level with the extreme anterior tip of the notochord ; the third (2) or *mandibular cavity* is much the largest and lies more dorsally and caudally ; while the fourth (3) or *hyoid cavity* lies still more caudally between the 1st and 2nd visceral clefts.

Shortly after the discovery of these cavities by Balfour (1878), Marshall (1881)

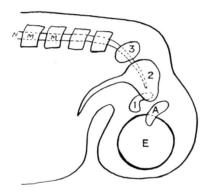

Fig. 289.—The Head Cavities of the Dogfish.
E, eye ; N, notochord ; M, somites ; A,1, 2, 3, the head cavities (after Platt).

concluded that the extrinsic ocular muscles supplied by the third nerve (superior, medial and inferior recti, inferior oblique) arose from the walls of the pre-mandibular cavity and suggested that the lateral rectus, innervated by the sixth nerve, arose from the walls of the mandibular and hyoid cavities. van Wijhe (1883), on the other hand, believed that the superior oblique and lateral rectus muscles arose respectively from the mandibular and hyoid cavities, a view endorsed by Platt (1891), Neal (1898–1918), Lamb (1902), and Dohrn (1904). The levator palpebræ is derived from the superior rectus, and the retractor bulbi from the lateral rectus : in this scheme they were therefore assumed to belong to the same segments as their parent muscles. Evidence for this arrangement can be obtained in higher forms (Ryder, 1897 ; in the tortoise, Johnson, 1913 ; in marsupials, Fraser, 1915 ; in the rabbit, Edgeworth, 1902) ; but it has been claimed that the lateral rectus may be in part derived from the mandibular somite, an arrangement which occurs in elasmobranch fishes (Neal, 1918). Edgeworth (1935), on the other hand, concluded that the primary source of all the ocular muscles is the pre-mandibular somite, and that in ganoids and plagiostomes the origins of the superior oblique and lateral rectus have been shifted back. From this it would follow that the IVth and VIth nerves are not segmental but are separated portions of the IIIrd, and that the extrinsic ocular muscles form a single morphological unit.

A considerable amount of work has been done on higher species and several writers have observed the presence of three head-cavities (pre-mandibular, mandibular and hyoid) in various species of amphibians (Marcus, 1910) and reptiles (Oppel, 1890 ; Filatoff, 1907 ; Johnson, 1913) ; two (pre-mandibular and mandibular) in birds (Rex, 1905 ; Adelmann, 1926 ; Wedin, 1953); but the only cavity consistently found in reptiles, birds and marsupials has been the pre-mandibular (Edgeworth, 1907 ; Fraser, 1915 ; Parker, 1917 ; Adelmann, 1926 ; Gilbert, 1954). In placental mammals they have proved much more elusive and most investigators have failed to identify them (Corning, 1899 ; Bonnet, 1901 ; Edgeworth, 1923–35 ; Leser, 1925 ; Gilbert, 1947–50 ; and others). Indeed, the only reports of their presence in this class have been in man. In him several such cavities lined by epithelium were observed by Zimmermann (1899) and by Gilbert (1950–57) in the pre-mandibular condensation of mesoderm on each side of the head (Fig. 290). These cavities which are transitory,

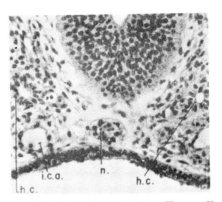

FIG. 290.—THE HEAD CAVITIES IN A HUMAN EMBRYO.

A transection through the head of a human embryo of 28 somites. One head cavity, h.c., appears on either side, slightly dorsal and lateral to the internal carotid artery, i.c.a. n, notochord ($\times$ 300) (Perry W. Gilbert).

appearing and vanishing within a few hours when the embryo is 26 to 28 days old, are situated lateral and dorsal to the internal carotid arteries and were interpreted by Gilbert as being homologous with the pre-mandibular cavity of elasmobranchs, reptiles, birds and marsupials. They never coalesce to form the large cavities seen in the lower vertebrates and are probably non-segmental in type but are merely mechanically determined owing to the rapid expansion of the mesoderm in this region at this time, possibly because there is a space to be filled (Wedin, 1955; Gilbert, 1957). Gilbert concluded that the pre-mandibular condensations in which the head cavities of the human embryo briefly appeared ultimately gave rise to the extrinsic ocular muscles innervated by the third nerve.

Whatever their phylogenetic relationships, it seems clear that the extrinsic ocular muscles are derived from mesodermal condensations situated on each side of the head. For long the teaching of Lewis (1910) has been accepted that all the muscles were ultimately derived from a single common pre-muscle mass appearing at about the 7 mm. stage and, as it extended anteriorly around the globe, splitting into the rudiments supplied by the three ocular motor nerves about the 11 mm. stage, so that by the 14 mm. stage all the individual muscles could be distinguished. The unprecedentedly rich material of early embryos available in the Carnegie Institution of Washington, however, has led Gilbert (1952–57) to abandon the concept that the whole of this musculature in placental mammals (including man) is derived from a single primordium on each side of the head and to suggest that they arise from three independent but closely related (bilateral) condensations. In this view the origin and development of the extra-ocular muscles of man follow a pattern conforming in its essential features with that found in elasmobranchs, reptiles, birds, marsupials and the cat.

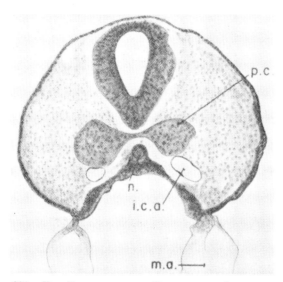

FIG. 291.—THE PREMANDIBULAR MESODERMAL CONDENSATION.

An oblique transection through the head of a 19-somite human embryo. The conspicuous premandibular condensations (p.c.) which first appear in embryos of 14 somites are connected across the midline by a bridge of prechordal mesoderm ; the condensations are accentuated by heavy shading. i.c.a., internal carotid artery ; m.a., mandibular arch ; n, notochord (Perry W. Gilbert).

It would appear that the earliest sign of the differentiation of the extrinsic ocular muscles is a pair of *premandibular condensations* of mesodermal cells derived from the prechordal plate lying on either side between the primitive carotid artery and the cephalic vein, medial to the semilunar ganglion at the level of the cephalic end of the notochord. In man they appear about the 24th day as two ovoid condensations of mesoderm, one on either side united by a bridge across the midline cephalad to the termination of the notochord (Fig. 291) ; Iwasaki (1954) recognized the primordium about the same time in Japanese embryos. About the 29th day (6 to 7 mm. stage) the bridge becomes tenuous and ruptures and eventually disappears (8–9 mm.). In this condensation three processes grow antero-laterally towards the optic vesicle, the primordia of four ocular motor muscles. The primordium of the superior rectus appears first (6–7 mm.), that of the medial rectus and the common primordium of the inferior rectus and inferior oblique at a later stage (9–10 mm.) (Figs. 292 and 293).

Lateral to each premandibular condensation two separate condensations subsequently form in the maxillo-mandibular mesoderm which arches upwards and forwards from the dorsal aspect of the mandibular arch over the eye. The first of these *maxillo-mandibular condensations* to appear, the primordium of the lateral rectus, is situated medially and caudally. It forms about the 4–5 mm. stage and reaches the periphery of the optic vesicle about the 9–11 mm. stage. It would seem probable, however, that this muscle has a dual origin since its distal end is formed from the intermediate mass of maxillo-mandibular mesoderm.[1] The second maxillo-mandibular condensation appears in an extension of this mesoderm above the optic vesicle at the

FIGS. 292 and 293.—THE EXTRINSIC OCULAR MUSCLES
(P. Gilbert, Carnegie Institution of Washington).

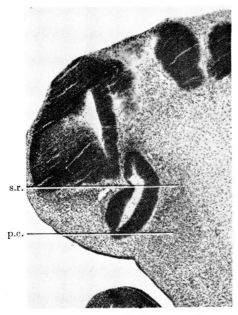

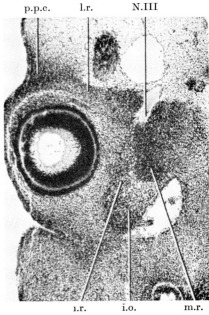

FIG. 292.—Parasagittal section through the head of an embryo of 4·9 mm. From the premandibular condensation, p.c., an arm of mesoderm, the primordium of the superior rectus, s.r., has extended cranio-laterally over the dorso-medial surface of the optic vesicle.

FIG. 293.—Frontal section through the head of an embryo of 13 mm., showing the early condensations of the lateral rectus, l.r., medial rectus, m.r., inferior rectus, i.r., continuous distally with that of the inferior oblique, i.o. N.III, third nerve ; p.p.c., posterior peripheral condensation.

6–7 mm. stage ; this is the primordium of the superior oblique muscle. Growing towards the periphery of the optic vesicle, the primordium swings sharply ventrally, laterally and caudally to reach the globe at the 13–14 mm. stage.

The nerves grow from the brain into their respective condensations some time after the latter have been formed—the oculomotor (7–8 mm. stage), the abducens (8–9 mm.) and the trochlear (10–12 mm.).

[1] It would seem that this portion is the homologue of the *muscle E* of elasmobranch fishes described by Platt (1891) and said to degenerate by Lamb (1902), Johnson (1913) and Fraser (1915), but considered to contribute to the lateral rectus in this species by Dohrn (1904), and Neal (1918) as well as in the chick (Adelmann, 1927), the cat (Gilbert, 1947), and man (Gilbert, 1957).

By the 6th week (13·5 mm.) the muscles are very obvious as bilateral masses lying close to the optic stalk (Figs. 292–3), and the four recti have met peripheral condensations forming in the maxillo-mandibular mesoderm beneath the surface ectoderm at the margin of the optic cup. These blend with the scleral condensation being formed at the same time so that shortly thereafter (19–20 mm.) the scleral condensation has consolidated near the region of the future insertions of the muscles and has extended to the limbus, the process extending posteriorly therefrom, in the opposite direction to the development of the muscles. At this stage, therefore, the ocular muscles form a divided cone of condensed mesodermal tissue blending anteriorly with the developing rudiment of the sclera, but at the apex of the cone the mesoderm as yet shows no sharp line of demarcation from the loosely arranged orbital stroma, nor is there any evidence of fascia or the presence of muscular sheaths (Figs. 294–7).

By the end of the 2nd month (37–40 mm. stage) when the eye is about 1·0 mm. in diameter, the elongated cells of the developing muscles have formed myofibrils (Leplat, 1958) and striations have begun to appear, but the muscle bellies, although still poorly demarcated except at their insertions, can be defined only with a certain amount of difficulty since they blend with the surrounding mesodermal tissue, a tendency particularly evident at the apex of the cone (Fink, 1956). Even at this early stage, however, the general arrangement of the muscles and their relationship with the globe closely resemble those seen in the adult. From the earliest stage the medial rectus is stronger and more fully developed than the lateral, a relationship which Poyales (1917) and Casanovas Carnicer (1951) associated with the frequent development of internal strabismus. The insertions of the obliques blend with those of the adjacent recti and their angulation with the globe varies between 40° and 45° (Fink, 1956). The trochlea appears at the orbital margin before ossification occurs in the frontal bone (20–21 mm.) and is conspicuously but not completely developed 7 days later (30 mm.) (Gilbert, 1957) (Figs. 296–9).

The last of the muscles to be differentiated is the levator palpebræ superioris. It makes its appearance between the 22 and 30 mm. stages when some of the fibres on the medial aspect of the superior rectus separate off (Reuter, 1897; Henckel, 1898; Gilbert, 1957) (Fig. 295). At the 60 mm. stage this muscle is fully developed and lies on the inner side of the superior rectus; it then grows laterally on a slightly higher plane overlapping the inner edge of the rectus (75 mm.) and finally (4th month) lies above it. The secondary origin and late appearance of the levator explain the fact that it is so often congenitally defective, an anomaly which may be associated with a similar failure in the development of the superior rectus.

The subsequent development of the muscles merely shows minor changes (Fink, 1953–56). During the 3rd month when the diameter of the globe is 3 mm. the muscle cone is about 5 mm. long (Fig. 298). The muscles them-

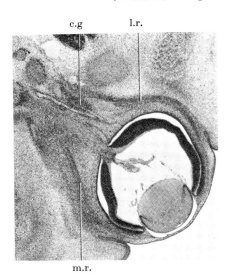

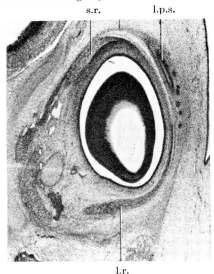

Fig. 294.—Transverse section through the head of an embryo of 25·3 mm. The peripheral condensations into which the four rectus muscles insert have spread over the optic vesicle to form part of the sclera. The section shows the lateral, l.r., and medial recti, m.r., and the ciliary ganglion, c.g.

Fig. 295.—Transverse section through the head of an embryo of 32 mm. The levator palpebræ, l.p.s., has split off from the superior rectus, s.r., and extended downwards into the upper lid. l.r. lateral rectus muscle. Fibres are present in all the muscles at this stage.

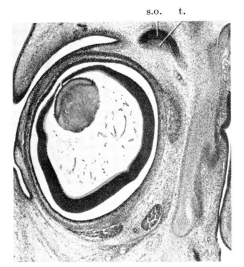

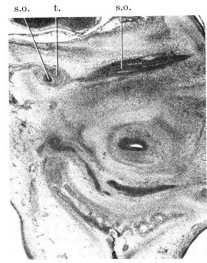

Fig. 296.—Transverse section through the head of an embryo of 32 mm. The section cuts the tendon of the superior oblique muscle, s.o., longitudinally at the trochlea, t. The eye is now clothed with a well-defined sclera into which all the six extrinsic muscles find insertion.

Fig. 297.—Section through the head of an embryo of 32 mm., showing the superior oblique muscle, s.o., with its tendon in the trochlea, t.

FIGS. 298 and 299.—THE ORBIT OF THE 3-MONTH FŒTUS (F. Vrabec).

III

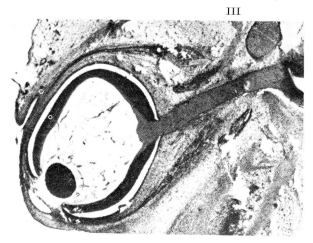

FIG. 298.—Horizontal section showing the optic nerve running centrally and entering the brain above the recessus opticus. The medial and lateral recti are well developed and at the lateral side of the optic nerve the ciliary ganglion and the third nerve (III) are well seen.

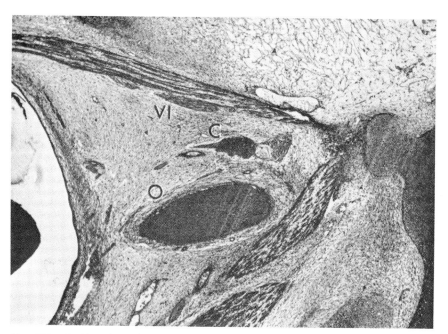

FIG. 299.—Section through the apex of the orbit, showing the lateral rectus with the sixth nerve (VI) ; C, ciliary ganglion ; O, optic nerve.

15—2

FIGS. 300 and 301.—THE INTERMEDIATE DEVELOPMENT OF THE
EXTRA-OCULAR MUSCLES IN THE ORBIT (W. Fink).

N, optic nerve ; M, muscle ; R, orbital reticulum.

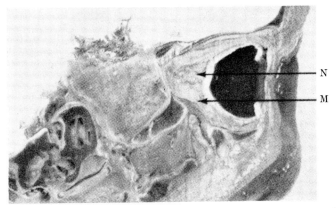

FIG. 300.—In a 4-month fœtus. The mesoderm shows evidences of early condensation in the vicinity of the muscles, especially near their insertions where they are more fully differentiated than in the posterior third of the orbit. Some indication of Tenon's capsule is seen near the insertions of the muscles.

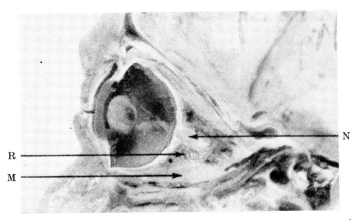

FIG. 301.—In a 5⅓-month fœtus. The mesodermal condensation is more definite even at the origin of the muscles. The condensation surrounding the globe begins to be evident in its anterior half near the insertion of the muscles. Supporting reticulum and some fat are present in the orbit.

selves are thicker in comparison with their length than in the later stages of growth, the insertions of the recti are well defined but their origins are less definitely demarcated (Fig. 300). The insertions of the obliques are now separated from those of the recti, being situated nearer to the equator, and the reflected portion of the superior oblique is round and tendinous making an acute angle of 30° with its parent belly. By the 4th month when the length of the muscle-cone is 10 mm., the muscles become narrower, their

Figs. 302 and 303.—The Late Development of the Extra-ocular
Muscles in the Orbit (W. Fink).

N, optic nerve ; M, muscle ; R, orbital reticulum.

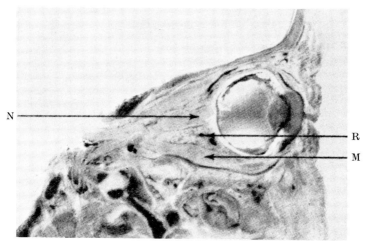

Fig. 302.—In a 7⅓-month fœtus. The muscles, their sheaths and expansions
are fully formed as well as Tenon's capsule, while the fascial covering begins to be
evident surrounding the optic nerve.

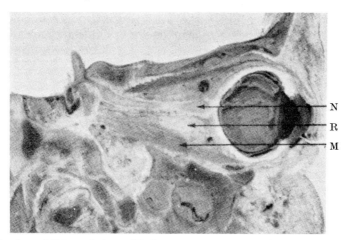

Fig. 303.—In a full-term fœtus. All the structures, although more delicate than
in the mature stage, are evident.

origins at the apex of the orbit become clearly defined, and the borders of
their bellies are clearly demarcated and readily separable from the surrounding tissue (Figs. 299 and 300). By the 8th month their insertions take on a
tendinous appearance, and the same tendencies of lengthening and narrowing
are evident until at term, when the length of the muscle-cone is 25 mm., the
individual muscles show the characteristics of the mature state except that

they are still somewhat shorter, thicker and broader and the insertions of the recti more anterior than in the fully mature condition (Figs. 301–3). The (sensory) spiral nerve-endings appear just before birth (Okamoto, 1960).

During their development the orientation of the muscles around the globe alters little apart from the considerable change in the angle formed at the trochlea between the proximal and distal portions of the superior oblique muscle as the orbit increases in size, a change probably due to the advancement of that portion of the frontal bone to which the trochlea is attached. Thus in embryos of 17 mm., this angle is obtuse but it subsequently becomes increasingly less so until in the embryo of 3 months the trochlear angle appears to be acute (approximately 30°) increasing again to 50° at 9 months.

THE ORBITAL FASCIA AND MUSCLE SHEATHS

Initially the extrinsic ocular muscles are separable with difficulty from the surrounding mesoderm from which they are differentiated by condensation, and it is not until the 3rd month of gestation that a mesodermal condensation can be detected separating this from the surrounding tissue (Fink, 1956). This process commences near their insertions and proceeds slowly so that by the 6th month a definite but poorly defined sheath is evident surrounding the anterior half of the muscle bellies ; during the 8th month the sheaths and their expansions are readily identified, a process of differentiation which proceeds during the 9th month until birth.

TENON'S CAPSULE appears to be developed in association with the extrinsic muscles as a prolongation of this system rather than as an independent condensation of the peri-ocular mesoderm (Winckler, 1937–38 ; Casari, 1953). The first signs of its formation were noted by Casari at the 45 mm. stage as a thin irregular line of mesodermal condensation outside the scleral condensation in the region of the insertions of the rectus muscles and the equator ; during the 3rd month it is quite obvious (Fink, 1956). Its differentiation proceeds posteriorly until by the 5th month the posterior portion has a definite consistency and can be seen to become continuous with the mesodermal coverings of the optic nerve (Goldstein, 1923) (Figs. 300–2).

The supporting RETICULUM OF THE ORBIT is meantime becoming differentiated. Fink (1956) noted early evidences of its presence during the 4th month ; during the 6th month it is relatively well developed and some deposits of fatty tissue are seen within its meshes, a process of differentiation which proceeds progressively until term, when the orbital fascia is fully developed and differentiated from the muscle sheaths, although more delicate in its structure than in the mature state.

Adelmann. *J. Morph.*, **42**, 371 (1926) ; **44**, 29 (1927).
Balfour. *A Monograph on the Development of Elasmobranch Fishes*, London (1878).
Bodemer. *J. Morph.*, **102**, 119 (1958).
Bonnet. *Anat. Hefte*, **16**, 231 (1901).
Casanovas Carnicer. *Arch. esp. Morf. Valencia*, **8**, 75 (1951).
Casari. *Arch. Anat.* (Strasbourg), **35**, 203 (1953).

Corning. *Morph. Jb.*, **27**, 173 ; **28**, 28 (1899) ; **29**, 94 (1900).
Dohrn. *Mitt. Zool. Stat. Neapol.*, **17**, 1 (1904).
Edgeworth. *J. Anat. Physiol.*, **37**, 73 (1902) ; **57**, 313 (1923).
  Quart. J. micr. Sci., **51**, 511 (1907) ; **56**, 167 (1911).
  Phil. Trans. B, **217**, 39 (1928).
  The Cranial Muscles of Vertebrates, Camb. (1935).
Fawcett. *J. Anat. Physiol.*, **44**, 207, 378 (1909–10).
Filatoff. *Morph. Jb.*, **37**, 289 (1907).
Fink. *Amer. J. Ophthal.*, **36** (2), 10 (1953) ; **42** (2), 269 (1956).
Fraser. *Proc. Zool. Soc. Lond.*, **2**, 299 (1915).
Froriep. *Hb. d. Vergl. u. exper. Entwicklungslehre d. Wirbeltiere*, Jena, **2** (1906).
Gaskell. *The Origin of Vertebrates*, London (1908).
Gilbert. *J. Morph.*, **81**, 151 (1947) ; **90**, 149 (1952) ; **95**, 47 (1954).
  Anat. Rec., **108**, 517 (1950).
  Contrib. Embryol. Carneg. Instn., **36**, 59 (1957).
Goldstein. *Arch. Ophthal.* (Chicago), **52**, 327 (1923).
Henckel. *Anat. Hefte*, **10**, 487 (1898).
Iwasaki. *Acta Soc. ophthal. jap.*, **58**, 878 (1954).
Johnson. *Amer. J. Anat.*, **14**, 119 (1913).
Kingsbury. *J. Morph.*, **42**, 83 (1926).
von Kölliker. *Entwicklungsgeschichte d. Menschen*, Leipzig (1861).
Lamb. *Amer. J. Anat.*, **1**, 185 (1902).
Leplat. Dejean, Hervouët and Leplat's *L'embryologie de l'œil et sa tératologie*, Paris, 461 (1958).
Leser. *Brit. J. Ophthal.*, **9**, 154 (1925).
Levi. *Arch. mikr. Anat.*, **55**, 341 (1900).

Lewis. Keibel and Mall's *Manual of Human Embryology*, Phila., **1**, 505 (1910).
Marcus. *Beitr. z. Kenntnis d. Gymnophionen. IV. Zur Entwicklungsges. d. Kopfes. Festschr. R. Hertwig*, **2**, 373 (1910).
Marshall. *Quart. J. micr. Sci.*, **21**, 72 (1881).
Neal. *Bull. Mus. comp. Zool.*, Harvard, **31**, 147 (1898).
  J. Morph., **25**, 1 (1914) ; **30**, 433 (1918).
Okamoto. *Jap. J. Ophthal.*, **4**, 12 (1960).
Oppel. *Arch. mikr. Anat.*, **36**, 603 (1890).
Parker. *J. Anat.*, **51**, 181 (1917).
Platt. *J. Morph.*, **5**, 79 (1891).
  Anat. Anz., **6**, 251 (1891).
Poyales. *Anat. Rec.*, **13**, 375 (1917).
Reuter. *Anat. Hefte*, **9**, 365 (1897).
Rex. *Morph. Jb.*, **33**, 107 (1905).
Ryder. Norris and Oliver's *System of Diseases of the Eye*, London, **1**, 64 (1897).
Schultze. *Grundriss d. Entwicklungsges d. Menschen*, Leipzig (1896).
von Schumacher. *Anat. Anz.*, **31**, 142 (1907).
Spöndli. *Ueber d. Primordialschädel d. Säugethiere u. d. Menschen*, Zürich (1846).
Todd and Lyon. *Amer. J. phys. Anthrop.*, **7**, 325 (1924).
Wedin. *J. Morph.*, **92**, 303 (1953).
  Acta anat. (Basel), **18**, 30 (1953).
  Embryonic Segmentations in the Head, Malmö (1955).
Whitnall. *The Anatomy of the Human Orbit*, Oxon. (1921).
van Wijhe. *Ueber d. Mesodermsegmente u. d. Entwickelung d. Nerven d. Selachier Kopfes*, Amsterdam (1883).
  Zool. Anz., **9**, 657 (1886).
Winckler. *Arch. Anat.* (Strasbourg), **24**, 295 (1937).
  Ann. Oculist (Paris), **175**, 368 (1938).
Zimmermann. *Arch. mikr. Anat.*, **53**, 481 (1899).

THE LIDS, CONJUNCTIVA AND LACRIMAL APPARATUS

THE LID-FOLDS

During the first month of development the optic vesicle is covered merely by a thin layer of surface ectoderm following the unbroken contour of the surface of the embryo. Thereafter, however, during the 2nd month (von Ammon, 1858 ; von Kölliker, 1861), about the 16 mm. stage (Mann, 1928), active cellular proliferation of the adjacent mesoderm results in the formation of a circular fold of mesoderm (covered on both sides by ectoderm) which encircles the gradually protruding eye (Figs. 304 and 310). This fold constitutes the rudiments of the eyelids which elongate over the eye, fuse for a period of some $2\frac{1}{2}$ months during its development, and eventually separate.

The mesodermal portion of the upper lid is developed from the fronto-nasal process in two parts (medial and lateral) and occasionally a notch or coloboma may mark their imperfect union in the adult ; the lower lid is a similar upgrowth of the maxillary process. The covering layer of ectoderm becomes skin on the outside and conjunctiva on the inside, the inner layer being directly continuous with the corneal epithelium, while the tarsal plate and the connective and muscular tissues of the lid are derived from the mesodermal core of the folds. Initially circular, short and rounded, the upper

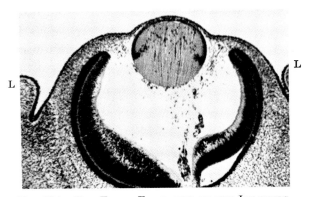

FIG. 304.—THE EARLY FORMATION OF THE LID-FOLDS.

In an embryo of 18 mm. The mesodermal condensation is seen on either side of the optic cup to form the emerging circular lid-fold, L (A. N. Barber).

and lower portions of the folds elongate, and gradually approximate so as to cover the eye, the marginal epithelium eventually fusing in the horizontal line over the centre of the cornea during the 9th week of gestation. The process of fusion of the lids by an epithelial seal begins at the two extremities at the 31 mm. stage (Ask, 1908) and is complete at the 35 mm. stage (Contino, 1907) (Figs. 305–6). The lids remain adherent for a variable period—until

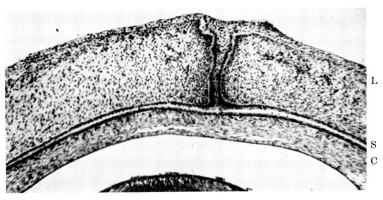

FIG. 305.—FUSION OF THE LIDS.

In a foetus of 9 weeks (35 mm.). Note the narrow conjunctival sac (S) between the lids (L) and the cornea (C) (A. N. Barber).

FIGS. 306 and 307.—DEVELOPMENT OF THE LIDS (A. N. Barber).

OM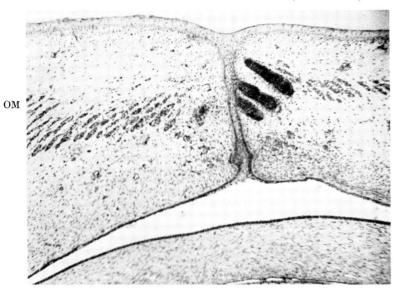

FIG. 306.—In a fœtus of 4 months (80 mm.). The meibomian glands are seen developing from epithelial ingrowths near the fused margins as well as the orbicularis muscle (OM).

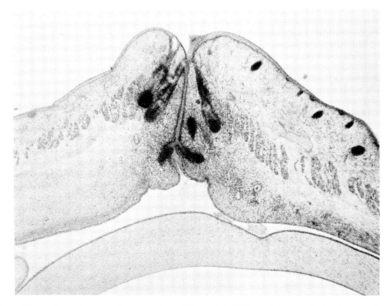

FIG. 307.—In a fœtus of 6 months. The epithelial seal is partly broken and the lids are beginning to open, while the glandular structures are well formed.

the end of the 5th month (Mann, 1928), the 6th month (Barber, 1955), or even the 7th month (Leplat, 1958)—whereafter separation begins on the nasal side, a process which is usually completed during the 6th or 7th month but may be delayed until the 9th month (330–390 mm., Leplat, 1958) (Fig. 307). Very rarely the process is incomplete at birth, a condition normally found in rabbits, mice and kittens.

The mechanism determining the separation of the lids has been the subject of some discussion and it is possible that several factors contribute to the process. The first to speculate on the problem was Contino (1907) who suggested that three factors were operative : the action of the secretion of the tarsal glands, the progressive keratinization of the epithelium forming the epithelial seal, and (to a less extent) the mechanical action of the levator palpebræ muscle. These conclusions were accepted by Ask (1908) and to these factors Addison and How (1921) added the effect of the proliferation of the stratum germinativum of the underlying skin. Subsequently some authors have stressed the effect of glandular secretion (Alferow, 1931) but most have attributed the major role to progressive keratinization and histolysis of the epithelial cells, a process which has been studied in animals (particularly rats) in which the separation of the lids is easily observed some days after birth (Guieysse-Pellissier, 1937 ; Burrows, 1944 ; Dordi, 1947 ; Viard, 1955 ; and others). Keratinization starts towards the nasal side of the lid, at first on the cutaneous aspect, then on the conjunctival, carving out triangular defects in the epithelial plug, the apices of which eventually meet. Tusques (1951–52) found that the process could be accelerated (in rats) by the administration of thyroxine, and Eayrs (1951) that it was retarded by the sex hormones, methyl thiouracil and (on the homolateral side) by cervical sympathectomy.

THE PLICA SEMILUNARIS

While the lids are fusing at the end of the 2nd or the beginning of the 3rd month, at about the 33 mm. stage, the plica semilunaris develops at the inner aspect of the globe as a crescentic epithelial fold containing mesodermal elements. At the 11th to 12th week blood vessels penetrate to it and it is well formed at the beginning of the 4th month (Contino, 1907 ; Yamazaki and Osumi, 1954 ; Leplat, 1958) (Fig. 308).

THE CARUNCLE

The caruncle is developed independently at the end of the 3rd month after the lids have fused (Figs. 308–9). Classically it has been described as being formed by the cutting-off of the inner part of the margin of the lower lid by the development of the inferior canaliculus and has been therefore said to be absent in animals with no lacrimal passages (Ask, 1907–8 ; Broman and Ask, 1910). Papamiltiades (1947), however, found that it is developed at the end of the 3rd month by cellular proliferation of the epithelium of the posterior surface of the medial part of the lower lid near its upper free border ; such an independent origin resembles that of the plica semilunaris (Leplat, 1958). That this independent origin is the more correct view is seen in the fact that the caruncle develops normally in cases of congenital

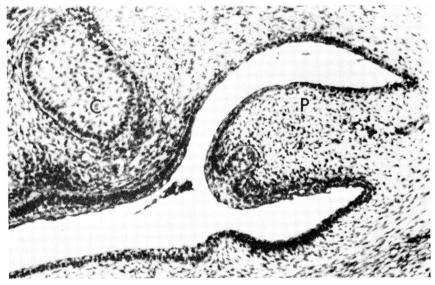

FIG. 308.—THE PLICA SEMILUNARIS.

At the 3rd month. P, plica ; C, lacrimal canaliculus (× 160) (F. Vrabec).

absence of the canaliculi[1] ; moreover, in cases of reduplication of either the canaliculi or the caruncle, the other structure is normal. The fine lanuginous lashes and sebaceous glands with which it is characterized develop as down-growths of the surface epithelium during the 4th month, but the adenoid tissue and crypts do not appear until about the time of birth or immediately thereafter.

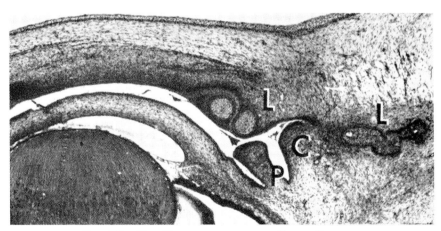

FIG. 309.—THE DEVELOPMENT OF THE INNER CANTHUS.

In a fœtus at the end of the 3rd month, while the lids are still fused and the anterior chamber is shallow. L, lacrimal canaliculi ; C, caruncle ; P, plica (F. Vrabec).

[1] See Part 2, p. 929.

THE MESODERMAL STRUCTURES

The mesodermal structures which comprise the tissues of the lids are derived in the case of the upper lid from the paraxial mesoderm of the fronto-nasal process, of the lower lid from the visceral mesoderm of the maxillary process. The differentiation of the tissues commences shortly after the fusion of the lids and is essentially completed before they separate.

The ORBICULARIS MUSCLE is part of the facial musculature (platysma) developed from the mesoderm of the second visceral arch. Muscle cells begin to migrate from this arch at the 10 to 12 mm. stage, and by the 16 mm. stage they have spread over the mandibular arch to reach the face and have begun to surround the eye. By the 40 mm. stage, soon after the lids have fused, the first rudiments of the palpebral portion of the muscle are detectable in the mesoderm midway between the dermal and palpebral surfaces ; the muscle itself is well formed by the 11th week (55 mm.), before the appearance of the cilia and the palpebral glands (Fig. 306). It is interesting that the growth of the ciliary follicles cuts off the fibres of the marginal muscle of Riolan and the posterior edge of this bundle of fibres is limited by the growth of the tarsal glands ; at the 62 mm. stage it is isolated from the main mass of the orbicularis muscle. Towards the end of the 3rd month the anlage of the tarsus is recognizable as a condensation of connective tissue (Goto, 1951) and is well formed in the upper lids by the 7th month (Fig. 307). Elastic fibres are first visible in the substance of the lid about the 5th month and are almost fully developed by the 8th month except in the pretarsal area where they do not appear until the 9th month (Lehtinen, 1951).

THE SURFACE EPITHELIUM

The surface epithelium is initially present in the embryo as a single layer but at a very early stage (5 to 7 mm.) a few scattered flattened cells appear on its superficial surface ; these are particularly prominent in the neighbourhood of the lens pit. These cells are the forerunners of the EPITRICHIAL LAYER, and at the end of the 2nd month of gestation the epidermal layer becomes duplicated by the formation of a complete layer of irregular epitrichial cells lying superficially to the basal layer of cubical cells (Fig. 310). During the 3rd month three layers appear, the constituents of which are formed by proliferation of the basal cells : (a) an outer layer of two strata of epitrichium, (b) a middle layer of two or three strata of irregular cells which forms the future stratum mucosum, and (c) a single layer of cubical cells lying deeply, the forerunners of the future stratum germinativum. During the 5th month the superficial layers begin to show keratinization in the lids and during the 6th month the epitrichial layer disappears over the hairy parts of the body, being retained only in special localities where it proliferates to form the thick stratum corneum of the palms, the soles and the nails.

The rudiments of the hairs appear about the end of the 3rd month, the hair bulbs emerging as outgrowths of the stratum corneum and growing obliquely into the subjacent corium ; the papillæ are derived from the latter while the hairs are formed from the overlying epidermis. Initially the hairs lie under the epitrichium and when this layer disappears about the end of the 5th month the hairs become free to form the first crop of LANUGO covering the entire surface of the fœtus to become fully developed during the 7th month. This initial growth is shed shortly before or shortly after birth.

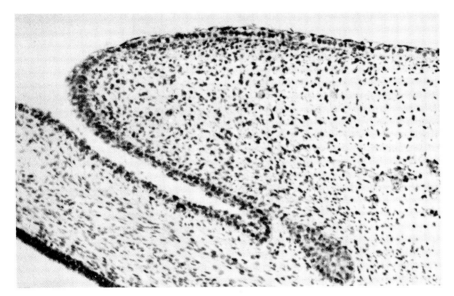

FIG. 310.—THE LID-BUDS AND CONJUNCTIVAL SAC.

In an embryo of 2 months, showing the cubical cells of the epithelium covered by the irregular epitrichial layer. Above is the lid-fold and at the apex of the conjunctival sac is seen the solid outgrowth of the lacrimal gland (F. Vrabec).

THE LANUGO HAIR becomes visible first in the region of the eyebrows where the primordia of the hairs appear precociously at the end of the 3rd and the beginning of the 4th month of gestation, to be replaced by stiffer bristles just before birth. Initially the lanugo covers the entire forehead and the direction of the fine hairs of which it is composed is determined by the rate of growth of the stratified elements of the epidermis. Their direction is hereditarily determined as a dominant characteristic (Abel, 1935 ; Routil, 1939 ; Löffler, 1940) and the configuration of the hairs of the eyebrows remains the same from their fœtal origin to the end of life. Two main types of arrangement are seen (Kiil, 1948–52 ; Breitinger, 1955) (Figs. 311 and 312):

(a) a *frontal (glabellar) hair-stream*, making a curve from the inner canthi upwards and outwards symmetrically over the supra-orbital region ;

(b) a *parietal (bregmatic) hair-stream* directed from the upper parietal angle in the region of the obelion running forwards and downwards over the forehead to the supra-orbital region where it diverges downwards and outwards on either side. This latter arrangement is a specially acquired human characteristic seen in man and not in the anthropoids.

The direction of the hair-stream determines the shape and morphology of the eyebrows and where the streams meet, frontal whorls commonly occur which may give rise to prominent whorls in the eyebrows. Their arrangement is hereditarily determined, controlled by complex factors not yet understood (Devi, 1959) ; it is interesting that monozygous twins always show a concordant arrangement.

On the CONJUNCTIVAL ASPECT of the palpebral folds the mucous membrane develops similarly. The goblet cells (in the rabbit) increase in number after the opening of the palpebral fissure (Ueda, 1959), while the folds of the fornices (in man) are not obvious until the last month of gestation.

FIGS. 311 and 312.—TYPICAL HAIR-STREAMS IN THE FŒTUS (after Breitinger).

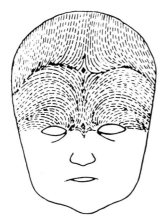 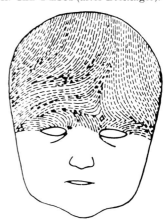

FIG. 311.—Frontal hair-stream.   FIG. 312.—Parietal hair-stream.

THE APPENDAGES AND GLANDS OF THE LIDS

These are all derived as ingrowths from the surface epithelium and, in their case also, the essential period of development is during the time when the lids are fused.

The FOLLICLES OF THE CILIA are derived from solid cylindrical bud-like ingrowths from the basal epithelial cells at the outer edge of the fused lid-margins, growing downwards and obliquely into the underlying mesoderm. Those of the upper lid appear just after fusion of the lids has occurred at the 37 mm. stage ; those of the lower lid about the 40 mm. stage ; while at a somewhat later period (90 mm.) hair-shafts are visible in the follicles (Figs. 307, 313–16). The lashes seem to be shed twice during intra-uterine life, at the beginning and end of the 7th month (Contino, 1907).

From the walls of the follicles the ducts of the GLANDS OF MOLL AND ZEIS are formed as epithelial ingrowths during the 4th month, those of Moll preceding those of Zeis, and again, as occurs in the case of the lashes, those of the upper lid preceding those of the lower. In each case the acini appear a little later (Fig. 307).

The MEIBOMIAN (TARSAL) GLANDS develop similarly at a somewhat later stage (70–80 mm.) by epithelial budding from the basal epithelial cells of the inner edge of the fused lid-margins and around them the mesoderm of the lids becomes condensed (Contino, 1907 ; Klee, 1920) (Figs. 306–7).

FIGS. 313 to 316.—THE DEVELOPMENT OF THE APPENDAGES OF THE LIDS (after Ida Mann).

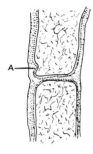

FIG. 313.—A 37 mm. fœtus.

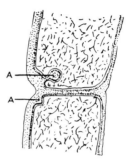

FIG. 314.—A 50 mm. fœtus.

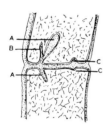

FIG. 315.—A 73 mm. fœtus.

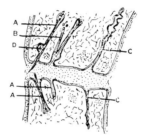

FIG. 316.—A 160 mm. fœtus.

A, lash follicle ; B, gland of Moll ; C, tarsal gland ; D, gland of Zeis.

Initially they are composed of solid columns of cells which soon develop a lumen from which acini secreting sebaceous material are formed during the last month of gestation.

THE LACRIMAL GLAND. The lacrimal gland emerges during the 22 to 25 mm. stage from the basal cells of the conjunctiva lining the temporal portion of the upper fornix (Speciale-Cirincione, 1909 ; Keibel and Mall, 1912) (Fig. 317). The proliferation of these cells results in the formation of 5 to 8 solid branching outgrowths extending upwards and anteriorly towards the equator of the globe within the surrounding mesoderm from which the glandular supporting tissues are derived. Further proliferation results in an increase in both the size and number of these solid cords, ten of which may have appeared by the 4th month (Figs. 318–9). Although initially solid, they rapidly develop a lumen by a breakdown of the central cells (55–60 mm. stage), the walls thereafter consisting of two layers of cells. During the 5th month the developing tendon of the levator palpebræ superioris cuts the gland into two parts ; the early buds form the deep or orbital portion while the secondary buds, which appear somewhat later (40–60 mm.), develop into the palpebral lobe.

FIGS. 317 to 319.—THE DEVELOPMENT OF THE LACRIMAL GLAND (F. Vrabec).

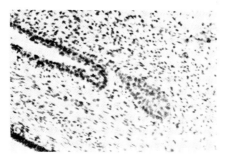

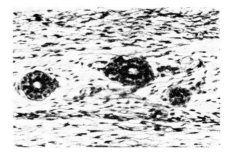

FIG. 317.—In a 24 mm. embryo. The gland develops as a solid outgrowth from the basal cells of the conjunctival fornix.

FIG. 318.—In a 50 mm. fœtus. The solid outgrowths become canalized by a breakdown of the central cells.

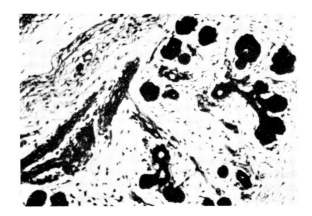

FIG. 319.—In a fœtus of 4 months. From the initial collecting channels with their central lumen solid buds of cells continue to grow.

It should be noted that even at birth the lacrimal gland has not attained its full development, a process which continues up to the age of 3 to 4 years (Kirchstein, 1894). Thereafter, until the age of 40 years, the glandular epithelium decreases in height and the interstitial and adenoid tissues increase, while in later life the glandular substance gradually atrophies (Götz, 1908). It is to be remembered that as a general rule the newborn infant does not weep. Reflex weeping may appear shortly after birth but may be delayed for several weeks (Kirchstein, 1894 ; Axenfeld, 1899) ;

psychic weeping is usually delayed for several months presumably owing to lack of the requisite central nervous connections, and, indeed, some people never experience emotional weeping (Collins, 1932).   Charles Darwin, exploring the subject to write his classical book, *The Expression of Emotion in Man and Animals* (1890), investigated the matter and found the onset of weeping to vary between 20 and 104 days after birth ; his own child showed reflex weeping 77 days after it was born and psychic weeping on the 139th day.

The ACCESSORY LACRIMAL GLANDS (of Krause) are similarly formed as ectodermal invaginations from the conjunctiva ; according to Mann (1928) they are the first epithelial ingrowths to be detected, being evident in the fornices and on the plica as epithelial buds penetrating the underlying meso- derm at the 55 mm. stage.   Other writers have failed to find them until a much later period, about the 6th or 7th month (Falchi, 1905 ; Ask, 1910 ; 170 mm., Leplat, 1958).   Even at birth, however, these glands are few in number and appear to be formed at very varying stages of development.

Exceptionally, *serous glands* resembling those of Moll or the accessory lacrimal glands of Krause develop on the caruncle, but they usually disappear in adult life (Terson, 1893 ; Alt, 1900 ; Ask, 1908 ; Contino, 1909).   *Sebaceous glands* resembling tarsal glands and hair follicles equipped with sebaceous glands resembling those of Zeis are, however, common in this structure.   Papamiltiades (1947) described the presence of small mucous glands after the 7th month of gestation.

The INFRA-ORBITAL GLAND (OF HARDER) is a transitory structure in man, appearing in late foetal life in the infero-lateral fornix and soon disappearing again (Löwenthal, 1910) ; it is homologous with the gland of Harder which is a characteristic of all vertebrates from amphibians to the higher primates.[1]

THE LACRIMAL PASSAGES

The lacrimal passages are developed along the line of the cleft between the lateral nasal and the maxillary processes (Figs. 279–82).   It was origin- ally supposed that this cleft was converted into a tube by the fusion of its boundaries (von Baer, 1828 ; Erdl, 1846), but Born (1876) showed that it was developed by the canalization of a solid rod of ectodermal cells found beneath the surface in this line.   Its development has subsequently been studied by a number of writers.[2]   We have seen that, as it grows rapidly upwards, the maxillary process overlaps the paraxial mesoderm around the eye, leaving a fold of thickened ectoderm buried in the mesoderm between itself and the lateral nasal process (Figs. 281–2).   As this ectodermal fold extends downwards into the underlying mesoderm it initially forms a sulcus (the NASO-OPTIC FISSURE) but this soon becomes detached from the surface to form an irregular solid rod of cells situated between the future medial

[1] Vol. I, p. 493.

[2] Legal (1882), Ewetzky (1888), Stanculeanu (1900), Rochon-Duvigneaud (1900), Monesi (1904), Matys (1905–6), Fleischer (1906), Cosmettatos (1906), Contino (1907), Ask (1908), Riquier (1911), Lang (1911), Schaeffer (1912), Ask and van der Hoeve (1921), Iwata (1927), Speciale-Cirincione (1929), Ehlers (1930), Nishi (1933), Politzer (1935), Fischer (1936), Dusseldorp *et al.* (1937), Leplat (1958), Kautzky and Pichler (1938), Cassady (1952), Gaini (1954) and Seo (1958).

FIGS. 320 TO 322.—DIAGRAMMATIC REPRESENTATION OF THE DEVELOPMENT OF THE LACRIMAL PASSAGES (after Iwata and Ask).

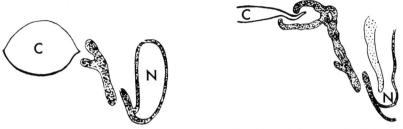

FIG. 320.—An embryo in the 6th week.   FIG. 321.—A fœtus in the 12th week.

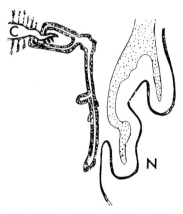

FIG. 322.—A fœtus of 3½ months.
C, conjunctival sac ; N, nasal cavity.

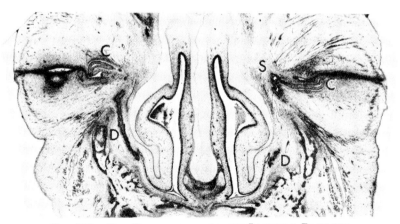

FIG. 323.—THE DEVELOPMENT OF THE LACRIMAL PASSAGES.

At the end of the 4th month. The canaliculi, C, are seen, the upper on the left, the lower on the right, leading into the lacrimal sac, S (on the right). These structures are seen to be canalizing. The naso-lacrimal duct, D, is seen throughout most of its extent on the right and in its termination on the left still separated from the nasal cavity (G. Renard).

FIGS. 324 and 325.—THE DEVELOPMENT OF THE CANALICULI (F. Vrabec).

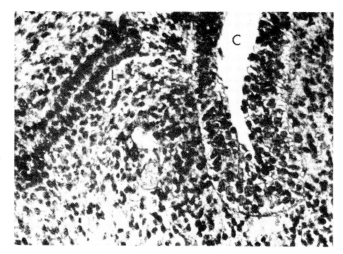

Fig. 324.—In an embryo of 25 mm. The solid epithelial tube of the canaliculus, L, is approaching but does not reach the conjunctival sac, C.

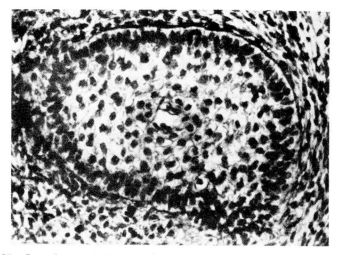

FIG. 325.—In a fœtus of the 3rd month. The beginnings of canalization of the canaliculus by lysis of the central cells is seen.

canthus and the nasal cavity ; the epithelial cord thus formed represents the rudiments of the lacrimal passages in the 15 mm. embryo. According to Leplat (1958), however, during the 6th week a second rod of epithelial cells appears to emerge from the primitive nasal cavity and by progressive elongation the adjacent extremities of these epithelial cords become approximated although they remain separate for some time before fusing

(Figs. 320–2). The cells forming the upper extremity of the uppermost rod of cells then proliferate to form two bud-like outgrowths which, on elongation, diverge to form a bifurcation closely applied to the internal angle of the developing inner canthus ; these are the rudiments of the lacrimal canaliculi, in the formation of which the epithelium of the lids plays no part. They reach the epithelium of the lid-margins at the 35 mm. stage and at the same time the upper portion of the rod of cells becomes thickened to form the rudiments of the lacrimal sac (Figs. 309, 323–7).

During the 3rd month the central cells of the solid rod begin to disintegrate, the disintegration at first being segmental in distribution so that

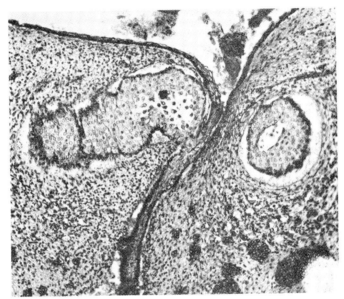

Fig. 326.—The Development of the Canaliculi.
In a fœtus of 4 months. The process of canalization is proceeding (F. Hervouët).

isolated cavities appear which eventually unite to form a continuous central lumen ; the originally solid naso-lacrimal passages thus become canalized (Figs. 323–6). This canalization begins at the upper or ocular end of the rod and progresses downwards, while the same process occurs in the epithelial outgrowth from the primitive nasal cavity so that the completed canal thus formed opens into the inferior meatus. The lysis of the central cells at the point of union of the two epithelial rods which finally establishes the oculo-nasal communication takes place at the end of the 6th month but may be delayed up to weeks or months after birth. The folds and so-called " valves " of the lacrimal passages are inconstant not only in number but in form and situation, anomalies which may well be explained by irregular

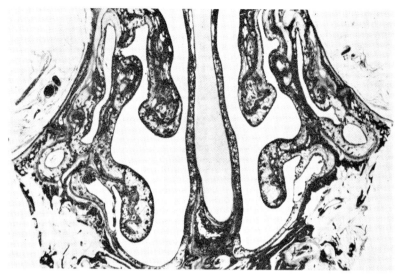

FIG. 327.—THE NASO-LACRIMAL PASSAGES IN A FULL-TERM INFANT.
Under the inferior turbinate the lower end of the naso-lacrimal duct is seen in cross-section separated from the nasal cavity on each side by a still unruptured membrane (J. V. Cassady).

canalization (Rochon-Duvigneaud, 1900 ; Leplat, 1958) (Fig. 322). Although the lumina of the canaliculi become patent during the 4th month, the lacrimal puncta do not open onto the lid-margins until just before the lids separate during the 7th month. The lower end of the duct, however, is frequently separated from the cavity of the inferior meatus at birth by a membrane consisting of the apposed mucosal linings of the nasal fossa and the lower end of the duct, an obstruction which makes this portion of the duct balloon out under the inferior turbinate bone. Cassady (1952) found this condition present in 73% of full-term still-born fœtuses (Fig. 327).

Abel. *Z. Morph. Anthrop.*, **33**, 261 (1935).
Addison and How. *Amer. J. Anat.*, **29**, 1, (1921).
Alferow. *Anat. Anz.*, **71**, 113 (1931).
Alt. *Amer. J. Ophthal.*, **17**, 234 (1900).
von Ammon. *v. Graefes Arch. Ophthal.*, **4**, 1 (1858).
Ask. *Anat. Anz.*, **30**, 197 (1907).
    Anat. Hefte, **36**, 189 (1908) ; **40**, 491 (1910).
Ask and van der Hoeve. *v. Graefes Arch. Ophthal.*, **105**, 1157 (1921).
Axenfeld. *Klin. Mbl. Augenheilk.*, **37**, 259 (1899).
von Baer. *Ueber Entwickelungsges. d. Thiere*, Königsberg, **1** (1828).
Barber. *Embryology of the Human Eye*, St. Louis (1955).
Born. *Morph. Jb.*, **2**, 577 (1876).
Breitinger. *Homo*, **6**, 149 (1955).

Broman and Ask. *Dtsch. Südpolarexped.*, **12** (1910).
Burrows. *Yale J. Biol. Med.*, **17**, 397 (1944).
Cassady. *Arch. Ophthal.* (Chicago), **47**, 141 (1952).
Collins. *Brit. J. Ophthal.*, **16**, 1 (1932).
Contino. *v. Graefes Arch. Ophthal.*, **66**, 505 (1907) ; **71**, 1 (1909).
Cosmettatos. *Arch. Augenheilk.*, **55**, 362 (1906).
Devi. *Amer. J. hum. Genet.*, **11**, 35 (1959).
Dordi. *Arch. ital. Anat. Embriol.*, **52**, 136 (1947).
Dusseldorp, Courtis, Damel, Gallino *et al.* *Acta I Cong. argent. Oftal.*, **1**, 25 (1937).
Eayrs. *J. Anat.* (Lond.), **85**, 330 (1951).
Ehlers. *Acta ophthal.* (Kbh.), **8**, 305 (1930).
Erdl. *Die Entwickelung d. Menschen*, Leipzig (1846).

Ewetzky. *v. Graefes Arch. Ophthal.*, **34** (1), 23 (1888).

Falchi. *Arch. ital. Biol.*, **44**, 412 (1905).

Fischer. *Z. Augenheilk.*, Suppl. 22 (1936).

Fleischer. *v. Graefes Arch. Ophthal.*, **62**, 379 (1906).

Gaini. *Arch. ital. Otol.*, **65**, 299 (1954).

Goto. *Acta Soc. ophthal. jap.*, **55**, 869 (1951).

Götz. *Untersuch. von Tränendrüsen aus verschiedenen Lebensaltern* (Diss.), Tübingen (1908).

Guieysse-Pellissier. *Bull. Histol. Techn. micr.*, **14**, 73 (1937).

Iwata. *Folia Anat. jap.*, **5**, 51 (1927).

Kautzky and Pichler. *Morph. Jb.*, **81**, 286 (1938).

Keibel and Mall. *Manual of Human Embryology*, Phila., **2** (1912).

Kiil. *J. Hered.*, **39**, 206 (1948); **43**, 247 (1952).

Kirchstein. *Ueber die Tränendrüse der Neugeborenen* (Diss.), Berlin (1894).

Klee. *Arch. mikr. Anat.*, **95** (1), 65 (1920).

von Kölliker. *Entwicklungsgeschichte d. Menschen*, Leipzig (1861).

Lang. *Anat. Anz.*, **38**, 561 (1911).

Legal. *Morph. Jb.*, **8**, 353 (1882).

Lehtinen. *Ann. Acad. Sci. fenn. Anthropol.*, **23**, 1 (1951).

Leplat. Dejean, Hervouët and Leplat's *L'embryologie de l'œil et sa tératologie*, Paris, 444 (1958).

Löffler. *Hb. d. Erbbiol. d. Menschen*, Berlin, **3**, 403 (1940).

Löwenthal. *Bib. Anat.*, **19**, 301 (1910).

Mann. *The Development of the Human Eye*, Camb. (1928).

Matys. *Z. Augenheilk.*, **14**, 222 (1905); **16**, 303 (1906).

Monesi. *Klin. Mbl. Augenheilk.*, **42** (1), 1 (1904).

Nishi. *J. Kumamoto med. Soc.*, **9**, 877 (1933).

Papamiltiades. *C.R. Ass. Anat.*, **34**, 418 (1947).

Politzer. *Z. Anat. Entwickl. Gesch.*, **105**, 329 (1935).

Riquier. *Monit. zool. Ital.*, **22**, 56 (1911).

Rochon-Duvigneaud. *Arch. Ophtal.* (Paris), **20**, 241 (1900).

Routil. *Z. Rassenk. u. ges. Forsch. am Menschen*, **9**, 48 (1939).

Schaeffer. *Amer. J. Anat.*, **10**, 313 (1910); **13**, 1 (1912).
J. Morph., **21**, 613 (1910).

Seo. *Acta Soc. ophthal. jap.*, **62**, 1747 (1958).

Speciale-Cirincione. *v. Graefes Arch. Ophthal.*, **69**, 193 (1909).
Ann. Ottal., **57**, 435 (1929).

Stanculeanu. *Arch. Ophtal.* (Paris), **20**, 141 (1900).

Terson. *Les glandes lacrymales, conjonctivales et orbito-palpébrales* (Thèse), Paris (1893).

Tusques. *C.R. Soc. Biol.* (Paris), **145**, 404 (1951); **146**, 729 (1952).

Ueda. *Folia ophthal. jap.*, **10**, 1072 (1959).

Viard. *Arch. Anat. micr.*, **44**, 344 (1955).

Yamazaki and Osumi. *Rinsho Iho*, **48**, 5 (1954).

THE VASCULAR SYSTEM

As occurs in the vascular system generally, the development of the blood vessels of the orbit—and, indeed, of the whole of the body—is characterized by the unexpected appearance of new vessels, the gradual dwindling or even the complete elimination of some that were once prominent in order to serve temporary needs, the elaboration of others and the formation of new linkages and anastomoses to serve new needs so that the final design bears little resemblance to the previous configuration.

The complex development of the vessels of the head (and orbit) has not been fully worked out, and has, indeed, claimed little attention. Studies have been made by Tandler (1902) and Moffat (1961) in the rat, by Fuchs (1905) in the rabbit, and by Mall (1904), de Vriese (1905), Beevor (1909), Evans (1912), Streeter (1918), Congdon (1922), Padget (1948–54) and Krause (1956) in man. This account is essentially derived from the work of Dorcas Padget.

The Arteries

The first of the early vessels to become established in the embryo are the two (bilateral) primitive aortæ which appear about the time at which the head-fold begins to form (1·4 mm. stage) (Fig. 328); passing first cephalically and then looping dorsally to form the FIRST (AORTIC) PHARYNGEAL ARCH, they run caudally on either side of the notochord giving off dorsal segmental branches in the intervals between the developing mesodermal somites ; eventually the primitive dorsal aortæ fuse to form a single permanent descending aorta. By the time 14 somites have formed, the

FIGS. 328 and 329.—THE VASCULAR SYSTEM IN THE EARLY EMBRYO (modified from Felix).

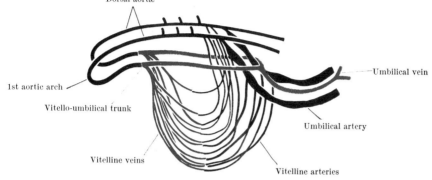

FIG. 328.—In the 6 somite (1·35 mm.) stage.

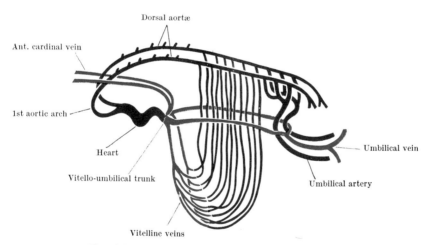

FIG. 329.—In the 14 somite (2·6 mm.) stage.

ventral portions of the primitive aortæ have fused to form a single heart to the cephalic end of which the arteries are connected and to the caudal end the veins (Fig. 329).

At about the same time venous channels make their appearance returning blood to the heart ; the first of these are the two ANTERIOR CARDINAL HEAD VEINS which run caudally from the region of the optic vesicle, one on each side of the cephalic part of the neural tube, to the sinus venosus of the heart near the junction of the umbilical veins (draining the placenta) and the vitelline veins (draining the yolk sac) (Fig. 329).

As development proceeds several channels spring from the primitive ventral aortæ, skirt the fore-gut on either side in the branchial arches, and

Figs. 330 and 331.—Scheme of the Aortic Arches (after Cunningham).

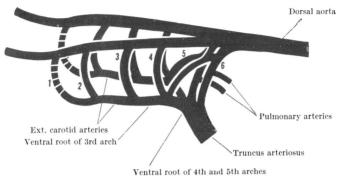

Fig. 330.—In a 9 mm. embryo. 1–6, aortic arches ; the 1st has atrophied.

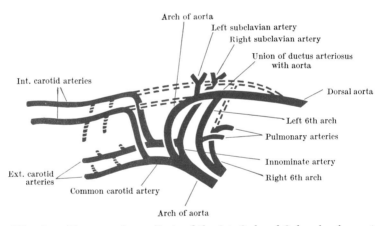

Fig. 331.—In a 15 mm. embryo. Parts of the 1st, 2nd and 3rd arches have atrophied, as well as the dorsal part of the right 6th and the dorsal root of the right 4th and 5th arches.

terminate in the primitive dorsal aortæ ; altogether six PHARYNGEAL ARCH ARTERIES (including the original first arch) are thus formed on each side (Fig. 330). As the later arches situated most caudally appear, the older more cranially situated ones partially disappear : at the 5 mm. stage the first 4 and the 6th arch are present, and at the 7 mm. stage the first two arches have begun to disintegrate and the transitory 5th arch has been formed. At a later stage the dorsal roots of the 3rd arches on both sides and the 4th and 6th arches on the right side partially disappear ; the definitive arteries which persist and supply the region of the head are formed from the vessels which remain (Fig. 331).

The evolution of the main vessels of ophthalmological interest is seen in Figs. 332–38 ; as so often occurs in the development of the vascular system it forms a complicated story of partial disappearances, new developments and multiple junctions (Streeter, 1918 ; Congdon, 1922 ; Padget, 1948–54 ; Krause, 1956). The left 5th arch artery persists as the arch of the aorta ;

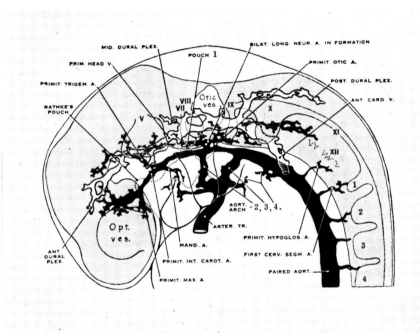

FIG. 332.—THE EARLY VASCULAR SYSTEM OF THE HEAD.

In a human embryo of 4 mm. The third aortic arch has formed. The primitive internal carotid supplies the optic vesicle, the forebrain and the midbrain.

Veins in white, arteries in black. V–XII, cranial nerves ; 1, 2, 3, 4, cervical segments (D. H. Padget).

the ventral portion of the 3rd arch artery on either side forms the common carotid artery which thus seems to arise from the aortic arch itself ; while a continuation of this, linking up with persisting remnants of the 1st and 2nd arch arteries, forms the external carotid artery. Finally, the 3rd arch itself is prolonged forwards as a continuation of the dorsal aorta to form the internal carotid.

In the description of the development of the vessels of the orbit and lids, the two main systems concerned—the internal and the external carotid

systems—will be considered separately, the first derived from the 3rd
pharyngeal arch artery and the remnants of the dorsal roots of the 1st and
2nd, and the latter from the ventral roots of the 1st and 2nd arch arteries.

The internal carotid system. The main vascular supply to the orbit—
the ophthalmic artery—is derived from the internal carotid system. The
emergence of the definitive vessel is both complicated and late, and in its
formation two vessels merge, the development and partial disappearance of

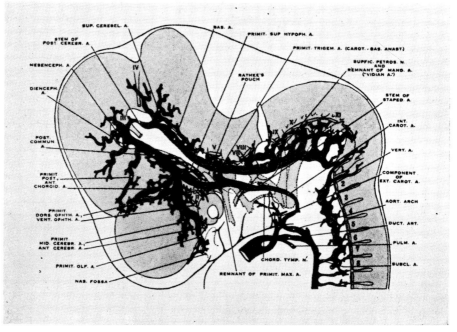

Fig. 333.—The Early Arterial Supply to the Head.
In a human embryo of 11·5 mm. II–XII, cranial nerves. 1–8, cervical segments
(D. H. Padget).

which must now be considered—the primitive ophthalmic system and the
transient stapedial artery.

In the very young embryo (20 somites) the primitive internal carotid
artery, as we have seen,[1] terminates in a plexus at the caudal aspect of the
emerging optic vesicle (Figs. 239, 332–3). By the 4 mm. stage the main
trunk has given off two branches and has divided into two terminal divisions.
The latter are not of immediate ocular concern : (a) a cranial division (which
supplies the olfactory area and gives rise eventually to the anterior and
middle cerebral arteries), and (b) a caudal division which supplies the region

[1] p. 183.

of the mesencephalon. The two branches, however, participate in the blood supply of the eye (Fig. 334) :

(i) The TRANSIENT MAXILLARY ARTERY is a small vessel which initially sends a tiny (hypothalamic) branch to supply the base of the developing optic vesicle ; soon, however, it loses all connection with the optic region and eventually anastomoses with the maxillo-mandibular division of the stapedial artery (vide infra).

(ii) The PRIMITIVE DORSAL OPHTHALMIC ARTERY is a larger vessel which emerges from the parent carotid trunk just at its terminal point of bifurcation. From this vessel is given off the hyaloid artery which enters the optic cup through the embryonic fissure,[1] while its terminal portion (the common temporal ciliary artery) supplies the plexus investing the dorsal and outer aspects of the cup.

At this early stage (9 mm.), therefore, apart from the temporary supply from the primitive maxillary artery, the developing eye is supplied by branches of the primitive dorsal ophthalmic branch of the internal carotid artery.

Between the 7 and 12 mm. stage a second vessel arrives in this area— the PRIMITIVE VENTRAL OPHTHALMIC ARTERY—derived from the cranial division of the internal carotid ; this supplies the ventral and medial aspects of the plexus around the optic cup. As the optic stalk elongates both the primitive dorsal and ventral ophthalmic arteries are drawn out in length and, at about the 16–18 mm. stage, the stem of the primitive dorsal artery annexes the distal end of its companion ventral artery to form the common nasal ciliary artery (Fig. 335). This secondary anastomosis takes place under the optic nerve so that for a time there is an arterial ring around the nerve ; between the anastomoses, however, the common nasal ciliary vessel soon disappears so that the definitive main ophthalmic trunk passes from the ventral to the dorsal side of the optic nerve. At the same time, while the rapidly expanding brain draws the cerebral arteries away from the optic region, the main ophthalmic stem (originally the dorsal ophthalmic artery) migrates caudally down the internal carotid by a series of " anastomotic loops " to occupy its final position just caudal to the eye and lateral to Rathke's pouch. At this stage (16–18 mm.), therefore, the definitive arterial supply to the eye is evident, now entirely arising from the (dorsal) ophthalmic trunk, as the ophthalmic artery, the stem of which is derived from the primitive dorsal ophthalmic artery ; it has three branches, the common temporal ciliary (which eventually becomes the long posterior temporal) and the hyaloid artery derived from their parent vessel, and the common nasal ciliary (which eventually becomes the long posterior nasal), initially the distal part of the ventral ophthalmic branch of the internal carotid. It will be noted that at this stage the area of supply of this ophthalmic system is essentially ocular.

[1] p. 190.

FIGS. 334 and 335.—THE EARLY ARTERIAL SUPPLY TO THE HEAD (D. H. Padget).

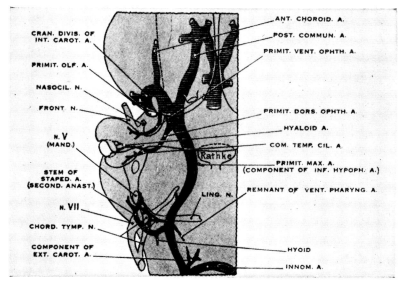

FIG. 334.—In a human embryo of approximately 14 mm. Both dorsal and ventral ophthalmic arteries are elongated and from the dorsal has developed the hyaloid artery.

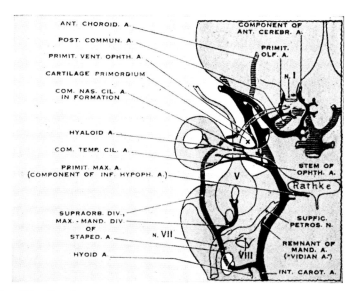

FIG. 335.—In a human embryo of approximately 18 mm. The primitive stem of the ophthalmic artery has appeared. A secondary anastomosis joins its hyaloid branch to the primitive ventral ophthalmic artery which is subsequently interrupted. The stapedial artery has formed its two primary divisions—the supra-orbital and maxillo-mandibular arteries.

A second artery now enters into the picture which initially is entirely responsible for the blood supply to the orbital region—the STAPEDIAL ARTERY. It arises from the carotid as a derivation of the second (hyoid) pharyngeal arch and, piercing the stapes primordium, forms two divisions which follow the main branches of the trigeminal nerve : the *supra-orbital division* follows the 1st (ophthalmic) division of this nerve to the orbital region, while the *maxillo-mandibular division* accompanies the 2nd and 3rd divisions of the nerve to their respective territories of supply (the maxillary and mandibular processes) (Figs. 335–7). At the 20 mm. stage the stem of the ophthalmic artery anastomoses with the supra-orbital division of the stapedial artery and annexes its distal part. The main peripheral trunk (the lacrimal artery) runs to the primordium of the lacrimal

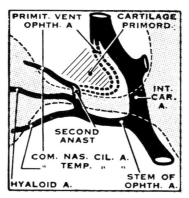

FIG. 336.—THE EVOLUTION OF THE OPHTHALMIC ARTERY.

In an embryo of 18 mm., showing the formation of the three primary ocular branches, the common nasal ciliary, the common temporal ciliary, and the hyaloid arteries (D. H. Padget).

gland, and from it two branches emerge, a medial and a lateral, following respectively the frontal and naso-ciliary branches of the 1st division of the trigeminal nerve and constituting the corresponding definitive arteries. It is thus evident that by the annexation of this portion of the stapedial artery the ophthalmic artery acquires orbital as well as ocular branches, the former, indeed, being the most conspicuous in the adult.

The further fate of the stapedial artery is interesting (Figs. 337, 338). The external carotid, through its internal maxillary branch, annexes the maxillo-mandibular division of the stapedial to form the first part of the middle meningeal artery. The proximal part of the orbital division of the stapedial (that is, the part proximal to its anastomosis with the ophthalmic) forms the second part of the middle meningeal ; while the stem of the stapedial artery obliterates itself at the stapes and its lower division is transferred to the external carotid system to form the definitive internal maxillary artery.

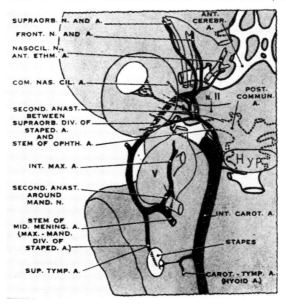

Fig. 337.—In a human embryo of 20 mm. The supra-orbital division of the stapedial artery, the stem of which is dwindling, has developed several orbital branches and is being annexed by the ophthalmic artery. Note the arterial ring by means of which the ophthalmic artery passes round to the dorsal side of the optic nerve.

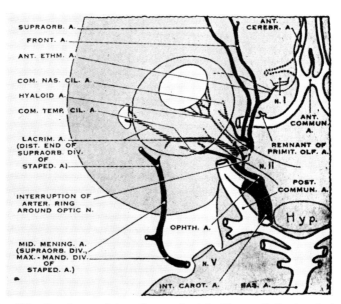

Fig. 338.—In a human fœtus of approximately 40 mm. Following the interruption of the cranio-ventral segment of the arterial ring around the optic nerve and the supra-orbital division of the stapedial artery, the ophthalmic artery assumes its adult configuration. The supra-orbital division of the stapedial artery is seen forming the lacrimal artery and the anterior branch of the middle-meningeal.

This complex development of the orbital arteries explains the occurrence of an anastomosis in the adult between the lacrimal and middle meningeal arteries at the lateral end of the sphenoid fissure, as well as certain anomalous arrangements which occasionally occur—the origin of the lacrimal artery from the middle meningeal, of the middle meningeal from the ophthalmic, or the replacement of the ophthalmic by the middle meningeal.[1]

The external carotid system emerges from the ventral parts of the first two pharyngeal arch arteries. By the 16 mm. stage, coincidently with the formation of the common carotid artery, most of its branches of distribution are identifiable. As we have seen, it reinforces itself by annexing the maxillo-mandibular division of the stapedial artery from the internal carotid system in the formation of the internal maxillary artery.

The Veins

A basic knowledge of the development of the venous system of the head has only been recently acquired. The story resembles that of the arteries— the appearance of vessels, the diminution or even the disappearance of most and their replacement by new vessels evolved to meet new needs, and the linkage by anastomoses of different stem-vessels often followed by the disappearance of the connecting channels to suit changed needs, so that the final arrangement seen in the adult bears little resemblance to that found in the embryo. In comparison with the arterial system, however, the veins show a much more complex evolution which starts later than arterial differentiation, goes through more complicated stages, and does not cease at birth, for the configuration characteristic of the adult differs in certain important respects from the picture seen in the newborn.

Partly because of the complexity of the subject, partly because the basic scheme can be understood only when the stages of venous development in man are compared with embryonic and adult patterns in lower vertebrates, and partly because of the multitude of variations encountered, the literature on the embryology of the veins of the head in man is sparse, generally unilluminating, and often contradictory. The pioneering report of Mall (1904) was followed by the classical studies of Markowski (1911–22) and Streeter (1915–18), but an adequate basic scheme had to wait for the admirable and exhaustive researches of Dorcas Padget (1956–57) from the Carnegie Institution of Washington ; we will discuss her findings and adopt her terminology. It would be out of place here to describe the development of the venous system of the entire head ; we will confine ourselves to discussing that part of the system which is of ophthalmological interest, merely noting shortly the main trends in the ontogeny of the great vessels and the cerebral sinuses such as are necessary for an understanding of the development of the venous outflow from the eye, the orbit and the face.

We have already seen that at an early stage of development the neural tube is covered by a continuous endothelial plexus (the future pial plexus) from which both arteries and veins evolve (Fig. 332). Initially this is drained by a primordial channel lying directly on the neural tube (pial in

---

[1] See Vol. II, p. 473.

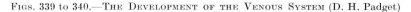

FIGS. 339 to 340.—THE DEVELOPMENT OF THE VENOUS SYSTEM (D. H. Padget)

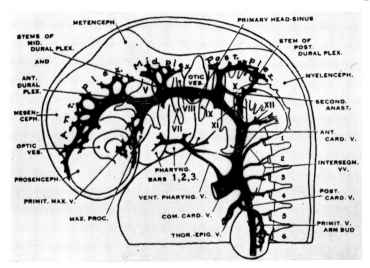

FIG. 339.—In an embryo of 5 mm. The endothelial plexus drains through many short channels into a superficial venous plexus divided into three sections, anterior, middle and posterior, which drain through the (paired) primary head-sinus which in turn empties into the anterior cardinal vein. The maxillary vein drains both optic and olfactory regions. V to XII, cranial nerves. 1 to 6, cervical segments.

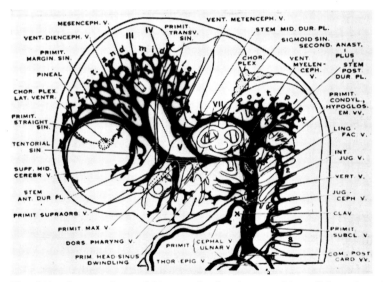

FIG. 340.—In an embryo of 18 mm. As the pharyngeal bars differentiate, the middle and posterior dural plexuses form the sigmoid sinus, while ventral to the labyrinth the head-sinus dwindles.

location) which is transient ; at a very early period, before the stage of 28 somites, the endothelial plexus drains dorso-laterally through many short vessels into a SUPERFICIAL VENOUS PLEXUS (the primitive dural plexus) divided into three sections, anterior, middle and posterior, corresponding to the three initial cerebral divisions, the prosencephalon, the metencephalon and the myelencephalon. This plexus drains through a paired PRIMARY HEAD-SINUS (dural in location) running caudally, medial to the Vth and Xth nerves but lateral to the other cranial nerves, to become continuous with the ANTERIOR CARDINAL VEIN (Fig. 339). It will be remembered that the anterior cardinal vein draining the head meets the posterior cardinal vein from the body to form the common cardinal vein (the duct of Cuvier) which enters the sinus venosus of the primitive heart (Fig. 329). The anterior cardinal vein thus forms the primitive internal jugular vein, a vessel which represents the primary jugular vein of vertebrates ; this configuration is characteristic of adult reptiles.

THE INTERNAL JUGULAR SYSTEM AND THE CEREBRAL SINUSES

Several important changes then rapidly occur in the evolution of this relatively simple system. The first change concerns the rapid development of the otic vesicle. A venous connection appears between the middle and posterior dural plexuses dorsal to the otic capsule (Fig. 340) ; this, accepting the responsibility for most of the blood-flow and joining up with

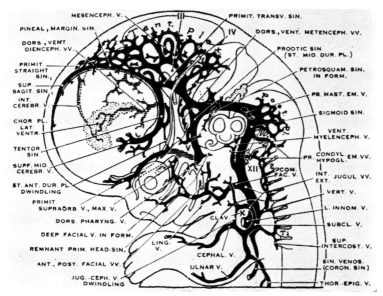

FIG. 341.—THE DEVELOPMENT OF THE VENOUS SYSTEM (D. H. Padget).

In an embryo of 24 mm. The middle stem of the primary head-sinus becomes the pro-otic sinus which empties into the new sigmoid sinus.

the posterior stem of the primary head-sinus, becomes the SIGMOID SINUS. Meantime, the corresponding portion of the primary head-sinus ventral to the labyrinth dwindles and disappears, and the middle stem of the primary head-sinus (now no longer part of the direct venous stream and with its blood-flow reversed) becomes the PRO-OTIC SINUS (Fig. 341). From it is evolved a series of plexiform elements extending medially to meet corresponding channels from the other side ; from these at about the 40 mm. stage develops the CAVERNOUS SINUS, while at the same time a ventral channel connects this complex with the jugular vein below its foramen to form the new INFERIOR PETROSAL SINUS (Fig. 342). The peculiar trabecular configuration of the adult cavernous sinus is due to its plexiform origin across the mid-line at the level of the hypophysis enmeshing the IIIrd, IVth and VIth cranial nerves and the internal carotid artery.

More anteriorly the expansion of the cerebrum causes similar changes. The anterior dorsal plexus becomes consolidated so that the prosencephalon becomes surrounded by definite channels—the SUPERIOR SAGITTAL SINUS superiorly, the MARGINAL SINUS dorsally, and the TENTORIAL SINUS ventrally ; while the accelerated growth of the basal nuclear masses of the brain and the choroid plexus results in the emergence of the Galenic system of intracerebral venous drainage. The last of the major sinuses to appear is the SUPERIOR PETROSAL which has become defined by the 80 mm. stage. The communication between this sinus and the cavernous sinus is a late secondary development which occurs, if at all, after birth and is usually absent in mammals. By the 80 mm. stage the basic arrangement of the venous sinuses is thus recognizable ; subsequent changes depend chiefly upon the continued expansion of the cerebral and cerebellar hemispheres and the relatively late ossification of the skull which determine the configuration of certain anastomoses in the dura. It is interesting, however, that at term cerebral drainage is into the transverse sinus by way of the gradually elongating embryonic tentorial sinus ; the final anastomoses between the cerebral veins and the cavernous sinus are a later event (Fig. 343).

THE OPHTHALMIC VENOUS SYSTEM

The first offshoot of the internal jugular system concerns the venous drainage of the optic vesicle. At a very early stage (20 somites) a PRIMITIVE MAXILLARY VEIN appears as a branch of the primary head-sinus, draining the endothelial plexus surrounding the vesicle from its ventro-caudal aspect as well as the olfactory region and the emerging maxillary process ; by the 5 to 8 mm. stage this vessel is well developed and receives a tributary from the embryonic fissure in the ventral aspect of the optic stalk, probably representing the future central vein of the retina (Fig. 339). Into the maxillary vein all the intrinsic veins of the eye drain initially, including the choriocapillary net and the annular vessel. At a later stage (11–14 mm.) a second vessel, the PRIMITIVE SUPRA-ORBITAL VEIN emerges on the dorsal aspect of the vesicle and, running between the frontal and naso-ciliary branches of the ophthalmic nerve, also drains this part of the endothelial plexus into the anterior dural stem of the head-sinus (Fig. 340) ; it will be remembered that the dorsal part of the perivesicular plexus is more retarded in its appearance than the ventral.[1] The subsequent development of these veins is complicated,

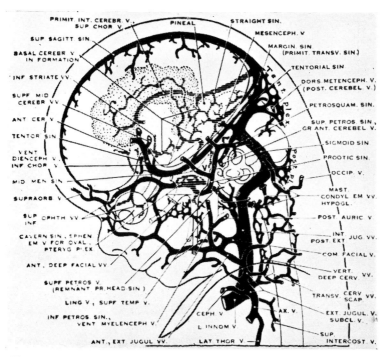

FIG. 342.—THE DEVELOPMENT OF THE VENOUS SYSTEM (D. H. Padget).

In a fœtus of 80 mm. From the pro-otic sinus a series of channels extends medially to form the (central) cavernous sinus which connects with the jugular vein to form the inferior petrosal sinus. Cerebral growth and expansion of the otic capsule are responsible for a new superior petrosal sinus.

recalling the dramatic changes that occur in the ophthalmic artery. In general, the maxillary vein loses many of its tributaries to the external jugular system and becomes the inferior ophthalmic vein ; the supra-orbital vein, initially the laggard in development and the smaller in size, becomes the superior ophthalmic vein, is permanent and eventually constitutes the main drainage-vessel of the orbit, but its proximal end disappears and, after the two vessels have anastomosed, the proximal portion of the otherwise shrunken maxillary vein becomes the outlet of all the orbital veins into the cavernous sinus. Up to the 14 to 17 mm. stage the course of the two vessels

[1] p. 186.

is direct into the primary head-sinus and they are separate. The shifting
and unequal growth of the brain and orbit, however, wedge the proximal part of the supra-orbital vein against the tissues surrounding the
IVth and Vth nerves so that its course necessarily becomes progressively
more devious and circuitous. Meantime, a secondary anastomosis between it and the maxillary vein has occurred, and by the 40 mm. stage

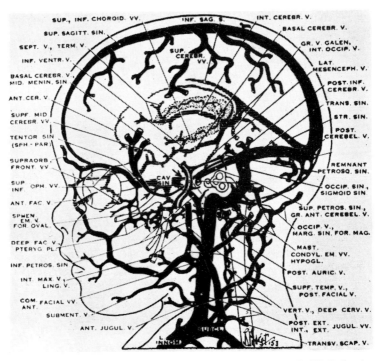

FIG. 343.—THE DEVELOPMENT OF THE VENOUS SYSTEM (D. H. Padget).

In an infant. Further expansion of the cerebral and cerebellar hemispheres determines
the configuration of the dural anastomoses. Cerebral drainage is still through the transverse
sinus by way of the tentorial sinus.

the proximal stem of the mechanically strained supra-orbital vein has
disappeared; its distal branches, however, remain permanently as the
SUPERIOR OPHTHALMIC VEIN constituting the main orbital drainage system.
By this time the primitive maxillary vein, originally confined to the
maxillary process and later invading, cranially and caudally, the territory
of the other two divisions of the Vth nerve, has lost most of its tributaries to
the facial veins (Figs. 339–43), so that its distal portion is reduced to comparatively small remnants which persist as the INFERIOR OPHTHALMIC VEIN with
relatively insignificant infra-orbital, facial, ethmoid and nasal tributaries.
Its proximal stem, however, taking over the blood from the superior

ophthalmic vein, forms the large COMMON OPHTHALMIC VEIN draining into the pro-otic sinus (Fig. 341). With the dwindling of this sinus after the 40 mm. stage and the development of its central derivation, the cavernous sinus, the latter forms the outlet for the ophthalmic system. With the development of this sinus the common vein is shortened so that the two ophthalmic veins may appear in the adult to enter the cavernous sinus separately; and since the final channel is the maxillary stem, the superior vein, although its course is dorsal and then lateral to the orbital structures, leaves the orbit at the lowest medial extremity of the orbital fissure and joins the cavernous sinus ventral to all the orbital structures. Even at term, however, there is apparently no direct or sizable connection at the cavernous sinus between the ophthalmic veins and those draining the cerebrum as commonly occurs in the adult.

THE EXTERNAL JUGULAR SYSTEM AND THE FACIAL VEINS

The emergence of the external jugular system is delayed long after the internal jugular system is fully functional but eventually, and particularly in mammals below the primates, it takes over much of the territory drained by the latter. Initially it is represented by the VENTRAL PHARYNGEAL VEIN which drains the mandibular and hyoid arches and joins the common cardinal vein (Fig. 339); before the 14 mm. stage this vessel has migrated cranially to drain into the anterior cardinal vein as the LINGUO-FACIAL VEIN (Fig. 340). Although this vessel is thus primarily a tributary of the internal jugular, it is taken over secondarily by the external jugular vein at a later stage when the internal jugular system dwindles in favour of the external. About the 24 mm. stage the linguo-facial anastomoses with a postero-lateral tributary of the maxillary vein near the outer labial angle to form a new ANTERIOR FACIAL VEIN taking much of its blood-flow; the orbital portion of the maxillary is thus considerably diminished in importance and at its cranial end, near the bridge of the nose, it anastomoses with the primitive supra-orbital (superior ophthalmic) vein (Fig. 341). At the same time the linguo-facial receives a tributary from the superficial temporal region, the POSTERIOR FACIAL VEIN. At this stage the embryonic linguo-facial vessel may now be called the definitive COMMON FACIAL VEIN, and the lateral tributary of the diminishing maxillary vein, the DEEP FACIAL VEIN (Fig. 342). Meantime, at the 60 to 80 mm. stage the EXTERNAL JUGULAR VEIN, the last of the great vessels to appear, emerges as a tributary of the primitive cephalic vein in the arm forming the definitive subclavian vein, and annexes the common facial and its tributaries, a process associated with a considerable degree of regression of the internal jugular system (Figs. 342 and 343).

The Lymphatics

The development of LYMPHATIC VESSELS was first thoroughly studied by Huntington and McClure (1907–08) who claimed that they appeared in the mesoderm as clefts which became confluent and communicated secondarily with the venous system, a view maintained by Kampmeier (1912), Huntington (1914) and Zimmermann (1940). Sabin (1902–12), on the other hand, believed that they were initially formed by budding from the veins and that the ramifications of the lymphatic system were determined by progressive endothelial sprouting in a centrifugal direction from the venous diverticula that constituted the major lymphatics, a view now more generally accepted (see Yoffey and Courtice, 1956). Five such diverticula are formed, two jugular lymphatic sacs from the internal jugular veins, two iliac sacs from the common iliac veins, and a single median retroperitoneal diverticulum from the inferior vena cava, forming the cisterna chyli. From the first pair the lymphatics of the lids develop.

Lymph nodes are developed as aggregations of *lymphoblasts* in the mesodermal tissue surrounding the lymphatic plexuses derived from the primary lymphatic sacs. Such aggregations can be detected at the 30 mm. stage and the nodes are identifiable at 50 mm., but complete histological differentiation into cortex and medulla does not occur until after birth. Initially they are " hæmolymph " nodes containing a proportion of erythroblasts, but in the later stages of development they are solely lymphocytopoietic.

THE NERVES

THE MOTOR NERVES

The VOLUNTARY MOTOR CRANIAL NERVES are developed in the cranial part of the neural tube from the most medial column of neuroblasts which constitutes the somatic efferent column and is serially continuous with the cells which give rise to the spinal motor nerves of the anterior column of the cord. They include the ocular motor nerves (the IIIrd, IVth and VIth cranial nerves) innervating the extrinsic muscles of the eye, and the XIIth (hypoglossal) nerve which innervates the musculature of the tongue. These nerves innervate the muscles (presumably) derived from the cranial somites. We have already discussed the metameric origin of the ocular muscles and have seen that, although the matter is by no means settled, in all probability the three ocular motor nerves are derived from the mesodermal condensation associated with the premandibular cavity[1] ; if this be the correct interpretation of this difficult problem, the IVth and VIth nerves are not individually segmental but are separated portions of the IIIrd.

However that may be, the nucleus of the IIIrd nerve appears earliest, being visible at the 8 to 9 mm. stage in the mesencephalic nasal plate (Fig. 344) ; almost simultaneously (9 mm. stage) the nucleus of the IVth nerve is recognizable as a small group of cells lying on the outskirts of the mantle

[1] p. 221.

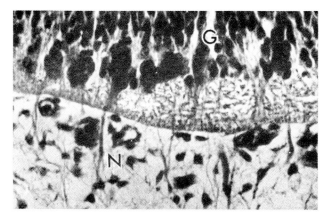

FIG. 344.—THE EMERGENCE OF THE IIIRD CRANIAL NUCLEUS.

In an embryo of 8 mm. The neuroblasts migrate from the germinal layer, G, towards the external surface. The nerve fibres, N, are seen running through the periaxial cranial mesoderm. (Heidenhain's hæmatoxylin ; × 373) (F. Vrabec).

layer of the neural tube situated in the lateral wall of the narrow communication between the metencephalon and the mesencephalon which forms the isthmus (E. R. A. Cooper, 1946–47). The nucleus of the VIth nerve rapidly follows (10 mm. stage), appearing in the somatic efferent column in the posterior part of the midbrain. By the 15 mm. stage the trunk of the IIIrd nerve is seen as a projection on the surface of the midbrain, between the 6th

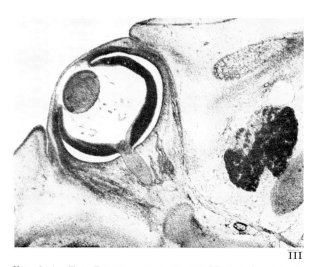

III

FIG. 345.—THE DEVELOPMENT OF THE MOTOR APPARATUS.

In an embryo of 23 mm. The trunk of the third nerve (III) is seen travelling from the brain to the muscle. The muscles are seen attached to the scleral condensation (marked in the anterior part of the globe but hardly distinguishable from the surrounding mesoderm posteriorly) (G. Leplat).

and 7th week the IVth nerve is apparent, and by the 8th week the abducens is recognizable. By the 23 mm. stage the IIIrd nerve is visible as a relatively large trunk running along the deep surface of the developing ocular muscles (Fig. 345). By the end of the 8th week all these nerves have reached their respective muscles (Sakamoto, 1953).

The dorsal origin and peculiar course of the IVth nerve with its decussation between the tectum and the developing cerebellum have never been adequately explained (see Kappers *et al.*, 1936) (Figs. 346–8). It would appear that the course of the nerve is

FIGS. 346 and 347.—THE REGION OF THE ISTHMUS (E. R. A. Cooper).

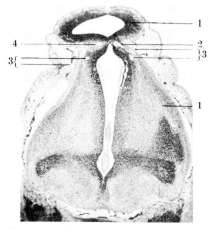

FIG. 346.—In a 13 mm. embryo (× 20).

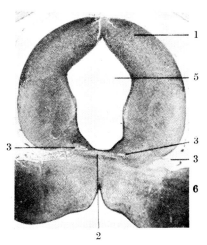

FIG. 347.—In a 37 mm. fœtus (× 13).

1, alar plate ; 2, decussation of trochlear nerves ; 3, trochlear nerves ; 4, superior medullary velum ; 5, mesencephalon ; 6, superior cerebellar peduncle.

determined by developmental occurrences in the region of the isthmus which originates as the constriction between the developing rhombencephalon and the mesencephalon. Frazer (1928) suggested that the nucleus of the trochlear nerve originally lay in series with the oculomotor and other somatic efferent nuclei in the basal plate of the isthmus and that, when this structure migrated to form the lateral wall of the isthmus, it carried the nucleus with it. It was pointed out by E. R. A. Cooper (1946–47) that the fibres reach the dorsal surface between the mesencephalic basal plates and the cerebellar rudiment—a relatively easy course in place of a ventral pathway which would have to traverse the dense mass of fibres of the superior cerebellar peduncle occupying the basal plate.

THE FACIAL (VIIth) CRANIAL NERVE belongs to the 2nd (hyoid) pharyngeal arch and supplies the muscles of facial expression (including those around

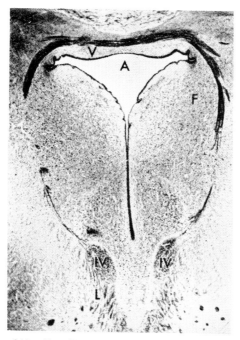

FIG. 348.—THE DEVELOPMENT OF THE IVTH NERVE.

In a fœtus of 6 months. The IVth nucleus (IV) is shown giving off the fibres (F) of the IVth nerve which decussate dorsally in the anterior medullary velum (V). A, aqueduct of Sylvius ; L, medial longitudinal bundle with outlying cells of the IIIrd nucleus (Agduhr's stain ; × 18) (F. Vrabec).

the orbit) which are derived from this arch. The main motor nucleus is part of the visceral efferent column lying in the posterior portion of the metencephalon, close to the nucleus of the VIth nerve and serially homologous with the motor nuclei of the glosso-pharyngeal (3rd pharyngeal arch) and vagal nerves (4th, 5th and 6th pharyngeal arches). It has been suggested that the fibres supplying the muscles of the lids were ultimately derived from the IIIrd nucleus (Mendel, 1887) ; but it would appear more likely that they originate in a small subgroup of the main nucleus lying more dorsally in the visceral column (the superior facial nucleus) (Harman, 1903 ; Bruce and Pirie, 1908 ; Villiger, 1912 ; Vraa-Jensen, 1942). It is interesting that during development after the fibres have formed, the VIIth nucleus migrates, passing dorsally around the VIth nucleus so that the fibres, trailing after their parent cells, pursue a curious and complicated course, running dorsally and looping ventrally in the brain-stem before they emerge on the ventral aspect close to the nucleus itself. Kappers (1920) explained this on neurobiotactic grounds,[1] the curious and apparently purposeless loop being due to the migration of the facial towards the nucleus spinalis of the trigeminal from which its afferents are derived.

THE SENSORY NERVES

The sensory nerves to the head, associated with the Vth, VIIth, IXth and Xth cranial nerves are developed essentially from cells of the neural crest, the ridge of ectoderm which flanks each lateral margin of the neural plate,[2] and are thus serially homologous with the posterior root ganglia of the cord (Halley, 1955) ; in addition, however, it would seem that a contribution is derived from thickenings of ectoderm (placodes) overlying their sites of origin (Batten, 1957).

THE SENSORY ELEMENTS OF THE Vth (TRIGEMINAL) NERVE which assumes responsibility for the entire sensory supply for the ocular region (and, indeed, for practically all the face) are derived from the cells of the most anterior portion of the neural crest supplemented by cells from the localized surface ectodermal thickenings related to the ocular region and the first pharyngeal arch. These cells migrate to form the mass of the *semilunar ganglion* placed caudal and lateral to the primary head vein (the anterior cardinal vein) where they are apparent in the 4 mm. embryo (Lopez Marin, 1952). This large collection of neuroblasts is initially arranged as a small anterior and a larger posterior group which eventually fuse. The former, which determines the 1st or ophthalmic division of the nerve and innervates the fronto-nasal (paraxial) process (including the distribution of the naso-ciliary nerve and its anterior ethmoid branch) is a non-branchial component corresponding to the profundus nerve which innervates the cephalic end of the embryos of the lower vertebrates. The latter is the nerve of the 1st pharyngeal arch, and is distributed to the two (visceral) segments of this arch, one to the maxillary (2nd division) and the other to the mandibular (3rd division) process. According to Sakamoto (1952) the ophthalmic nerve is recognizable as early as the 5th week as a projection from the semilunar ganglion (Fig. 349). The naso-ciliary and frontal nerves and the lacrimal nerve are visible at the 6th and 7th week respectively, and all three are fully developed by the 13th week.

[1] Vol. I, p. 699; Vol. II, p. 769.   [2] p. 25.

The cells of the *mesencephalic nucleus of the trigeminal* are probably elements from the neural crest which have become included in the neural plate ; they are unique in the body since, although primary sensory neurons, they do not migrate to the periphery but remain in the brain-stem forming an " endoneural " afferent ganglion (Johnston, 1909 ; Kidd, 1910 ; Willems, 1911 ; Piatt, 1945 ; Pearson, 1949). The cells migrate forwards from the metencephalon so that the nucleus itself differentiates in the midbrain (Windle and Fitzgerald, 1942) ; it serves as a proprioceptive centre for the muscles of mastication supplied by the Vth nerve (May and Horsley, 1910 ;

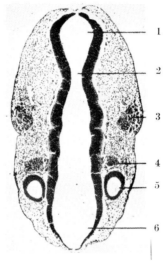

FIG. 349.—SECTION THROUGH THE HEAD END OF A 4 MM. EMBRYO (× 37)
(E. R. A. Cooper).

1, mesencephalon ; 2, isthmus rhombencephali ; 3, trigeminal ganglion and nerve ;
4, acoustic ganglion ; 5, otic vesicle ; 6, 4th ventricle.

Allen, 1919 ; Kidd, 1922 ; S. Cooper *et al.*, 1953), probably also for the extrinsic muscles of the eye (Freeman, 1925–27 ; Weinberg, 1928 ; Byrne, 1929 ; S. Cooper and Fillenz, 1952) and possibly from the mimetic muscles of the face (Bruesch, 1944 ; Pearson, 1945).

THE SENSORY ELEMENTS OF THE VIIth (FACIAL) NERVE are related to the 2nd pharyngeal arch, developed in part from the neural crest and in part from a small ectodermal placode related to this arch. They are closely related to the sensory elements of the VIIIth nerve and together the two groups form a single acoustico-facial primordium with which are incorporated cells from the wall of the otocyst. The anterior cells of this mass separate from the rest at an early stage (6 mm.) and migrate peripherally to form the geniculate ganglion on the main motor trunk of the facial nerve ; the central processes of these cells enter the central nervous system to terminate in the visceral afferent column, while their peripheral processes form the chorda tympani and the greater superficial petrosal nerves.

THE AUTONOMIC NERVES

The precise origin of the autonomic system is still in doubt although all authorities are agreed that it is ectodermal in nature. It has been contended that it derived from cells from the neural tube which have migrated along the anterior roots (Kuntz, 1934), but it is now generally accepted that its constituent cells arise from the neural crests[1] (Müller and Ingvar, 1923 ; Harrison, 1937–38 ; Yntema and Hammond, 1947).

THE SYMPATHETIC SYSTEM is constituted by cells from the thoracic and lumbar regions of the cord, reinforced by migrating cells from the cervical and lumbo-sacral regions, all of which travel peripherally to form a continuous chain with segmental enlargements dorsal to the paired dorsal aortæ, each column extending cranially along the aorta into the cervical region (the *sympathetic chains*). Nerve fibres (which eventually medullate) with their cells of origin in the visceral efferent columns of the central nervous system terminate in these sympathetic ganglia (*pre-ganglionic fibres*), while the non-medullated axons of the sympathetic neuroblasts are distributed peripherally as visceral nerves to the heart, lungs and abdominal organs or to the blood vessels, sweat glands and arrectores pilorum. Those supplying the orbit and eye travel along the carotid artery which they leave to enter the orbit about the 20 mm. stage.

Elements in the sympathetic chain derived from cells identical with the other sympathetic neuroblasts have a different fate ; since they stain characteristically with chromic salts, these para-ganglionic cells are called *chromaffin cells*. In the embryo they are scattered widely over the sympathetic system, but the only group which normally persists into adult life develops in the posterior abdominal wall medial to each gonad ; here in relationship with the cœlomic epithelium they give rise to the suprarenal glands.

THE CRANIAL PARASYMPATHETIC SYSTEM arises from pre-ganglionic fibres derived from cells in the visceral efferent column which pass out of the central nervous system along the IIIrd, VIIth, IXth and Xth cranial nerves to terminate in the ciliary, the spheno-palatine, the otic, the sub-maxillary and sublingual ganglia (Figs. 294, 299, 350).

The origin of the cells of the CILIARY GANGLION and therefore of the post-ganglionic fibres to the eye has given rise to considerable controversy. The adult gland in man contains some sympathetic cells, a few sensory cells from the Vth, but the major part of its cellular population is parasympathetic in nature. Phylogenetically the ganglion is essentially autonomic and associated solely with the IIIrd nerve. In fishes, amphibians and reptiles it has no connection with the Vth or sympathetic nerves, and the same relation exists in most mammals (Schwalbe, 1879 ; Peschel, 1893 ; Apolant, 1896 ; Christensen, 1936), while scattered ganglionic cells are often seen along the course of this nerve (Ganfini, 1911 ; Mobilio, 1912).[2]

[1] p. 26.   [2] For full discussion, see Vol. II, p. 859.

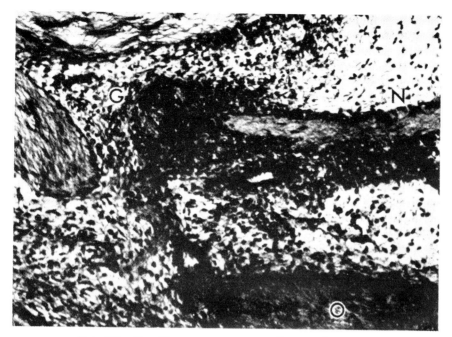

FIG. 350.—THE DEVELOPMENT OF THE CILIARY GANGLION.

In a fœtus of the 3rd month. The ganglion cells, G, are seen migrating into the orbit and from the anterior border of the ganglion a ciliary nerve, N, issues. O, optic nerve (H. & E. ; × 160) (F. Vrabec).

The source of these cells has given rise to considerable speculation. Some authors consider that the cells of all the cranial autonomic ganglia arise by migration along the course of the pre-ganglionic fibres (Stewart, 1920) ; others maintain that in addition they arise from the trigeminal also (Kuntz, 1934) ; while others believe that they migrate exclusively along the Vth (ciliary), the VIIth (facial) and the IXth cranial nerves (Cowgill and Windle, 1942). On the one hand, it has been said that the ciliary ganglion can arise independently of the semilunar ganglion (Yntema and Hammond, 1947) ; on the other, that it arises from its ophthalmic segment (Cowgill and Windle, 1942). The question in the meantime must be left undecided.

Allen. *J. comp. Neurol.*, **30**, 169 (1919).
Apolant. *Arch. mikr. Anat.*, **47**, 655 (1896).
  Arch. Anat. Physiol., Physiol. Abt., 344 (1896).
Batten. *J. Anat.*, **91**, 174, 471 (1957).
  J. comp. Neurol., **108**, 393 (1957).
Beevor. *Phil. Trans. B*, **200**, 1 (1909).
Bruce and Pirie. *Rev. Neurol. Psychiat.*, **6**, 685 (1908).
Bruesch. *J. comp. Neurol.*, **81**, 169 (1944).
Byrne. *Amer. J. Physiol.*, **88**, 151 (1929).
Christensen. *J. Anat.* (Lond.), **70**, 225 (1936).
Congdon. *Contrib. Embryol. Carneg. Instn.*, **14**, 47 (1922).
Cooper, E. R. A. *Brain*, **69**, 34, 50 (1946).
  Brit. J. Ophthal., **31**, 257 (1947).

Cooper, S., Daniel and Whitteridge. *J. Physiol.*, **120**, 471, 491, 514 (1953).
Cooper, S., and Fillenz. *J. Physiol.*, **118**, 49P (1952).
Cowgill and Windle. *J. comp. Neurol.*, **77**, 619 (1942).
Evans. Keibel and Mall's *Manual of Human Embryology*, Phila., **2**, 570 (1912).
Frazer. *J. Anat.* (Lond.), **63**, 7 (1928).
Freeman. *Arch. Neurol. Psychiat.* (Chicago), **14**, 111 (1925).
  J. nerv. ment. Dis., **65**, 381, 387 (1927).
Fuchs. *Anat. Hefte*, **28**, 1 (1905).
Ganfini. *Arch. ital. Anat. Embriol.*, **10**, 574 (1911).
Halley. *J. Anat.* (Lond.), **89**, 133 (1955).

Harman. *Trans. ophthal. Soc. U.K.*, **23**, 356
  (1903).
Harrison. *Anat. Anz.*, **85**, Erg., 3 (1937–38).
Huntington. *Anat. Rec.*, **2**, 19 (1908).
  Amer. J. Anat., **16**, 259 (1914).
Huntington and McClure. *Anat. Rec.*, **1**, 36
  (1907) ; **2**, 1 (1908).
Johnston. *J. comp. Neurol.*, **19**, 593 (1909).
Kampmeier. *Amer. J. Anat.*, **13**, 401 (1912).
Kappers. *Die vergl. Anat. d. Nervensystems d.
  Wirbeltiere*, Haarlem, **1** (1920).
Kappers, Huber and Crosby. *The Compara-
  tive Anatomy of the Nervous System of
  Vertebrates*, N.Y. (1936).
Kidd. *Rev. Neurol. Psychiat.*, **8**, 594, 673, 749
  (1910).
  Brit. J. Ophthal., **6**, 49 (1922).
Krause. *Z. Anat.*, **119**, 311 (1956).
Kuntz. *The Autonomic System*, London (1934).
Lopez Marin. *Arch. Soc. oftal. hisp.-amer.*,
  12, 367 (1952).
Mall. *Amer. J. Anat.*, **4**, 1 (1904).
Markowski. *Bull. Acad. Sci. Cracovie, B,
  (Sci. nat.)*, 590 (1911) ; 1 (1922).
May and Horsley. *Brain*, **33**, 175 (1910).
Mendel. *Münch. med. Wschr.*, **34**, 902 (1887).
Mobilio. *Monit. zool. Ital.*, **23**, 80 (1912).
Moffat. *Anat. Rec.*, **140**, 217 (1961).
Müller and Ingvar. *Arch. mikr. Anat.*, **99**,
  650 (1923).
Padget. *Contrib. Embryol. Carneg. Instn.*, **32**,
  205 (1948) ; **36**, 79 (1957).

Anat. Rec., **119**, 349 (1954).
  Amer. J. Anat., **98**, 307 (1956).
Pearson. *Anat. Rec.*, **91**, 294 (1945).
  J. comp. Neurol., **90**, 1 ; **91**, 147 (1949).
Peschel. *v. Graefes Arch. Ophthal.*, **39** (2), 1
  (1893).
Piatt. *J. comp. Neurol.*, **82**, 35 (1945).
Sabin. *Amer. J. Anat.*, **1**, 367 (1902).
  Anat. Rec., **6**, 335 (1912).
Sakamoto. *Acta Soc. ophthal. jap.*, **56**, 1355
  (1952) ; **57**, 146 (1953).
Schwalbe. *Jena. Z. Naturwiss.*, **13**, 173
  (1879).
Stewart. *J. comp. Neurol.*, **31**, 163 (1920).
Streeter. *Amer. J. Anat.*, **18**, 145 (1915).
  Contrib. Embryol. Carneg. Instn., **8**, 5
  (1918).
Tandler. *Morph. Jb.*, **30**, 275 (1902).
Villiger. *Brain and Spinal Cord*, Phila.
  (1912).
Vraa-Jensen. *The Motor Nucleus of the Facial
  Nerve*, Copenhagen (1942).
de Vriese. *Arch. Biol.* (Liège), **21**, 357 (1905).
Weinberg. *J. comp. Neurol.*, **46**, 249 (1928).
Willems. *Le Névraxe*, **12**, 7 (1911).
Windle and Fitzgerald. *J. comp. Neurol.*, **77**,
  597 (1942).
Yntema and Hammond. *Biol. Rev.*, **22**, 344
  (1947).
Yoffey and Courtice. *Lymphatics, Lymph
  and Lymphoid Tissue*, London (1956).
Zimmermann. *Illinois med. dent. Monog.*, **3**,
  1 (1940).

THE NOSE AND NASAL SINUSES

We have already seen[1] that the first evidence of the development of
the nose is the bilateral ectodermal thickenings which form the olfactory
placodes ; these appear at the 5 to 6 mm. stage (Streeter, 1945) and rapidly
become buried by the growth of the surrounding mesoderm to form the
olfactory pits, bounded medially by the fronto-nasal process and laterally
by the lateral nasal process. We have also traced the upward and medial
growth of the maxillary processes below the optic vesicle and the olfactory
pits, at first to meet the lateral nasal process and then to progress medially
underneath it, so that, with the disappearance of a plug of ectoderm, the
two olfactory pits become continuous with the PRIMITIVE NASAL CAVITY.
After the rupture of the bucco-pharyngeal membrane, this again becomes
continuous with the foregut to form the PRIMITIVE BUCCAL CAVITY, an
extensive single chamber bounded by the ectoderm of the stomatodæum
above and below by the endoderm of the foregut.

With its continued forward and medial growth, the maxillary process
next overlaps the lower part of the fronto-nasal process to meet with its
fellow of the opposite side and form the tissues of the upper lip and the

[1] p. 211.

alveolar process of the maxilla, while along the line of its fusion with the lateral nasal process the anlage of the lacrimal passages is laid.[1] As they grow forwards and medially the maxillary processes depress the fronto-nasal process to form the primitive nasal septum, the free lower surface of which forms the primitive palate (Frazer, 1931 ; Boyd, 1933 ; Streeter, 1948).

The next step in development is the medial growth of the palatal process from the inner aspect of each maxillary process ; these eventually fuse with the primitive palate and the downgrowing nasal septum and with each other, dividing the anterior part of the primitive buccal cavity into two, the nasal cavity and the mouth. On the lateral side of the former ectodermal elevations appear which become invaded by mesoderm and ultimately differentiate into osteogenic tissue, forming the superior, middle and inferior conchæ.

THE ACCESSORY NASAL SINUSES appear late in fœtal life or after birth (Turner, 1901 ; Coffin, 1905 ; Schaeffer, 1910 ; Fawcett, 1911). They are developed from the nasal mucous membrane as ectodermal buds which push their way into the surrounding mesoderm. The first to become evident is the maxillary sinus which, indeed, is the only one to be more than a mere rudiment at birth ; it appears as a depression in the nasal wall just below the middle concha and grows laterally into the maxilla but does not reach its full development until the time of the permanent dentition. The sphenoid bud appears before birth, is a small but definite cavity at birth, and at the age of 5 years has reached the pre-sphenoid bone ; it undergoes two periods of rapid growth about the age of 10 and at puberty. The ethmoid cells are present as epithelial dimples during the last month of fœtal life ; at birth they are still very rudimentary. From the diverticulum destined to form the anterior ethmoid sinus the frontal sinus develops ; it invades the frontal bone during the 1st or 2nd year of life, grows slowly during the years of childhood, develops rapidly at puberty and is not fully formed until a period varying from 20 to 25 years of age. All the sinuses, indeed, increase in size during the period of skeletal growth and there is some evidence that this is rendered possible by the active destruction of the surrounding bone by the mucous membrane.

Boyd. J. Anat. (Lond.), **67**, 409 (1933).
Coffin. Amer. J. med. Sci., **129**, 297 (1905).
Fawcett. J. Anat. Physiol., **45**, 378 (1911).
Frazer. A Manual of Embryology, London (1931).

Schaeffer. Amer. J. Anat., **10**, 313 (1910).
J. Morph., **21**, 613 (1910).
Streeter. Contrib. Embryol. Carneg. Instn., **31**, 27 (1945) ; **32**, 133 (1948).
Turner. Accessory Sinuses of the Nose, London (1901).

[1] p. 241.

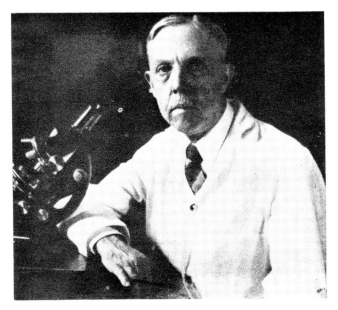

FIG. 351.—PIERRE MASSON
[1880–1959].

CHAPTER IX
THE OCULAR PIGMENT

It will be seen in the subsequent discussion that the origin of pigment cells remained for many years an enigma. The investigator who first made order out of chaos and evolved a comprehensive theory based on prolonged and painstaking research, tracing their origin from the nervous system, was PIERRE MASSON [1880–1959] ; for this reason we are introducing this chapter with his photograph (Fig. 351). Masson was born in Dijon in France where he pursued his early medical studies ; thereafter he went to Paris and eventually worked at the Pasteur Institute with Borrel under the directorship of Metchnikoff. After an interlude in the Army during the First World War, he became titular professor in pathological anatomy at Strasbourg and in 1926, the year in which his original and now classical observations on the origin of melanophores were published, he was appointed to a similar position in the department of pathology in the University of Montreal where he took a large part in organizing the service of pathological anatomy then being instituted in the Faculty of Medicine and where he worked until his retirement. Masson was a histologist of genius and an artist who revelled in the " magic of colours " obtainable with the multitude of staining agents then becoming available ; his name is perpetuated in Masson's stain for collagen ; and to him the greens and the yellows were based upon the colours of " une vieille Chartreuse ". His main work concerned the histopathology of tumours, a number of which (benign genital mesothelioma, spermatocytoma, appendicular neuroma, glomus tumours, and many others) he designated for the first time. His book, *Diagnostic des Tumeurs* (1923) has been described as a revelation for the pathological world of his generation both because of the elegance of its presentation and writing, and for its broad philosophical treatment of the morphogenesis of neoplasias in association with general biology. Not the least of the advances for which he was responsible was his work on pigmented tumours and for this as well as his many contributions to the science of his choice his name will always be remembered in French-Canadian medicine long after the charm and vivacity of his personality have been forgotten.

MELANIN ($\mu\epsilon\lambda\alpha\varsigma$, black) seems to be formed as a biological adaptation for the absorption of radiant energy[1]; it is therefore typically found in the skin and the eye, especially in races that are exposed to tropical conditions. To a less extent it is met with in internal organs such as the central nervous system (substantia nigra, pia mater), or in association with nerves (especially the sympathetic) in the heart and great vessels, the retroperitoneal and mesenteric tissue, and the gut.

---

[1] The primary function of melanin as an absorbent of radiant energy is occasionally modified ; thus it is used for the purpose of protection in *Sepia* to cover its retreat from enemies, when it is extruded from the ink-sac, a diverticulum of the rectum (Turchini and Ladreyt, 1921). The changes in colour undergone by some animals to harmonize with their environment or to make themselves more conspicuous are similar although less dramatic examples of this secondary biological function. (See Vol. I, p. 82.)

THE DISTRIBUTION OF MELANIN IN THE EYE

In the eye itself melanin is found primarily in two tissues : (1) in the pigmented layer of the *neural epithelium* (of the retina, ciliary body and iris), and (2) in the *uveal tract*. Its density and distribution in the former locality are very constant ; in the latter they are very variable.

Although in the dark and yellow races the iris is heavily pigmented before birth (Usher, 1920 ; Mijsberg, 1948), we have already noted that in the white races the pigment develops after birth,[1] and that, depending on the extent of its development, the adult iris may be light blue with its architecture delicately outlined, or dark brown with the intricacy of the pattern obscured. A *yellow colour* in the pattern of the iris is not uncommon. This has usually been regarded as a diluted brown pigment (Galloway, 1912), but Davenport (1927) considered that it resembled a golden yellow pigment related to, but not identical with melanin, such as is met with in the skin of the Mongolian. The dramatic and variegated colour-displays seen in the irides of invertebrates and many fishes, amphibians and birds, are due to carotenoids such as occur in man in the corpus luteum, the adrenals and the pigment epithelium of the retina (Kühne, 1879 ; Lo Cascio, 1923).[2]

From the stroma of the uveal tract chromatophores may migrate into the ciliary muscle and the inner layers of the sclera, and not infrequently they travel along the perivascular channels in the anterior region of the sclera to appear subconjunctivally as pigmented areas in association with the anterior ciliary vessels and nerves. These localized pigment deposits are not congenital, but appear after about 6 weeks (Augstein, 1912). Uveal pigment may also be found physiologically in the optic nerve, owing to the migration of chromatophores into the mesodermal septa and the tissues of the lamina cribrosa (Müller, 1872 ; Berger, 1882 ; Oguchi, 1909 ; Scheerer, 1922). This type of pigmentation is more common and pronounced in darker races (Japanese, Ogawa, 1906) and among animals (Hoffmann, 1883 ; Ogawa, 1905).

Pigment in the *conjunctiva*, while in association with the eye, comes into the category of the pigment of the skin. In the white races of mankind it is normally absent except in the basal epithelial cells in a ring round the limbus, but in the dark races it is found also in the basal cells of the conjunctival epithelium and in the loose episcleral tissue.

In the eyes of animals there is usually more pigment in this situation ; according to Hauschild (1910) it is either more abundant in the conjunctiva, in which case the sclera is pigment-free, or in the sclera when the conjunctival pigment is represented by a ring round the corneal margin. The same writer has divided the racial distribution in man into three types :

1. *Negroid type* (Negroes, Melanesians), with deep pigmentation in the superficial layers of the conjunctiva and round poorly-branching cells in the iris. Pergens (1898) noted a marked peri-corneal pigment ring in the Negroes of the Congo.

[1] Vol. II, p. 169.   [2] Vol. I, p. 88.

2. *Mongolian type* (Chinese, Japanese, Malayans, Indians), with deep pigmenta-tion in the basal cells of the conjunctiva and finely branched pigment cells in the iris. Steiner (1905) noted that the natives of Java showed a mottling of pigment over the conjunctiva.

3. *European type*. The iris pigment is of finely branched cells, and the conjunctiva is white with very reduced sporadic pigment practically entirely confined to a peri-limbal pigment ring in the basal cells of the epithelium which is evident in 0·3% of people (H. Virchow, 1910 ; Redslob, 1922). As animals are inbred and become domesticated the ocular pigment tends to diminish ; a similar tendency seems to be evident among the races of mankind.

THE NATURE AND ORIGIN OF MELANIN

In general melanin is granular in form and ranges in colour from pale yellow to black, the darker melanins tending to take the form of rods while the more lightly coloured melanins usually appear as small spheres (Rawles, 1948 ; Tousimis and Fine, 1959). Its chemical composition has been found to vary greatly, partly because it is difficult to obtain in the pure state and partly because it is probable that the term includes several distinct but related bodies. The elementary composition has been found to vary for carbon from 48·95 to 60·02%, for hydrogen 3·05 to 7·57%, for nitrogen 8·1 to 13·77%, and the sulphur value is usually high (Abderhalden, 1915). Lo Cascio (1915) gave the following figures for the melanin of the choroid :

C, 54·45% ; H, 5·88% ; N, 12·35% ; O, 26·08% ; S, 1·77% ; Fe, 0·101%.

In a previous volume we have discussed the origin of melanin[1] and shown that it is formed as an end-product in the enzymic oxidation of a number of alternative groupings in the protein molecule (tyrosine, phenyl-alanine, tryptophane, etc.), the main enzymes involved being phenylalanine hydroxylase and tyrosinase ; whatever the metabolic pathway, the processes involved are essentially similar.[2] It is now generally accepted that colour-less substances of the nature of 3,4-dihydroxyphenylalanine (dopa) are brought by the blood stream to specific cells in which they are oxidized and turned into coloured pigment ; a cell which synthesizes melanin in this way is called a MELANOBLAST (βλαστός, a sprout) (or CHROMATOBLAST). The pigment is formed in association with the Golgi apparatus, an origin demon-strated by the fractional destruction of the cell's constituents by graded x-radiation (Güttes, 1953 ; Moyer, 1960). A cell which contains the formed pigment is called a MELANOPHORE (φόρος, a bearer) or CHROMATOPHORE.

Melanin is closely allied to adrenaline for the two substances are derived from the same precursors and form alternative end-products in the catechol metabolism. When the pigment cells are stimulated to proliferate so that there is an increase of the oxi-dative ferment, a pigmented tumour is the result or a generalized melanomatosis ; when, owing to cachexia or some dyscrasia of the adrenals, these glands fail to utilize

[1] Vol. I, p. 118.
[2] Bloch (1917), Figge (1940), Hogeboom and Adams (1942), Herrmann and Boss (1945), Lerner (1950), and others.

the chromogenic substance for the manufacture of adrenaline, an increase in pigment is the result, as is seen in Addison's disease, the effects of which appear in the skin generally and even in the epithelial cells of the cornea (Meesmann, 1920) ; and if there is no enzyme present, pigment cannot be formed and the condition of albinism results.

THE NATURE AND ORIGIN OF PIGMENT CELLS

Associated with the eye, four types of pigmented cell exist : (1) the most characteristic are the large chromatophores of the uveal tract, flat cells with an infinite variety of branched processes frequently forming a syncytium and with granular pigment scattered throughout[1] ; (2) in the iris, small round clump cells occur devoid of processes,[2] in which the pigment is rod-shaped and concentrated near the nucleus ; these bear a considerable resemblance to (3) the cells of the pigmentary epithelium of the retina.[3] Finally (4), pigmented cells occur in the conjunctiva resembling those seen in the skin. About the nature and ultimate origin of the retinal pigment cells from the central nervous system there is no dubiety ; but the nature and origin of chromatophores have given rise to a great deal of controversy.

Originally von Recklinghausen (1882) thought that the pigmented cells of "nævi" arose from endothelium ; but his view was contested by Unna (1893) who put forward the hypothesis that pigmented cells were confined to the epithelium, and that the cells of pigmented tumours were derived directly or indirectly from this layer. His views received wide acceptance, notably by Kromayer (1893–1905) and Wieting and Hamdi (1907), who considered that the uveal pigment migrated from the retinal epithelium. In a similar way Kornfeld (1920–21), in a series of striking researches, showed that in the skin of frog embryos the subepithelial sheet of pigment was formed by the migration of epithelial cells through the basement membrane into the layers of the corium. Krompecher (1908–23) further contended that the epithelial cells not only became morphologically similar to connective tissue elements, but also assumed their function, producing collagenous fibrils (" desmoplasia "). In very extended researches, however, Ribbert (1911) developed the opposite theory that pigmentation depended upon a specialized connective tissue (mesoblastic) cell, the chromatophore, and he maintained that pigmentation and the formation of pigmented tumours were functions of the mesoderm. Acton (1922), basing his conclusions largely on comparative morphology, summarized the arguments of this school : he considered that the pigmentation of fishes, amphibians and reptiles arose from a subepithelial mesodermal sheet, from which diffusion of pigment into the epidermis may occur secondarily, and that this sheet is represented in the white races of man in the choroid, the genital areas, and in pigmented moles. Three view-points thus arose : some considered the genesis of pigment ectodermal, some mesodermal, while others maintained that its origin might be in both these layers.

A large amount of chemical evidence was brought forward substantiating the first of these theories. Bloch (1917) found that epidermal cells alone gave a positive " dopa reaction " (the basal cells of the rete Malpighii, the basal cells of hair follicles, and the branched cells of Langerhans), while mesodermal cells were negative ; and his views were enthusiastically developed by many pathologists (Spencer, 1923 ; Dawson, 1925 ; and others). According to these, pigment was formed through the activity of

[1] Vol. II, Fig. 193.   [2] Vol. II, Fig. 194.   [3] Vol. II, Fig. 253.

epithelial cells only, which were therefore the only melanoblasts. These cells might migrate inwards towards the mesodermal layers, or they might discharge their pigment granules which thereafter underwent phagocytosis by connective tissue cells ; meso-dermal cells could therefore act as melanophores. This view received confirmation from the fact that when melanin is injected subcutaneously it undergoes phagocytosis in this way by connective tissue cells ; moreover, pigmentation produced artificially by ultra-violet light appears in the deeper germinal layers of the epidermis (Meirowsky, 1906–8). The only cases, in fact, where connective tissue cells and endothelial cells were found to show a positive " dopa reaction " were in neoplasic cells where con-ditions are abnormal and the amount of melanogen is enormously increased (d'Agata, 1922). So far as the skin is concerned, therefore, the chemical evidence pointed to the preponderant role of the epithelium in the elaboration of pigment where the specialized pigment cells developed *in situ* and had an intrinsic origin.

A completely new aspect to the question was introduced by the work of Masson (1926–31) on pigmented tumours of the skin. He showed in a very convincing way in work which has been amply corroborated (Foot, 1932 ; Laidlaw, 1932 ; Laidlaw and Murray, 1933), that the characteristic cells of nævi are neither epithelial nor meso-blastic, but *neuro-ectodermal* in origin. In the skin the medullated sensory nerves end in the dermis in Meissner's corpuscles, the cells of the sheath of Schwann becoming differentiated into a corpuscle of polyhedral, pigment-free cells, while the non-medul-lated nerves enter the epithelial layer and end in the corpuscles of Merkel-Ranvier. Masson traced the development of nævus cells in all stages from these two types of cell, and therefore considered these tumours as neo-formations of the neural end-apparatus, situated either among the epithelial cells or in the dermis beneath them. He visualized these neural cells around which the nerve fibres terminate as forming the normal melanoblast of the part, either the melanoblasts of the epidermis or the cells of Langerhans in the basal layers.

This hypothesis necessarily implies an extrinsic origin of the prospective pigment cells either of the skin or the eye, and suggests that they migrate from the central nervous system to the periphery as colourless cells which acquire pigment at a later stage. It would seem most likely that the central origin is the *neural crests* (Borcea, 1909 ; Harrison, 1910 ; Weidenreich, 1912). In urodele amphibians an extensive variety of transplantation, explantation and deficiency experiments by DuShane (1934–38) has made it clear that in these species the pigment cells are thus derived. Similarly, in the chick, the grafting experiments of Rawles (1940) showed that the area of the blastula potentially capable of giving rise to pigment cells corresponds exactly with the area capable of forming neural tissue, a potentiality which later be-comes restricted to the neural crest (Fig. 354). Dorris (1936–38), experimenting at a later stage of development, explanted strips of the neural fold anterior to the first somite in early chick embryos (6 to 10-somite stage) and found that branched pigment cells with actively amœboid potentialities developed not only in culture but also when the explant was grafted to the base of the limb of another embryo (Fig. 352). This work was confirmed by Eastlick (1939) who transplanted the limb buds of 40- to 70-hour chick embryos to the body-wall of the same and other breeds and found that if the transections left the neural crest intact the resulting limb was non-pigmented while if the cuts were made to include part of the neural crest pigmentation of the limb resulted (Fig. 353). Similar findings were obtained by Brihaye-van Geertruyden (1962) in transplanting the optic vesicles of guinea-pigs.

The origin of the pigment cells of amphibians, birds and mammals is thus un-doubtedly established. Comparative grounds suggest that all vertebrate pigment cells have a common embryological origin. We may therefore assume that the origin of melanoblasts is from the neural crest, a hypothesis now generally accepted (DuShane, 1948 ; Boyd, 1949 ; Niu, 1954–59 ; Rawles, 1947–59 ; and others) (Fig. 354).

Figs. 352 and 353.—The Production of Pigment from the Neural Crest
(after R. W. Raven).

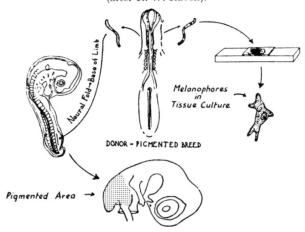

Fig. 352.—The experiments of Dorris. Neural folds of the donor embryo produce pigment cells in tissue culture and when grafted to the base of the limb-bud of another embryo.

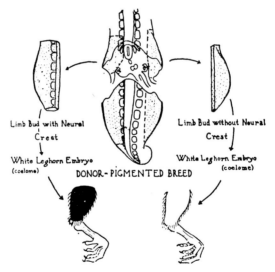

Fig. 353.—The experiments of Eastlick. The limb primordia are grafted with or without accompanying neural crest cells, depending upon the level of the cut made in removing the limb. If crest cells are included the limb develops pigment.

In the early developmental stages in amphibians the prospective melanoblasts cannot be differentiated morphologically or histologically from the other embryonic cells of the neural crest, but eventually they migrate as non-pigmented amœboid cells into the regions destined to become pigmented ; in most vertebrates the pigment develops when the cells have reached their final destination. The exact pathways of migration, however, are in most cases unknown. The systematic isolation of various

portions of the embryo at successive stages of development and the testing of the
capacity of such isolated tissue for the potentiality of producing pigment in grafts
have demonstrated that melanoblasts have reached their definitive location in all
parts of the chick embryo by the 4th day of incubation and in all parts of the mouse
embryo by the 12th day of gestation (Rawles, 1947) ; they have been found in the
fœtal skin of the Negro early in the 3rd month (Zimmermann, 1950).

Once these cells have reached their destination, the pattern of pigment laid down
would appear to depend upon an interaction between the melanoblasts themselves
and between them and their tissue-substrates.   Like any other embryonic cell the
melanoblast is endowed with a complement of genes which would appear to determine
its particular fate, while the physiological condition of the substrate may be influenced
by numerous environmental factors such as vitamins, temperature or light, among

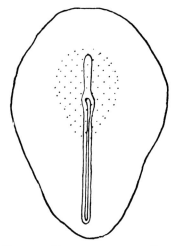

FIG. 354.—PIGMENT FORMATION IN THE CHICK EMBRYO.

The stippled area in the early embryo which corresponds to the region which produces
neural tissue in chorio-allantoic grafts is capable of giving rise to melanophores in host
feathers when grafted (after Rawles).

which one of the most important influences is hormonal control, particularly through
the hypophysis (Chavin, 1956).   It should be emphasized, however, that although
changes in the physiological condition of the substrate can modify or change the
melanoblastic response, including the amount of melanin produced, the specific
response is always in accordance with the genetic constitution (Rawles, 1948 ; Willeir,
1948).

THE CONJUNCTIVAL PIGMENTED CELLS

In the conjunctiva the pigmentation found in both normal and pathological conditions is in a similar case to all other pigmented areas of the
skin. Melanoblastic cells can be detected by a process of silver impregnation whereby the colourless mother substance is oxidized into melanin
(Masson, 1913) ; and using this method Redslob (1922) demonstrated that
the deeper cells of the limbal conjunctiva were invariably potential melanoblasts, as also were the corresponding cells of the caruncle, taking on a

deep pigmentation on oxidation. These cells correspond to the deep cells of Langerhans, the chromogenic agents in the skin.

This property may have some determining influence on the frequency of malignant neoplasms at the limbus or the caruncle. Since blood is required to supply one of the constituents necessary to elaborate melanin, the corneal epithelium is achromogenic ; but when vascularized pathologically it acquires this potentiality secondarily (Redslob, 1922).

THE UVEAL PIGMENTED CELLS

CHROMATOPHORES. So far as the uveal tract is concerned, however, difficulties in interpretation arose so long as the controversy existed between the advocates of the ectodermal and mesodermal hypotheses of the origin of

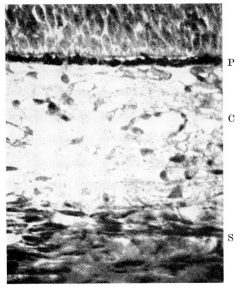

FIG. 355.—THE CHRONOLOGICAL DEVELOPMENT OF PIGMENT.

In a fœtus of 5 months. The pigmentary layer of the retina, P, is heavily pigmented but the choroid, C, shows no trace of pigmentation. The sclera, S, is below ($\times$ 262) (F. Vrabec).

melanoblasts. The advocates of the ectodermal theory contended that in the eye the retinal epithelium took the place of the epidermis of the skin and that the uveal tract corresponded to the corium ; it followed that the pigment of the choroid and iris was derived from the retina, either by the migration of cells or pigment (Lewis, 1903 ; Spencer, 1923 ; Knight, 1924 ; Dawson, 1925 ; and others) and, as an important corollary, that pigmented tumours in these tissues were carcinomata and not sarcomata.

This migration of retinal pigment cells into the choroid in embryonic life, however, is a purely hypothetical supposition, which has never been observed in fact. In the eye of the embryo rabbit, Güttes (1953) showed that the pigment of the epithelium appeared initially about the 13th to 14th day, while the first appearance of pigment in the uveal tissue was at 22 days. In man we have seen that the retinal pigment appears in the outer layer of the optic cup at about the 4th week of intra-uterine life, the choroidal not until the 5th, or even the 7th month of fœtal life, long after the formation of the barrier offered by the membrane of Bruch, and there is no evidence of migration from the one to the other (Fig. 355). Moreover, pigment appears first in the outer layers of the choroid where it is farthest from the retina (Wieting and Hamdi, 1907 ; von Szily, 1911 ; Redslob, 1925), and in animals provided with a tapetum the choroid outside this structure is normally pigmented while the retinal epithelium in this region is free from pigment. Further, we have seen that the mesodermal pupillary membrane atrophies before the ectodermal part of the iris has grown forwards to join it ; sometimes remnants of the atrophied tissue remain isolated on the anterior surface of the lens, and these, like other parts of the iris stroma, frequently become pigmented. It seems most improbable that any retinal pigment could have migrated to this region, with which it never had connection, even indirectly through the blood stream. Finally, cases of anophthalmos have been recorded wherein the eye was represented by mesodermal tissue alone without any epiblastic constituents, and the mesoblastic elements have been laden with pigment (van Duyse, 1899, in man ; Collins and Parsons, 1903, in a chick ; see Collins, 1926).

It is true that in the early stages of embryonic life the retinal epithelium is dopa-positive while the choroid is negative (Bloch, 1917), but Miescher (1922) showed that if the reaction is tested just at the stage before the choroidal pigment first appears, a positive reaction is obtained here also ; this proves the presence of the oxidizing ferment. With the silver impregnation method of Masson (1913), Redslob (1922) showed that the colourless mother substance (melanogen) was also present in the choroid during this time (6 to $6\frac{1}{2}$ months of fœtal life). Since, therefore, the two essential constituents are present in this tissue, it seems clear that the pigment is elaborated here. The only difference between the eye and the skin is that in the former melanogenesis is normally apparent during a short period only, while in the latter the potentiality is retained so that the skin may be activated at any time to produce more pigment (for example, in response to illumination). The only exception to this is in the malignant type of neoplasia in which the pigmented cells of the eye, normally dopa-negative after birth, revert to their embryonic activity and again become dopa-positive and resume the manufacture of melanin. The formation of pigment in tumours is thus merely an expression of changed metabolic activity and is in no sense essential to the character of the growth, a fact, as initially pointed out by R. Virchow (1863), in accordance with the great variation in the content of pigment from complete absence to intense concentration which is met with in primary and metastatic intra-ocular neoplasms.

The nature of the cells within the choroid wherein pigment is elaborated has again given rise to controversy. Rieke (1891) suggested that the uveal pigment was elaborated in fixed stromal cells, but the transformation of a non-pigmented to a pigmented mesenchymal cell apparently does not occur on tissue culture (Bisceglie, 1932). More recent experimental work on lower vertebrates has verified the origin of the melanoblasts from the neural crests.

Thus in grafting experiments in two different species of amphibia Barden (1942) showed that when optic vesicles of one species were transplanted into a host belonging to the other species, the migrant cells of the neural crest of the host became the iris pigment cells of the grafted eye so that the normal pattern of pigment characteristic of the host developed in the grafted eye. If, however, the neural crest of the host is removed the graft does not become pigmented. This would seem to demonstrate that in amphibians the uveal pigment is derived from the neural crest. Moreover, Ris (1941), noting the marked difference between the abundant and well-formed retinal pigment and the scanty pigmentation of the choroid in the fowl, found that on grafting fragments of the optic vesicle of the chick onto another chick embryo, pigment of the retinal type only was formed ; this would suggest that the retinal pigment epithelium apparently is incapable of forming pigment of the choroidal type. On the other hand, if a complete optic vesicle with a portion of the adjacent brain were grafted, a mass of melano-blasts of the uveal type spreads out in the choroid. Finally, it was shown by Brini (1949–53) who transplanted choroidal tissue from black Alsatian chick embryos to white Leghorns, that no pigmentation was seen if the experiment were done before migration of cells from the neural crests (10 to 11-somite stage), but occurred invariably thereafter.

These experiments would appear to show that in amphibians and birds the retinal and choroidal pigments have independent origins, the choroidal melanoblasts originating from the neural crest and the retinal pigment developing *in situ* in the ectodermal cells of the outer layer of the optic cup. No proof has yet been obtained in the higher vertebrates, however, that the same facts apply to mammals (King, 1937 ; Brini, 1953). Nevertheless, in view of the conclusive demonstration of the nervous origin of the cutaneous melanoblasts in mammals, it would appear logical to accept the hypothesis of a common origin of the melanoblasts of both the skin and the uvea.

The theory of a neural origin of the uveal chromatophores is supported by their nervous connections. In the chick the chromatophores are in close connection with the nerve-endings of the choroid from the beginning, and innervation of the cells always precedes the development of pigment (Nordmann and Stoll, 1947). In man these cells are also richly supplied with sympathetic nerves and it will be remembered that the sympathetic system is also derived from the neural crests (Münch, 1904 ; Lauber, 1908 ; Schock,

1910 ; and others)[1]. It is well known that interference with their nerve supply frequently alters the characteristics of these cells, a sympathetic paralysis, for example, frequently leading to their depigmentation, while they have been seen to change their shape, lose their characteristic processes, and become spherical (Komoto, 1915 ; Collins, 1926). Such an appearance bears a striking resemblance to the rapid pigmentary transformations determined by neural influences which occur in the integument of some lower animals, particularly the frog (Hogben and Winton, 1922–23), and can also be readily brought about in the iris of this animal if the nerves to the eye are sectioned (Kropp, 1927).[2]

The theory of the origin of the choroidal pigment from the neural crests receives further support from the impressive body of evidence which has now accumulated on the neurogenic origin of uveal melanomata. Since the nature of these depends on that of the chromatophores the same differences of view were put forward : that they were endothelial (v. Recklinghausen, 1882), mesodermal (Ribbert, 1897–1911 ; Acton,

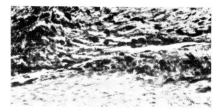

FIG. 356.—NÆVUS OF THE LONG POSTERIOR CILIARY NERVE.

Showing a proliferation of tumour cells from the cells of the sheath of Schwann and the accompanying pigment cells. Underneath is the ciliary nerve entering the tumour and above are the tumour cells (Theobald).

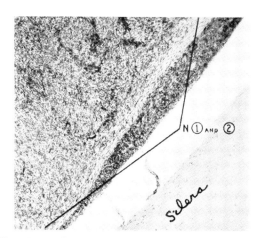

FIG. 357.—MALIGNANT MELANOMA OF THE CHOROID.

Proliferation of Schwann cells into bundles of tumour cells growing at right angles to the nerve at N (1) and (2) (G. Theobald).

[1] p. 268.   [2] See Vol. II, p. 854.

1922), a mixture of both (Fuchs, 1882 ; Coppez, 1901 ; Collins, 1926), or ectoderma (Unna, 1893 ; Krompecher, 1908–23 ; Wolfrum, 1909 ; Bloch, 1917–21 ; Kornfeld, 1920–21 ; Dawson, 1925). The work of Masson (1926–31) on the neurogenic origin of melanomata of the skin, however, transformed the situation and the researches of Theobald (1937) and Brihaye-van Geertruyden (1963) conclusively showed that both nævi and malignant melanomata of the uveal tract have a comparable ectodermal origin from proliferation of the cells of Schwann of the ciliary nerves as they traverse the ocular tissue, and are therefore derived from the neural crests (Figs. 356–7).

CLUMP CELLS. The origin of the clump cells first described by Koganei (1885) in the iris has also given rise to speculation. The perinuclear distribution of the rod-shaped pigmented granules so characteristic of the ectodermal cells of the retinal pigment epithelium led Fuchs (1885) and Elschnig and Lauber (1907) to suggest that they had migrated from the homologous ectodermal layers on the posterior aspect of the iris in a manner comparable to the wandering of the epithelial pigment cells into the retina in cases of chorio-retinitis. This view seems to be confirmed by the fact that they frequently remain dark in blue irides, and appear to have an arrangement radiating outwards from the three spurs (of Fuchs, von Michel, and Grunert) of the pigmentary epithelium and to be closely associated with the muscular derivatives of the ectodermal layers of this tissue (Salzmann, 1912 ; Wolfrum, 1922). Moreover, they are developed at a very early stage in embryonic life in association with the pigmentation of the ectodermal layers before chromatophores of the stroma are evident (Lauber, 1908) ; and in cases of partial albinism wherein the uveal pigment is absent these cells may be present (Lauber, 1908 ; Pearson, Nettleship and Usher, 1911). In Collins's opinion (1926) clump cells were simply metamorphosed chromatophores ; but while the uveal chromatophores do on occasion assume a spherical shape, this does not invalidate the arguments on which the probable ectodermal nature of the true cells of Koganei was determined.

A variant of the hypothesis of the mesenchymal origin of uveal pigment was put forward by Sondermann (1950–51) who suggested that the mesenchymal pigment of the eye is formed in the nuclei of the fœtal erythroblasts and is derived from their karyorrhexis. For this view, however, there seems little substantial evidence.

THE RETINAL PIGMENTED CELLS

The ectodermal retinal pigment (FUCHSIN) has long been considered to be different in type from the uveal pigment (melanin) (Kühne, 1879 ; Luna, 1920 ; Miescher, 1923), but it would seem that the differences are not fundamental. Apart from the small droplets of lipoid substances collected preferentially towards the base of the cells (Lo Cascio, 1923), biochemical investigations of homogenates in the chick suggest that the pigment in the retinal epithelium is produced by the enzymic oxidation of tyrosine to melanin, a reaction catalysed by tyrosinase (Miyamoto and Fitzpatrick, 1957). The mode of origin of the retinal and uveal pigments would therefore seem to be the same. In chick embryonic eyes Harrison (1951) found that two inductive factors were present in this layer, a growth factor and a pigment factor, separable by dialysis and fractional centrifugation ; these were found in young embryos (less than 24 somites). The pigment develops in the (ectodermal) cells in the outer layer of the optic vesicle ; its origin from the nervous system is therefore beyond doubt. That its appearance depends on

FIGS. 358 and 359.—THE DEVELOPMENT OF PIGMENT IN THE OUTER LAYER OF THE OPTIC CUP (G. Renard).

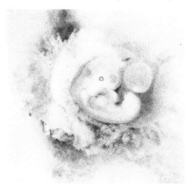

FIG. 358.—In an embryo of 8 mm.

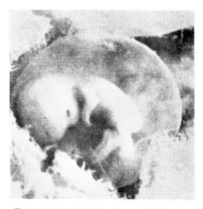

FIG. 359.—In an embryo of 12 mm.

the presence of blood-borne melanogenic substances is suggested by the fact that the outer layer of the optic cup becomes pigmented only when it is clothed by a vascular plexus.[1] This occurs in man at the 5·5 to 6 mm. stage, before the migration of the potential melanoblasts from the neural crests (Figs. 358 and 359). Moreover, the morphological differences between the two types of pigment are more apparent than real. In the uvea, pigment appears as round granules scattered uniformly throughout the cell ; in the pigment

[1] p. 101.

epithelium it tends to be concentrated around the nuclei, and its microscopic appearance varies—in the outer part of the cells it is round and granular somewhat resembling that found in the choroid, while towards the inner part it takes the form of crystalline needles about 1.5μ long (Raehlmann, 1907). It is interesting that in the iris of the cat Wolfrum (1922) found that the same type of cell could contain both morphological types and that the one would appear to replace the other. Moreover, in tissue-culture melanoblasts may contain pigment in solution in the cytoplasm of the cell or as particulate inclusions which may take the form of rods, granules or crystals (Raven, 1950). Electron-microscopic studies have shown that the granular pigment develops initially in tiny vacuoles in the basal zone of the epithelial cell without relation to the mitochondria (Yokoyama, 1961). Histological evidence indicates that all the pigment of the retinal epithelium is originally amorphous and granular (up to 6 weeks) and becomes crystalline only at a later date (Wieting and Hamdi, 1907 ; Redslob, 1925) ; the change is evident near the optic disc at 3 months, reaches the equator at 7 months, and the ora serrata at birth, but occasionally either form may persist (Raehlmann, 1907 ; Howard, 1917). It will be remembered, however, that electron-microscopic studies in vertebrates including man have shown that the granules of pigment in this layer assume a number of complicated formations and that their structure is very complex.[1]

It would seem, therefore, that from the embryological point of view *all the cells in the eye which elaborate melanin are of neural (ectodermal) origin* ; those of the pigmentary epithelium of the retina were originally the cells of the optic vesicle which migrated from the neural tube at an early stage ; it may well be that the clump cells of the iris represent a restricted and later migration of these cells into the neighbouring mesoblast ; while the uveal chromatophores are similarly ectodermal, the descendants of cells which have migrated from the neural crests.

Abderhalden. *Hoppe-Seylers Z. physiol. Chem.*, **96**, 1 (1915).
Acton. *Ind. J. med. Res.*, **9**, 464 (1922).
d'Agata. *Tumori*, **9**, 121 (1922).
Augstein. *Klin. Mbl. Augenheilk.*, **50** (1), 1 (1912).
Barden. *J. exp. Zool.*, **90**, 479 (1942).
Berger. *Arch. Augenheilk.*, **11**, 314 (1882).
Bisceglie. *Z. Zellforsch.*, **16**, 228 (1932).
Bloch. *Hoppe-Seylers Z. physiol., Chem.*, **98**, 226 (1917).
   Arch. Derm. Syph. (Wien), **135**, 77 (1921).
Borcea. *C.R. Acad. Sci.* (Paris), **149**, 688 (1909).
Boyd. *J. Anat.*, **83**, 74 (1949).
Brihaye-van Geertruyden. *Arch. Biol.* (Liège), **74**, 1 (1962).
   Docum. Ophthal., **17**, 163 (1963).

Brini. *Bull. Soc. Ophtal. France*, 474 (1949).
   Arch. Anat. micr., **42**, 67 (1953).
Chavin. *J. exp. Zool.*, **133**, 1 (1956).
Collins. *Trans. ophthal. Soc. U.K.*, **46**, 86 (1926).
Collins and Parsons. *Trans. ophthal. Soc. U.K.*, **23**, 244 (1903).
Coppez. *Arch. Ophtal.* (Paris), **21**, 1, 141 (1901).
Davenport. *Bibliog. genet.*, **3**, 443 (1927).
Dawson. *Edinb. med. J.*, **32**, 501 (1925).
Dorris. *Proc. Soc. exp. Biol. N.Y.*, **34**, 448 (1936).
   Arch. Entwickl.-Mech. Org., **138**, 323 (1938).
DuShane. *Science*, **80**, 620 (1934).
   J. exp. Zool., **72**, 1 (1935) ; **78**, 485 (1938).
   Spec. Pubs. N.Y. Acad. Sci., **4**, 1 (1948).

[1] Vol. II, p. 223.

van Duyse. *Arch. Ophtal.* (Paris), **19**, 412 (1899).

Eastlick. *Proc. nat. Acad. Sci.*, Wash., **25**, 551 (1939).

Elschnig and Lauber. *v. Graefes Arch. Ophthal.*, **65**, 428 (1907).

Figge. *J. cell. comp. Physiol.*, **15**, 233 (1940).

Foot. *Amer. J. Path.*, **8**, 309, 321 (1932).

Fuchs. *Das Sarcom d. Uvealtractus*, Wien (1882).

   v. Graefes Arch. Ophthal., **31** (3), 39 (1885).

Galloway. *Biometrika*, **8**, 267 (1912).

Güttes. *Z. Zellforsch.*, **39**, 168, 260 (1953).

Harrison, J. R. *J. exp. Zool.*, **118**, 209 (1951).

Harrison, R. G. *J. exp. Zool.*, **9**, 787 (1910).

Hauschild. *Z. Morph. Anthrop.*, **12**, 472 (1910).

Herrmann and Boss. *J. cell. comp. Physiol.*, **26**, 131 (1945).

Hoffmann. *v. Graefes Arch. Ophthal.*, **29** (2), 45 (1883).

Hogben and Winton. *Proc. roy. Soc. B.*, **93**, 318 ; **94**, 151 (1922) ; **95**, 15 (1923).

Hogeboom and Adams. *J. Biol. Chem.*, **145**, 273 (1942).

Howard. *Trans. Amer. ophthal. Soc.*, **15**, 244 (1917).

King. *Trans. ophthal. Soc. U.K.*, **57**, 97 (1937).

Knight. *J. Amer. med. Ass.*, **83**, 1062 (1924).

Koby. *Ann. Oculist.* (Paris), **160**, 119 (1923).

Koganei. *Arch. mikr. Anat.*, **25**, 1 (1885).

Komoto. *Trans. ophthal. Soc. U.K.*, **35**, 295 (1915).

Kornfeld. *Anat. Anz.*, **53**, 216 (1920–21).

Kromayer. *Arch. mikr. Anat.*, **42**, 1 (1893).
   Beitr. path. Anat., **22**, 412 (1897).
   Mh. prakt. Derm., **41**, 477 (1905).

Krompecher. *Beitr. path. Anat.*, **44**, 51, 88 (1908) ; **72**, 163 (1923).

Kropp. *J. exp. Zool.*, **49**, 289 (1927).

Kühne. Hermann's *Hb. d. Physiol.*, Leipzig, **3**, 235 (1879).

Kühne and Sewall. *J. Physiol.*, **3**, 88 (1880).

Laidlaw. *Amer. J. Path.*, **8**, 477 (1932).

Laidlaw and Murray. *Amer. J. Path.*, **9**, 827 (1933).

Lauber. *v. Graefes Arch. Ophthal.*, **68**, 1 (1908).

Lerner. *Zoologica*, **35**, 27 (1950).

Lewis. *Amer. J. Anat.*, **2**, 405 (1903).

Lo Cascio. *Clin. Oculist.*, **15**, 296 (1915).
   Ann. Ottal., **51**, 653 (1923).

Luna. *Arch. ital. Anat. Embriol.*, **18**, 146 (1920).

Masson. *C.R. Soc. Biol.* (Paris), **75**, 210 (1913).
   Ann. anat. path., **3**, 417, 657 (1926).
   Ann. Surg., **93**, 218 (1931).

Meesmann. *Klin. Mbl. Augenheilk.*, **65** (2), 316 (1920).

Meirowsky. *Mh. prakt. Derm.*, **42**, 541 ; **43**, 155 (1906) ; **44**, 111, 166 (1907).
   Frankfurt. Z. Path., **2**, 438 (1907–8).

Meirowsky, Freeman and Fischer. *Zoologica*, **35**, 29 (1950).

Miescher. *Klin. Wschr.*, **1**, 173 (1922).
   Arch. mikr. Anat., **97**, 326 (1923).

Mijsberg. *Acta néerl. morph.*, **6**, 281 (1948).

Miyamoto and Fitzpatrick. *Science*, **126**, 449 (1957).

Moyer. *Anat. Rec.*, **136**, 248 (1960).

Müller. *Gesammelte u. hinterlassene Schriften Anat. u. Physiol. d. Auges*, Leipzig, **1** (1872).

Münch. *Z. Augenheilk.*, **12**, 525 (1904).

Niu. *J. exp. Zool.*, **125**, 199 (1954).
   Gordon's *Pigment Cell Growth*, N.Y., 37 (1959).

Nordmann and Stoll. *Ophthalmologica*, **114**, 99 (1947).

Ogawa. *Arch. Augenheilk.*, **52**, 437 (1905) ; **55**, 106 (1906).

Oguchi. *Arch. Augenheilk.*, **63**, 160 (1909).

Pearson, Nettleship and Usher. *A Monograph on Albinism*, Cambridge (1911–13).

Pergens. *Ann. Oculist.* (Paris), **120**, 42 (1898).

Raehlmann. *Z. Augenheilk.*, **17**, 1 (1907).

Raven. *Ann. roy. Coll. Surg.*, **6**, 28 (1950).

Rawles. *Proc. nat. Acad. Sci. Wash.*, **26**, 86, 673 (1940).
   Physiol. Zool., **20**, 248 (1947).
   Physiol. Rev., **28**, 383 (1948).
   Gordon's *Pigment Cell Growth*, N.Y. (1959).

von Recklinghausen. *Ueber d. multiplen Fibrome d. Haut*, Berlin (1882).

Redslob. *Ann. Oculist.* (Paris), **159**, 523 (1922) ; **162**, 368, 921 (1925).

Ribbert. *Beitr. path. Anat.*, **21**, 471 (1897).
   Geschwülstlehre, Bonn (1904).
   Lhb. allg. Path. path. Anat., 4th ed., Leipzig (1911).

Rieke. *v. Graefes Arch. Ophthal.*, **37** (1), 62 (1891).

Ris. *Physiol. Zool.*, **14**, 48 (1941).

Salzmann. *Anat. u. Histol. des mensch. Augapfels*, Leipzig (1912).

Scheerer. *Klin. Mbl. Augenheilk.*, **69**, 583 (1922).

Schock. *Arch. vergl. Ophthal.*, **1**, 293 (1910).

Schultz. *v. Graefes Arch. Ophthal.*, **122**, 601 (1929).

Sondermann. *v. Graefes Arch. Ophthal.*, **150**, 580 (1950).
   Ophthalmologica, **122**, 166 (1951).

Spencer. *Brit. med. J.*, **2**, 907 (1923).
   Trans. ophthal. Soc. U.K., **46**, 74 (1926).

Steiner. *Zbl. prakt. Augenheilk.*, **29**, 293 (1905).

von Szily. *Arch. mikr. Anat.*, **77**, 87 (1911).

Theobald. *Arch. Ophthal.* (Chicago), **18**, 971 (1937).

Tousimis and Fine. *Amer. J. Ophthal.*, **48** (2), 397 (1959).
   Arch. Ophthal. (Chicago), **62**, 974 (1959).

Turchini and Ladreyt. *C.R. Soc. Biol.* (Paris), **85**, 905 (1921).

Unna. *Berl. klin. Wschr.*, **30**, 14 (1893).

Usher. *Biometrika*, **13**, 46 (1920).

Virchow, H. *Graefe-Saemisch Hb. d. ges. Augenheilk.*, 2nd ed., Leipzig, **1** (1), Chap. 2 (1910).

Virchow, R. *Die krankhaften Geschwülste*, Berlin (1863).

Weidenreich. *Z. Morph. Anthrop.*, **2**, 59 (1912).

Wieting and Hamdi. *Beitr. path. Anat.*, **42**, 23 (1907).

Willeir. *Spec. Pubs. N.Y. Acad. Sci.*, **4**, 321 (1948).

Wolfrum. *v. Graefes Arch. Ophthal.*, **71**, 195 (1909).

Klin. Mbl. Augenheilk., **69**, 591 (1922).

Yokoyama. *Acta Soc. ophthal. jap.*, **65**, 146, 796 (1961).

Zimmermann. *Zoologica*, **35**, 11 (1950).

SECTION IV

CHRONOLOGY
AND
POST-NATAL DEVELOPMENT

CHAPTER X

THE CHRONOLOGY OF DEVELOPMENT

In the previous chapters we have described the processes of development as they affect each part of the eye and adnexa. Such a topographical
arrangement is convenient to make a consecutive and integrated story of the
development of the different ocular tissues, but at this stage it may be
useful to correlate all these several events in their time-sequence in order
to appreciate more clearly the course of development as a whole and also to
relate them to the events which claim our interest elsewhere.

In general, the course of development may be divided into four periods
which, although they may not always be sharply delineated, are characterized by definite changes.

(1) The PRE-EMBRYONIC PERIOD may be taken to run during the first
three weeks after fertilization. It includes the formation of the morula (the
stage of cleavage), the formation of the blastula wherein different areas are
differentiated as the regions determining the presumptive organs, and the
formation of the gastrula, characterized by the establishment of the three
primary germ layers and the aggregation into the embryonic plate of the
organ-areas in the positions wherein they will subsequently undergo development. The period includes the implantation of the blastocyst into the uterine
wall and ends before the establishment of an intra-embryonic circulation,
with the appearance of the neural plate and the axial embryonic structures.

(2) The EMBRYONIC PERIOD which extends from the beginning of the 4th
week to the end of the 8th week. During this time the embryonic area
becomes folded into the form of the embryo and the organs undergo their
early development ; at the end of the period the main systems and organs
are established.

(3) The FŒTAL PERIOD, extending from the beginning of the 3rd month
until birth. At its commencement the embryo has reached a stage wherein
the main organs have been differentiated and the major features of the
external body have been established. Gross differentiation has now ceased
and the future process of development is one of minute differentiation and
continued growth. The distinction between embryonic and fœtal life is
arbitrary, but the commencement of the 3rd month is a convenient stage ;
the end of the period is variable and of physiological rather than embryological importance—for birth is a mere incident in a continued and
unitary process.

(4) POST-NATAL LIFE, which itself may be divided into two periods—
the first—the NEO-NATAL PERIOD—occupying approximately the first 4 to 6
months of life, during which some final differentiation still continues and

extra-uterine function is fully established ; and the second, terminating about the 20 to 25th year, characterized, apart from sexual development at puberty, by continued growth.

In the following summary the age of the embryo and its crown-rump length are recorded as if with mathematical precision ; *it cannot be stressed too strongly that this is entirely misleading*, particularly during the earlier stages when events proceed with great rapidity. The frequent difficulty of being uncertain of the time of the particular incident which determines fertilization invalidates a time-scale ; while measurements of length—again particularly in the early stages—are notoriously variable depending on such factors as the freshness of the embryo, the technique of fixation and the presence of pathological conditions. It is obvious that most human embryos available for examination are not normal. Streeter (1948), indeed, protested that the most accurate method of assessment is based on the examination of macaque embryos in the production of which the time of conception can be rigidly controlled, the freshness guaranteed, the methods of fixation standardized, and pathological processes eliminated. The figures in this chapter should therefore be interpreted merely as a guide to help to indicate the sequence of events and the reader is adjured to keep their inaccuracy constantly in his mind.[1]

1. The Pre-embryonic Period

Fertilization to the end of the 3rd week

1–3 days : The formation of the morula.
4th day : The commencement of the formation of the blastula.
7½–11 days : Implantation of the ovum in the uterine mucosa.

During this period the principal germinal layers begin to form ; at the 16th day the embryonic plate is still bilaminar ; thereafter the primitive streak appears and the mesoderm insinuates between the ectoderm and endoderm.

At the end of the 3rd week the neural plate and the neural groove have formed and the 1st pair of somites is evident (20th day).

2. The Embryonic Period

Beginning of the 4th to approximately the end of the 8th week

4TH WEEK : Events during this period are most accurately timed by the appearance of somites ; the following are approximate :

1st pair of somites	20th day	20 pairs	26th day
7 pairs	22nd day	25 pairs	28th day
10 pairs	23rd day	28 pairs	30th day
14 pairs	25th day		

7-somite stage (?22 days) : Beginning of the closure of the neural canal in its central part.

10-somite stage (?23 days) : The neural groove has closed up as far anteriorly as the mesencephalon.

14-somite stage (?25 days ; ?2·6 mm.) : The optic pits appear.

At this stage the otic placodes also appear, while the 1st two branchial pouches reach the ectoderm and the 3rd is forming. There is a single median heart with paired aortæ.

[1] See p. 45.

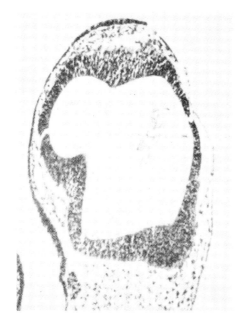

FIG. 360.—AN EMBRYO OF 2·5 MM.

The section is oblique and shows the optic vesicle emerging from the forebrain
on the left-hand side (W. A. Manschot).

19–25-somite stage (?26–28 days ; ?3·2 mm.) (Fig. 360) : The optic vesicles have
evaginated from the prosencephalon, and the primitive carotid artery terminates in a
plexus of endothelial tubes at the caudal aspect of the vesicle. At the same time the
lens placode is beginning to form.

The condensation of mesoderm determining the extrinsic ocular muscles becomes
evident.

The medullary tube is closed and the neural crests are detached from it ; the
notochord is differentiated from the ectoderm ; the beginnings of the vesicularization
of the brain are seen as well as the rudiments of the hypophysis.

The otic placode is fully developed and beginning to invaginate from the ectoderm ; the placodes of the cranial nerves begin to appear ; the olfactory placodes
become visible ; and the pharyngeal membrane disappears.

5TH WEEK (?3·4–8 MM.)

4–4·2 mm. : The primary optic vesicle has fully developed and cellular proliferation
of the neuro-epithelium of its distal part is proceeding with the earliest appearance of
the primitive and marginal zones of the presumptive retina. The lens placode is
thickening and behind it the otic placode is well formed.

The head-fold is formed ; three cerebral vesicles are now distinct. The cranial
nerves are appearing, as also is the semilunar ganglion.

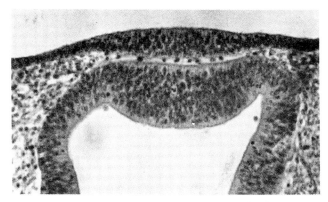

FIG. 361.—An Embryo of 4·8 mm. (R. O'Rahilly).

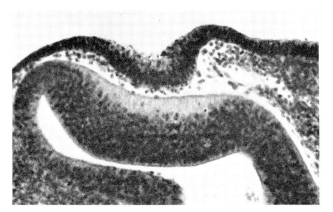

FIG. 362.—An Embryo of 5·3 mm. (R. O'Rahilly).

4·5 mm. : The peripheral portion of the optic vesicle is steadily thickening but its cavity is still widely open into the middle cerebral vesicle. The lens placode has markedly thickened.

The otic vesicle is now completely separated from the surface ; the hypophysial pouch is well formed ; four branchial pouches reach the ectoderm.

4·5–5 mm. (Fig. 361) : The optic vesicle begins to invaginate to form the optic cup. Cellular differentiation is now marked in the retina with the migration of the primitive cells into the marginal layer. At this stage the thickness of the retina is 0·07 mm. and of the marginal layer 0·02 mm. The lens pit is beginning to appear in the lens plate.

The ophthalmic artery emerges from the internal carotid.

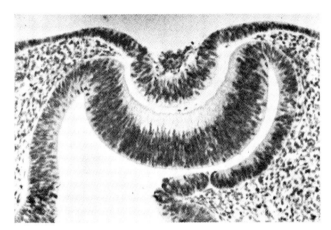

FIG. 363.—AN EMBRYO OF 6·3 MM. (R. O'Rahilly).

5·5–6 mm. (Figs. 362–3) : The optic cup is rapidly developing with the formation of the embryonic fissure. Vascularized mesoderm clothes the optic vesicle and the cerebral vesicles ; in the outer layer of the former melanin pigment appears. The hyaloid artery emerges from the primitive dorsal ophthalmic artery.

Five cerebral vesicles are now apparent as also is the olfactory placode. The sympathetic 'system migrates from the neural crest.

7 mm.: The optic vesicle is fully invaginated and the embryonic fissure is open throughout its whole length. The marginal zone of the retina is fully differentiated in the central area, and the outer layer of the optic cup is separated from the now fully developed vascular plexus by the cuticular portion of the membrane of Bruch. The lens pit has developed into a closed vesicle still in continuity with the surface ectoderm. The hyaloid artery has entered the posterior part of the embryonic fissure and reaches the posterior pole of the lens vesicle.

The cerebral hemispheres are recognizable and in the spinal cord the anterior horns and the anterior and posterior columns are apparent. The placode of nerve V has appeared and the olfactory placodes begin to dimple. The pharyngeal membrane absorbs and Rathke's diverticulum approaches the stomatodæum. Four branchial pouches have reached the ectoderm and a fifth is appearing. The inferior vena cava is forming and the skeleton of the base of the skull with the petrous portion of the temporal bone as well as the vertebræ are evident in the mesenchymal stage.

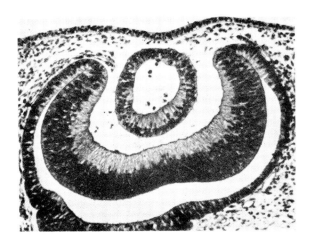

FIG. 364.—AN EMBRYO OF 8·8 MM. (R. O'Rahilly).

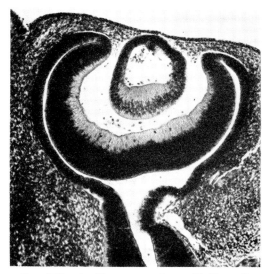

FIG. 365.—AN EMBRYO OF 9 MM. (G. Renard).

6TH WEEK (8–15 MM.)

8–9 mm. (Figs. 364–5) : In the retina the first stage of differentiation marked by the division into cellular and marginal zones is clear over a considerable area in the posterior part of the eye but the embryonic fissure is still open. The lens vesicle, now a hollow sphere, has detached from the ectoderm and its capsule is evident. The hyaloid artery takes part in the formation of the posterior part of the tunica vasculosa lentis ; the annular vessel is also developing, and the primitive dorsal ophthalmic artery ends over the dorsal aspect of the optic cup.

The facial fissures begin to close.

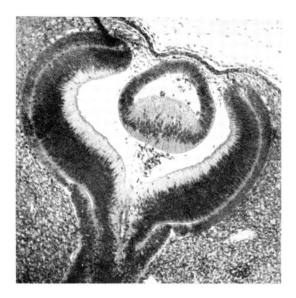

FIG. 366.—AN EMBRYO OF 10 MM. (A. N. Barber).

10 mm. (Fig. 366) : The thickness of the retina is now 0·13 mm., of which 0·055 mm. is occupied by the marginal layer. During the 10–13 mm. stage the nuclei of Müller's cells at the posterior pole are differentiated. The external layer of the optic cup is now richly pigmented. The cells of the posterior wall of the lens vesicle begin to elongate, and the lateral part of the tunica vasculosa lentis forms. The angle between the optic axes has been reduced from 180° to 160°.

The olfactory placode becomes invaginated, the rudiment of the naso-lacrimal passages appears as a solid cord of epithelial cells ; the otic vesicle has closed and has begun to differentiate.

11–12 mm.: The embryonic cleft begins to close in its mid-part. In the retina itself at the posterior pole the second stage of differentiation is inaugurated by the consolidation of the cells which have migrated into the marginal layer to form the primitive inner nuclear layer. In the lens vesicle the posterior cells are now forming fibres of considerable length and the cavity of the vesicle has become semilunar. The mesodermal cells which determine the future corneal endothelium begin their growth as a single layer under the surface epithelium.

The primitive ventral ophthalmic artery reaches the optic cup, and the lid-folds emerge.

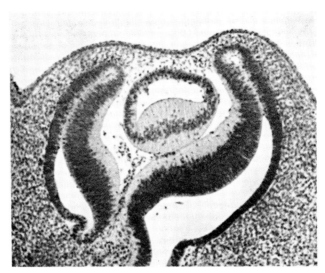

Fig. 367.—An Embryo of 13·2 mm. (R. O'Rahilly).

13–14 mm. (Fig. 367) : The embryonic fissure has closed except for a notch anteriorly at the margin of the optic cup and a small posterior opening. The optic nerve fibres are travelling proximally into the optic nerve. The cavity of the lens vesicle is now very much reduced and the lens capsule is completely formed, while the secondary vitreous begins to develop. The choriocapillaris is complete, while the vortex veins and the long posterior ciliary arteries are visible, and the annular vessel is fully formed.

A double layer of cells now appears in the surface ectoderm to form the corneal epithelium ; the mesoderm of the orbit begins to differentiate into the extrinsic muscles of the eye.

7TH WEEK (15–22 MM.)

15–16 mm.: The distal end of the embryonic fissure is completely closed, and differentiation into the outer and inner neuroblastic layers in the retina is effected by the appearance of the transient fibre layer of Chievitz at the posterior pole ; the optic nerve fibres are growing from the ganglion cells. The cuticular layer of Bruch's membrane appears. The cavity of the lens vesicle is now obliterated.

The rudiments of the lids have developed into definite folds forming a circular palpebral aperture and the muscle fibres of the orbicularis oculi begin to surround the eye. The angle between the optic axes has been reduced to 120°. The spheno-palatine, otic and semilunar ganglia are fully established.

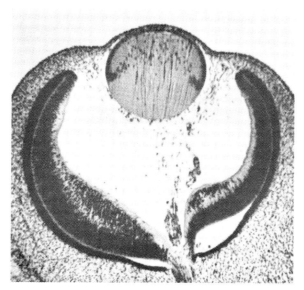

FIG. 368.—AN EMBRYO OF 18 MM. (A. N. Barber).

17–18 mm. (Fig. 368) : The primitive retinal layers are well formed in the posterior half of the globe ; the ganglion cells have differentiated and migrated inwards to the inner margin of the retina and their axons have reached the proximal part of the optic stalk in quantity ; some have reached the marginal zone of the neural tube. The cilia on the external limiting membrane of the retina are being replaced by proto-plasmic processes representing the future rods and cones ; the processes of Müller's fibres reach the limiting membrane. The thickness of the retina at this stage is 0·175 mm., of which the marginal layer (together with the cells of the inner neuroblastic layer which have migrated into it) occupies 0·08 mm.

The posterior cells of the lens vesicle have completely obliterated the cavity of the vesicle. The mesoderm determining the future stroma of the iris is beginning to take shape, and the scleral condensation becomes evident. The anterior portion of the tunica vasculosa lentis is forming ; and the common ciliary arteries are now present.

20–21 mm.: The proximal crescentic remnant of the embryonic fissure has finally closed. In the retina the two neuroblastic layers separated by the layer of Chievitz have reached the equator. At the 21 mm. stage the total thickness of the retina is 0·19 mm., of which the width of the original marginal layer (now containing Müllerian nuclei, ganglion cells and the future amacrine cells) measures 0·11 mm. The nerve fibres almost completely fill the inner layer of the optic stalk and are beginning to cross to form the optic chiasma ; the lateral geniculate body is appearing.

The surface ectoderm differentiates into the corneal epithelium and the posterior endothelium is separated from it by an acellular layer ; the scleral condensation is evident anterior to the equator. The nuclei of the primary lens fibres disappear ; the tunica vasculosa lentis is completed, and the vasa hyaloidea propria have appeared.

The anastomosis between the ophthalmic artery and the supra-orbital division of the stapedial has been effected. The lid-folds are gradually covering the eyes and although the lacrimal canaliculi are now present they have not reached the lid-margin.

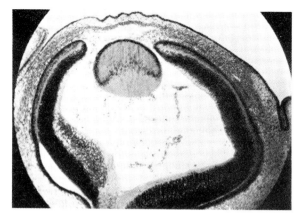

FIG. 369.—AN EMBRYO OF 26 MM. (A. N. Barber).

The fusion between the maxillary and lateral nasal processes is complete ; the external nares are well formed ; the conchæ are now to be recognized. The palatal processes are growing inwards from the maxillæ and rudiments of the teeth are present ; the submaxillary gland has budded out from the buccal mucosa. The maxilla, pre-maxilla and palate have begun to ossify.

8TH WEEK (22–30 MM.) (Fig. 369)

Retinal differentiation is rapidly proceeding ; the entire optic stalk is now occupied by nerve fibres, and the chiasma is fully formed. Three layers of epithelial cells are evident in the cornea. At the beginning of the week the mesoderm at the margin of the optic cup penetrates the acellular layer of the cornea to form the stroma of this tissue and the pupillary membrane is completely formed ; the beginnings of the anterior chamber can be discerned. The peri-ocular mesodermal condensation destined to form the sclera has reached the equator. In the lens the secondary fibres begin to form.

The anlage of the lacrimal gland has appeared and hairs are obvious in the region of the brows. Fibrillæ are now evident in the mesodermal condensations determining the extrinsic ocular muscles. All the ocular motor nerves have reached the extra-ocular muscles. Sympathetic cells are found in the adrenal. The full number of vertebræ is present, completing the cartilaginous skeleton ; bone is formed in the frontal and zygomatic bones and the squamous portion of the temporal.

3. The Fœtal Period

From the beginning of the third month until birth

9TH WEEK (30–40 MM.) : The eyeball is now about 1·0 mm. in diameter. At the posterior pole the layers of the retina are now :—external limiting membrane with filamentous prolongations, cone nuclei, outer neuroblastic layer, layer of Chievitz, inner neuroblastic layer, ganglion cells, nerve-fibre layer, internal limiting membrane.

The ciliary body begins to appear and the hyaloid system is reaching its maximal development. The secondary vitreous is now fully evident ; Y-sutures are apparent in the embryonic nucleus of the lens.

The lids have closed, obliterating the palpebral aperture, and the semilunar fold has appeared, while the canaliculi reach the surface epithelium of the lids. Muscular

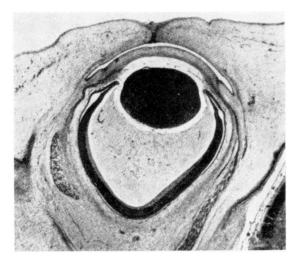

FIG. 370.—A FŒTUS OF 41 MM. (C. Dejean).

fibres are evident in the mesodermal elements which form the extra-ocular muscles, and the mesodermal condensations of the orbital walls are completed. The optic axes make an angle of 72° with each other.

10TH WEEK (40–50 MM.) (Fig. 370) : The ciliary body is progressively forming, the ciliary muscle is differentiating, and the zonule makes its appearance. In the cornea Bowman's membrane begins to become apparent and the scleral condensation is well formed.

The capsule of Tenon begins to appear in the equatorial region ; the fibres of the orbicularis oculi muscle appear in the lids, and membranous bone is being laid down in the orbital walls. At the end of the period the optic tracts have been formed.

11TH WEEK (50–60 MM.) : The macular area begins to differentiate. The uncrossed visual fibres appear at the chiasma ; and the differentiation of the occipital cortex into mantle and marginal zones is completed. The hyaloid system has reached its highest development.

The rectus muscles are well differentiated and the levator palpebræ separates itself from the superior rectus.

12TH WEEK (60–70 MM.) (Fig. 371) : The posterior region of the retina is now well differentiated, showing the following layers : rudimentary rods and cones, an outer nuclear layer consisting of a single layer of cone nuclei internal to which is a thick layer of undifferentiated oval nuclei, layer of Chievitz, a cellular layer 6–10 tiers deep containing amacrine and Müllerian nuclei, a layer of ganglion cells, and a nerve-fibre layer. The total thickness of the retina at 65 mm. is 0·143 mm., of which the original marginal layer occupies 0·08 mm. In the equatorial region the differentiation resembles that of the 21 mm. embryo at the posterior pole—there is a deep layer of cells the outer ones with oval nuclei (outer neuroblastic layer) and the inner with round nuclei (inner neuroblastic layer), and a relatively acellular marginal layer. The two neuroblastic layers separated by the fibres of Chievitz reach the ora serrata.

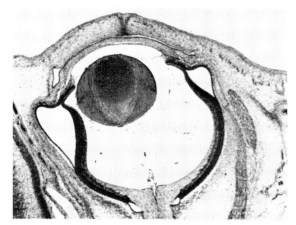

FIG. 371.—A FŒTUS OF 65 MM. (A. N. Barber).

At about the 65 mm. stage the axial growth of the rim of the optic cup forms the iris, while the glial framework of the optic nerve begins to differentiate. The sphincter pupillæ appears. The limbus is well demarcated and the canal of Schlemm emerges. At the same time the hyaloid system begins to atrophy.

In the lids the anlage of the tarsus is recognizable. At the end of the period the orbicularis muscle is well developed.

4TH MONTH (70–110 MM.) : The cytoplasm of the cone cells is now seen to protrude through the external limiting membrane. At the end of the period the outer plexiform layer begins to become differentiated at the posterior pole, so that the nuclei of the rods and cones are separated from the bipolar nuclei. The inner plexiform layer similarly separates the inner nuclear layer and the ganglion cells, and at the posterior pole is 4–6 cells thick. At the same time vascularization of the internal layers of the retina has begun. The dimensions of the retina are relatively unchanged—total thickness 0·165 mm. ; thickness of the original marginal layer 0·09 mm. The arrangement of the lower visual pathway now conforms to that seen in the adult.

During this month the globe increases in diameter from 3 to 7 mm., and the optic axes converge to 65°. The ciliary processes are fully formed and the middle layer of the choroid appears. During the month the sphincter muscle of the pupil consolidates and the posterior and lateral portions of the tunica vasculosa lentis regress. The secondary vitreous develops considerably, and elastic fibres are evident in the cornea.

The histological development of the lids commences with the appearance of lashes and glands, and the plica is well formed. The lacrimal canaliculi may become patent. The capsule of Tenon has now fully formed and the orbital walls are well developed. The cranial and spinal nerves become myelinated.

5TH MONTH (110–150 MM.) : During this period the differentiation of the retina has progressed with the formation of the inner nuclear layer, the inner plexiform layer and the obliteration of the layer of Chievitz except at the macula. Myelination is evident in the geniculate body, the differentiation of which is complete by the end of the month.

All the layers of the choroid are now visible and melanoblasts appear in its external part. The ciliary processes are fully formed, the meridional portion of the ciliary muscle is differentiating, and the fibres of the zonule run from the ciliary epithelium to the lens. The iris is fully developed and the marginal sinus has reached its maximal development. The increased curvature of the cornea is apparent, Bowman's membrane is easily recognizable and the scleral condensation has reached the posterior pole of the globe, while chromatophores appear in the lamina fusca.

The extrinsic ocular muscles have differentiated their tendinous insertions ; the dural sheath of the optic nerve can be distinguished.

6TH MONTH (150–200 MM.) : At the beginning of the period the outer nuclear layer of the retina is differentiated by the completion of the outer plexiform layer, and the foveolar depression is appearing. Myelination is recognizable in the optic tract, and the glial tissue of Bergmeister's papilla at the optic disc reaches its highest stage of development.

The sphincter muscle of the pupil is fully differentiated, oblique fibres are evident in the ciliary muscle, and the dilatator muscle of the pupil begins to form. Descemet's membrane has appeared ; the angle of the anterior chamber is forming peripherally. The choroid is becoming pigmented.

In the lids the tarsal glands and the lashes are well differentiated and the lids begin to open.

7TH MONTH (200–230 MM.) : In the retina the rod cells become differentiated, the fovea becomes obvious, while myelination of the fibres of the optic nerve reaches the chiasma. Bergmeister's papilla begins to atrophy.

The diameter of the globe is 10 to 14 mm. All the layers of the choroid are fully differentiated, while the pars plana of the ciliary body is evident and has reached the anterior third of the ciliary muscle. The pupillary membrane begins to atrophy, and the marginal sinus disappears. The hyaloid artery becomes impermeable.

The lacrimal canaliculi have opened onto the lid-margins and the tarsus is well formed in the upper lids.

8TH MONTH (230–265 MM.) : The outer nuclear layer is recognizable in the retina up to the ora, and all the layers are fully developed throughout ; the retinal vessels have reached the ora serrata. Myelination is proceeding distally along the optic nerve.

The fœtal nucleus of the lens is complete ; the hyaloid system is rapidly disappearing, a process finished by the middle of the month. The recurrent ciliary arteries vascularize the ciliary processes, making the circulation of the anterior segment of the globe complete.

The lids are separate throughout their length.

9TH MONTH (265–300 MM.) : In the retina the branches of the retinal arteries extend to the ora while the capillaries reach but do not penetrate the inner nuclear layer and, apart from the central area, the general structure of the retina is now complete ; at this time the relatively rudimentary central area is thicker than the remainder of the retina. The fundus itself (as seen in premature babies) lacks pigmentation so that the larger choroidal vessels are conspicuously seen. The periphery of the retina is grey or even white owing to lack of translucency and the vitreous, particularly around the region of the ora, is somewhat hazy and vitreous cells may be numerous.

The diameter of the globe increases to 16–17 mm., and the optic nerves make an angle of 71°. In the lens, the fibres of the infantile nucleus are beginning to appear. The pupillary membrane and the hyaloid vessels have disappeared and atrophy of the ectodermal tissue has led to the commencement of the physiological cup at the disc. The mesoderm in the angle of the anterior chamber has disappeared up to the peripheral end of the trabeculæ. The oblique fibres of the ciliary muscle are forming.

AT TERM. At birth the retina, apart from the fovea, is fully differentiated. The myelination of the optic nerve fibres has reached the lamina cribrosa but this process has not been completed in the upper visual pathways.

The uveal tract is differentiated apart from the oblique fibres of the ciliary muscle ; but the uvea as a whole is more cellular than in the adult. In white races pigment is usually absent from the iris. The corneal epithelium consists of four well-developed layers of cells. In the lens the infantile nucleus is of recognizable thickness and the coiled remnants of the hyaloid artery attached anteriorly to the lens capsule float freely in Cloquet's canal.

The orbit has a sharp bony margin circular in outline, closely fitting the globe, its marginal height being about half that of the face. The fossa for the lacrimal gland is deep and conical while that for the lacrimal sac faces anteriorly and is cylindrical in shape. The lacrimal gland is still undeveloped and no tears are secreted. The naso-lacrimal passages have reached the nasal fossa but are frequently still separated from the inferior meatus by a membrane.

4. The Post-natal Period

The changes which occur in the eye and its adnexa after birth may be divided into two types—(1) the continuation of differentiation and the commencement of functional activity, and (2) the growth of the eye as a whole.

POST-NATAL DIFFERENTIATION

At birth the *macular region* shows marked retardation in its development compared with the rest of the retina ; the acellular layer of Chievitz is still present and the cellular and plexiform layers have not conformed with the tendency found elsewhere in the retina to increase in area by thinning and spreading out. The ganglion cells and the outer nuclear layer, however, remain as a single row at the fovea, while the inner nuclear layer is thin ; the cones are short and ill-developed, a retardation which explains the absence of fixation at birth. Differentiation goes on for the first 4 months of life by which time the layer of Chievitz has practically disappeared, the ganglion cells and bipolars are represented only by a few scattered cells lying upon the nuclei of the cones, while the latter have increased in number and in length so that the external limiting membrane is curved to accommodate them. The migration of the retinal elements outwards from the fovea leads to the formation of the fibre layer of Henle and the development of the foveal pit, a tendency to some extent counteracted by the increase in the length of the cones in the central area. By the 4th month the fovea is fully differentiated, and on ophthalmoscopy the presence of a foveal reflex indicates the existence of the deep foveal pit. The *fundus* itself, however, still lacks the pigmentation characteristic of the adult, the choroidal vessels being distinctly seen with little pigmentation in the inter-vascular spaces, while the pigmented epithelium may give the background a stippled impression resembling a " pepper-and-salt " fundus. After the first 6 months the general picture approximates the appearance of the mature retina.

The *lamina cribrosa* at birth is not fully consolidated and does not become so until the infant is several months of age. The *upper visual pathways* begin to be myelinated about the time of birth ; the process proceeds from the occipital cortex downwards and is complete about the end of the 4th post-natal month.

As would be expected, the full development of the visual reflexes is delayed until their anatomical basis is established. A fixation reflex is present at birth, but it is only feebly developed, responding momentarily to a strong stimulus such as a bright light ; initially the movements of the eyes are independent, irregular and unconjugated, and they are not synchronized with movements of the lids. By the age of 5 to 6 weeks the conjugate reflex is sufficiently developed to allow the two eyes to follow a light over a considerable range. At about the 7th or 8th week the blinking reflex appears ; at 3 months the eyes will follow a small object and the transition from reflex to conscious fixation becomes apparent, but conjugate fixation does not become accurate until the age of 6 months by which time convergence is firmly established. Corrective fusion reflexes are fully operative towards the end of the first year of life (Worth, 1903). After about the age of 5 the reflexes thus tentatively conditioned begin to acquire the fixity characteristic of conditioned reflexes. It is interesting that the electroretinogram cannot be elicited by standard techniques during the first few days of life unless strong stimuli are employed after good dark adaptation (Horsten and Winkelman, 1960) ; the positive component (*b*-wave) is gradually built up during the first 6 months of life, and is not fully developed until the end of the first year (Heck and Zetterström, 1958).

In the *uveal tract* the whole of the tissue at birth is more richly nucleated than in the adult and the general histological picture does not become normal in this respect until the 2nd or 3rd year of life. The ciliary body continues to change for some time after birth. The pars plana elongates to some extent but the main post-natal change is in the ciliary muscle. The meridional fibres of this muscle are well formed at birth but the oblique fibres continue to develop for a variable time thereafter, often until the 5th year of life. The iris also undergoes important post-natal changes. At birth the dilatator muscle is ill-formed and while it retains its embryonic nature throughout life the muscle does not assume its full proportions until about the 5th year ; since this muscle is not functionally active until after birth, the pupil of the newborn is small. In the iris itself the pigment of the stroma develops after birth in white races so that initially this tissue is typically light blue in colour. Its anterior surface is covered by a fine diaphanous layer of endothelium which attenuates between the 1st and 2nd year of life, a process the extent of which has given rise to some controversy ; it is certain, however, that it disappears in the region of the crypts.

The final architecture of the stroma does not fully assume its adult form until after 7 years. The uveal pigment does not show a tendency to migrate along the intrascleral channels conducting the perforating vessels and nerves until towards the end of the first year of life.

The *angle of the anterior chamber* is filled with uveal trabeculæ. At birth the apex of the angle has reached the posterior portion of this meshwork behind the scleral spur and the canal of Schlemm, but the cleft formed by the angle extends after birth until its apex is level with the major circle of the iris considerably behind the trabecular fibres and it widens out to its full extent only between the ages of 2 and 4.

In the *cornea* the character of the stroma changes ; at birth the cellular elements are relatively numerous and during the first 2 or 3 years of post-natal life the number of corneal corpuscles gradually decreases and the fibrous elements proportionately increase. The corneal epithelium is typically composed of 4 layers at birth ; the 5th and 6th layers are added thereafter. It would appear also that the active transport of fluid out of the cornea is a function which is not fully effective until some days after birth (in the rabbit).

The cornea is relatively large at birth (v. Reuss, 1881 ; Königstein, 1884), and almost attains its adult size during the first and second years (v. Reuss, 1881 ; Grod, 1910 ; Kaiser, 1926) ; indeed, practically all its post-natal growth occurs in the second 6 months of life (Hymes, 1929), although some increase in size may be evident up to the end of the 2nd year (A. and S. Druault, 1946). In general terms it may be said that while the eyeball as a whole increases a little less than three times in volume from birth to maturity, the corneal segment plays a relatively small part in this ; the transverse diameter of the cornea increases (roughly) only from 10 mm. in the infant to a value slightly less than 12 mm. in the adult. Wilmer and Scammon (1950) give the comparative dimensions between the newborn and the young adult seen in Table II.

TABLE II

POST-NATAL DIMENSIONS OF THE CORNEA

	New-born mm.	Adult mm.
External diameter of horizontal base .	10·0	11·8
External diameter of corneal arc .	14·0	18·2
Internal diameter of corneal arc .	11·0	16·4
Mean thickness	0·8	0·9
Oblique thickness	1·1	1·6
External height	3·0	3·4
Internal height	1·1	2·7

The shape of the cornea also changes. In the newborn it is flatter than in the adult and, contrary to its condition in later years, it is more curved peripherally than centrally (von Reuss, 1881 ; Merkel, 1892). At birth the corneal curvature is almost spherical but during youth an astigmatism with the axis vertical (" with the rule ") tends to develop, and, indeed, does so in 68% of cases by the age of 4 and in 95% by the age of 7 years (Marin-Amat, 1956). As age advances it finally tends to flatten again, the vertical meridian usually more than the horizontal ; consequently astigmatism " against the rule " is frequently developed in emmetropic eyes, and if this condition is already present it tends to increase while astigmatism " with the rule " tends to diminish (Fischer, 1948).

The *lens* is unique in that it is the only tissue which *grows progressively throughout adult life*, a process which is peculiar to man and continues up to and beyond the 80th year. At birth the infantile nucleus has appeared, but the successive accretion of new fibres from the periphery determines the fully formed infantile nucleus up to the age of puberty ; thereafter a similar but slower accretion of fibres forms the lenticular cortex. This increase in the mass and volume of the human lens after puberty occurs approximately in a linear manner with age (Priestley Smith, 1883 ; Raeder, 1922 ; Scammon and Hesdorffer, 1937 ; Johansen, 1947 ; see Weale, 1962). Although the growth of the lens in animals ceases in comparative youth (Krause, 1934 ; Brown and Evans, 1935), in man the mass of the neo-natal lens (80 mg.) has increased two-fold at puberty and by a factor of 3 at the 70th year. This increment of growth applies also to the equatorial diameter but since the infantile lens is more nearly spherical than the adult, the equatorial diameter must grow at a greater rate than the sagittal during adolescence ; after puberty, however, the rates of growth of the two dia-meters are approximately equal. It is also to be noted that the refractive index of the lens rises as a function of age (Woinow, 1874 ; Freytag, 1908 ; Huggert, 1948). The rate of increase in the number of radial lamellæ is shown in Table III (Busacca, 1924), and the increase in its axial and equatorial diameters, as compounded from the data of Collins (1890), Dub (1891), von Pflugk (1909), and Alajmo and Sala (1932), is seen in Table IV.

TABLE III

No. of Radial Lamellæ in Lens

Fœtus 45 mm.	.	430	10 months	.	. 1814
Fœtus 4 months	.	1475	2 years	.	. 2121
Fœtus 6–7 months	.	1300	2nd decade	.	. 2173
At birth	.	. 1450	Adult	.	. 2058

The lens capsule, according to Druault (1913), increases in thickness during life to a very varying degree : the posterior capsule retains approxi-mately its neo-natal thickness while the anterior capsule grows much stouter,

becoming twice as thick in the adult at the anterior pole and three times
in the periphery.

TABLE IV

AXIAL AND EQUATORIAL DIAMETERS OF THE LENS

	Axis	Equatorial Diameter		Axis	Equatorial Diameter
6 months	3·8	4·5	12 years .	3·6	8·8
1 year .	2·46	7·46	30–40 years .		8·96
3–4 years	2·83	8·46	50–60 years .		9·44
5–6 years	3·2	8·4	70–80 years .	4·0–5·0	9·64

Attached to the posterior lens capsule are the coiled remains of the
hyaloid artery initially floating within the narrow confines of Cloquet's
canal ; after the 4th or 5th year of life the remnant hangs vertically downwards corkscrew-like from the posterior pole of the lens. During childhood
the process of atrophy tends to increase so that the whole structure may
eventually disappear although some traces may remain throughout life.

The *anterior chamber* is relatively deep at birth, but owing to the gradual
increase of size of the lens together with the flattening of the cornea, it
suffers a progressive diminution of depth amounting on the average to about
0·5 mm., a process which is evident throughout the whole of adult life.
Measurements in the literature are seen in Table V.

TABLE V

DEPTH OF ANTERIOR CHAMBER : VARIATION WITH AGE (IN MM.)

Raeder (1922)   20 to 40, 3·46 ; 40 to 60, 3·14 ; 60 to 80, 2·90
Lindstedt (1916)   15 to 30, 3·68 ; 31 to 80, 3·34
Rosengren (1931)   25 to 30, 3·57 ; 45 to 50, 3·32 ; 60 to 65, 3·12
Törnquist (1953)   19 to 21, 3·18 ; 34 to 36, 2·98 ; 49 to 51, 2·76 ; 64 to 66, 2·69
  (in males)
Calmettes *et al.* 12 to 15, 3·65 ; 20 to 30, 3·76 ; 30 to 50, 3·46 ; 50 to 80, 3·23
  (1958)

The *orbit* undergoes a considerable amount of change in post-natal
development. At birth the margin is sharp and almost circular in outline,
closely fitting around the globe. In the newborn the horizontal diameter
is slightly greater than the vertical ; at 3 months the height increases until
at the 5th year the vertical diameter approximates the horizontal (Parsons,
1921 ; Jöhr, 1953). During the years of childhood the expansion of the
brain with the corresponding growth of the bones of the calvaria as well as
the development of the bones of the face and nasal cavities mould the orbit
into a more oval or even square configuration, while the contour of the inner

angle is altered by the development of the bridge of the nose. Whitnall's (1921) measurements indicating the changes in the dimensions of the orbit throughout childhood are seen in Table VI. Table VII gives measurements of its increase in volume (Martin, 1928). At the age of 3 its dimensions are considerably less than those of the adult, the difference still exists at the age of 6, and although the eye, like the brain, attains its adult size much sooner than the rest of the body, it is not until the end of the most active period of cranial growth at puberty that the orbit approximately acquires its adult size and shape. The fact that growth continues until puberty accounts for the failure of the orbit to attain its normal size and for the development of some facial asymmetry if an enucleation of the eyeball is undertaken in childhood (Thompson, 1900 ; Taylor, 1939).[1]

TABLE VI

THE DIMENSIONS OF THE DEVELOPING ORBIT (Whitnall)

The measurements were made to the nearest half-millimetre, in the right orbits.
The " intra-orbital height " is the greatest height of the cavity, just within the margin.
The marginal width is taken medially to the point where the upper end of the posterior lacrimal crest meets the frontal bone.

AGE	MARGIN		INTRA-ORBITAL HEIGHT	DEPTH	
	Height	Width		Roof	Floor
6½ months foetus	15	16	17	23	19·5
8 ,, ,,	17·5	22	..	23	10
Birth	18	21	22	32	25
1½ years	30	32	33	46	40
3 ,,	28	32	30·5	42	38
4½ ,,	28	29	30	41	41·5
5 ,,	30	33	33	43	42·5
6 ,,	29	32	32	47	47
7 ,,	30·5	33	35	46	46
12 ,,	33	34	34	45	39
16 ,,	37	38	38	51	43
19 ,,	34	36	38	51	49
22 ,,	36	37	38	48	45·5
Adult Male	33	39	39	49·5	52·5
Adult Female	34	36	38	45	43·5

Some of the bones comprising the orbital walls show post-natal changes : at birth the metopic suture separates the two halves of the frontal bone while the centre of ossification of the crista galli does not appear until about the end of the 1st year of life. The sphenoid bone consists of three parts at

[1] See Coulombre and Crelin (1958) in the chick.

birth—a central body with the alisphenoid on either side, the fusion of which occurs towards the end of the 1st year ; while the dorsum sellæ does not ossify and fuse with the basi-occipital bone until the age of 25.

TABLE VII

THE VOLUME OF BOTH ORBITS IN ML.

At birth	.	. 10·3	Adult man	.	. 59·2
1 year	.	. 22·3	Adult woman	.	. 52·4
6–8 years	.	. 39·1			

The *palpebral aperture* increases gradually and regularly from birth to maturity (Hymes, 1929) (Table VIII).

TABLE VIII

LENGTH OF PALPEBRAL FISSURE (MM.)

(*In the male ; in the female it is under 2 mm. less*)

Birth	.	.	. 18·35	8–10 years	.	. 25·89
1–6 months	.		. 19·90	12–14 years	.	. 27·18
6 months–1 year		.	21·50	16–18 years	.	. 28·40
1–2 years	.		. 20·67	20–22 years	.	. 29·27
2–4 years	.		. 23·61	24–26 years	.	. 29·68
4–6 years	.		. 24·41			

The *lacrimal gland* is by no means fully developed at birth ; its evolution with age and the time of onset of the secretion of tears have already been noted.[1] At birth the accessory lacrimal glands are few in number. In the *lacrimal passages* the lysis of the central cells which results in canalization may be delayed for several weeks or even months after birth, while the lower end of the duct into the inferior meatus may be occluded by a membrane for a corresponding period.

POST-NATAL GROWTH OF THE GLOBE

Compared with the rest of the body, the eyeball grows relatively little after birth, and the post-natal growth is precocious. This is divisible into two stages : a period of relatively rapid growth up to the age of 3, a process particularly evident in the first year of life, followed by a slower phase between the ages of 3 and 14 years when the adult size is substantially attained. Thus the sagittal diameter is about 17 mm. at birth, increases rapidly to an average value of between 22·5 and 23 mm. at the age of 3, increases slowly by about 1 mm. between 3 and 14 years at an approximately regular rate of 0·1 mm. per year, whereafter little change takes place (Sorsby *et al.*, 1961). The eye thus attains its adult size at a much earlier age than the body as a whole ; while the body increases in volume 21-fold from birth to maturity, the eye increases only 3-fold and 70% of this

[1] p. 240

increment is attained by the age of 4 (Kaiser, 1926). The increase in the weight of the eyes involves a factor of 3·2, in body-weight of 20 (Weiss, 1897) : the weight of the two eyes compared with the rest of the body at birth is 1 : 419, while in the adult the ratio is 1 : 4,832. In this precocious development the eye is comparable to the brain and the other sense organs ; while the eye increases in weight approximately 3 times from birth to maturity, the brain increases 3·75 times, but the other sense organs suffer a smaller increment—the internal ear remains approximately constant in size between late fœtal and adult life, the olfactory mucosa increases in area by a factor of only 10%, and there is no increase in number of such sensory structures as the taste-buds.

The figures in Table IX are an average of the collated measurements in the literature.[1]

TABLE IX

THE GROWTH OF THE EYEBALL

		New-Born	Adult
Diameters :	outer sagittal .	17·5	24·14
(mm.)	transverse .	17·1	24·8
	vertical . .	16·5	23·5
Circumference :	sagittal . .	52·2	76·2
(mm.)	transverse .	53·0	76·9
	vertical . .	51·6	76·6
Volume : (ml.)	. . .	2·4	6·9
Weight : (G.)	. . .	3·0	7·5

The increase in growth, however, does not affect all the ocular structures to the same extent. In general the anterior segment (including the cornea) shows proportionately a smaller increase in size than the posterior segment (including the retina and vitreous) wherein the main growth occurs (Fig. 372). The result is a change in the shape of the globe. The eye of the newborn is more asymmetrical than that of the adult, the postero-temporal curve being more marked, so that the distance between the fovea and the disc is as great as in the adult condition ; the optic axis, therefore, cuts the retina between these two points and is displaced towards the fovea only later. There is also a difference in growth in proportion to the growth of the globe as a whole : the cornea, the lens, the retina, and the anterior and posterior

[1] DIAMETERS—von Jaeger (1861), Königstein (1884), Merkel (1892), Collins (1894), Weiss (1897), Schneller (1898), Halben (1900), Baratz (1902), Seefelder (1908), von Pflugk (1909), Nussbaum (1912), Scammon and Armstrong (1925), Sorsby and Sheridan (1960), Sorsby *et al.* (1961). CIRCUMFERENCE—Weiss (1897). VOLUME—Scammon and Armstrong (1925), Kaiser (1926), Wilmer and Scammon (1950). WEIGHT—Weiss (1897), Scammon and Armstrong (1925), Todd *et al.* (1940).

chambers decrease in proportionate size between birth and maturity, the uveal tract maintains a fairly constant relative proportion, while the sclera and vitreous body share a pronounced increase (Scammon and Wilmer, 1950).

The growth of the globe has an interesting effect on the refraction (Sorsby *et al.*, 1961). The axial elongation shows a considerable variation in different children and in a few the normal increase of the sagittal diameter of 0·1 mm. per annum may be substantially increased to as much as 0·6 mm. These different rates of axial elonga-

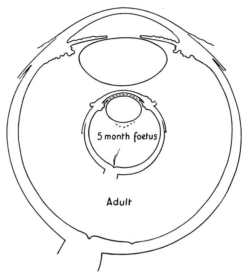

FIG. 372.—THE GROWTH OF THE FŒTAL EYE.

The comparison of the configuration of the 5 month fœtus and the adult. In the former the pupillary membrane, the posterior part of the tunica vasculosa lentis and the hyaloid artery are indicated. Note the striking difference in the shape of the lens and in the depth of the anterior chamber.

tion, however, tend to be masked by compensatory changes in the curvature of the cornea and the lens so that the total refraction usually remains relatively unchanged, the myopic tendency resulting from the increased axial length being matched by a flattening of the cornea and the lens ; in a minority, however, these compensatory changes lag behind with the result that the hypermetropia usually present at birth is decreased or gives place to the emergence of myopia. The growth of the eye does not thus represent the haphazard aggregation of a number of unrelated factors but is a co-ordinated process in which the divergence of one element from the mean tends to be counteracted by the influence of other elements, a tendency which is seen to some extent even in such children in whom full co-ordination does not occur. The fact that there is a high concordance not only in the total refraction but in all the six components which contribute to it in uniovular twins suggests that the controlling influence is essentially genetic (Sorsby *et al.*, 1962).

Alajmo and Sala. *Boll. Oculist.*, **11**, 130 (1932).

Baratz. *On the Growth of the Eye and its Peculiarities in the Suckling* (Thesis), St. Petersburg (1902).

Brown and Evans. *Trans. Amer. ophthal. Soc.*, **33**, 220 (1935).

Busacca. *Arch. ital. Anat. Embriol.*, **21**, 562 (1924).

Calmettes, Deodati, Huron and Béchac. *Arch. Ophtal.* (Paris), **18**, 513 (1958).

Collins. *Roy. Lond. ophthal. Hosp. Rep.*, **13**, 81 (1890).
Lancet, **2**, 1329 (1894).

Coulombre and Crelin. *Amer. J. phys. Anthrop.*, **16**, 25 (1958).

Druault, A. and S. *Ann. Oculist.* (Paris), **179**, 375 (1946).

Druault, M. *Ann. Oculist* (Paris), **149**, 288 (1913).

Dub. *v. Graefes Arch. Ophthal.*, **37**(4), 26 (1891).

Fischer. *Sorsby's Modern Trends in Ophthal.*, London, **2**, 54 (1948).

Freytag. *Die Brechungsindices d. Linse*, Wiesbaden (1908).

Grod. *Arch. Augenheilk.*, **67**, 251 (1910).

Halben. *In welchem Verhältnis wächst das menschliche Auge von der Geburt bis Pubertät ?* (Diss.), Breslau (1900).

Heck and Zetterström. *Ophthalmologica*, **135**, 205 ; **136**, 258 (1958).

Horsten and Winkelman. *Arch. Ophthal.* (Chicago), **63**, 232 (1960).

Huggert. *Acta ophthal.* (Kbh), Suppl. 30, (1948).

Hymes. *J. comp. Neurol.*, **48**, 415 (1929).

von Jaeger. *Ueber d. Einstellungen d. dioptrischen Apparates in mensch. Auge*, Vienna (1861).

Jöhr. *J. Génét. hum.*, **2**, 247 (1953).

Johansen. *Studies in the Inter-relation in Size between the Cornea and the Crystalline Lens in Man* (Thesis), Copenhagen (1947).

Kaiser. *v. Graefes Arch. Ophthal.*, **116**, 288 (1926).

Königstein. *v. Graefes Arch. Ophthal.*, **30** (1), 135, 141 (1884).

Krause. *Biochemistry of the Eye*, Baltimore (1934).

Lindstedt. *Arch. Augenheilk.*, **80**, 104 (1916).

Marin-Amat. *Bull. Soc. belge Ophtal.*, No. 113, 251 (1956).

Martin. *Lhb. d. Anthropologie*, Jena (1928).

Merkel. *Anat. Hefte*, **1**, 271 (1892).

Nussbaum. *Graefe-Saemisch Hb. d. ges. Augenheilk.*, 3rd ed., Leipzig, **2** (1), 1 (1912).

Parsons, F. G. *Trans. ophthal. Soc. U.K.*, **41**, 308 (1921).

von Pflugk. *Klin. Mbl. Augenheilk.*, **47** (2), 1 (1909).

Raeder. *v. Graefes Arch. Ophthal.*, **110**, 73 (1922).

von Reuss. *v. Graefes Arch. Ophthal.*, **27** (1), 27 (1881).

Rosengren. *Acta ophthal.* (Kbh), **8**, 99 (1930) ; **9**, 103 (1931).

Scammon and Armstrong. *J. comp. Neurol.*, **38**, 165 (1925).

Scammon and Hesdorffer. *Arch. Ophthal.* (Chicago), **17**, 104 (1937).

Scammon and Wilmer. *Arch. Ophthal.* (Chicago), **43**, 620 (1950).

Schneller. *v. Graefes Arch. Ophthal.*, **47**, 178 (1898).

Seefelder. *v. Graefes Arch. Ophthal.*, **68**, 275 (1908).

Smith, Priestley. *Trans. ophthal. Soc. U.K.*, **3**, 79 (1883).

Sorsby, Benjamin and Sheridan. *M.R.C. Spec. Rep. Series*, No. 301, London (1961).

Sorsby and Sheridan. *J. Anat.* (Lond.), **94**, 193 (1960).

Sorsby, Sheridan and Leary. *M.R.C. Spec. Rep. Series*, No. 303, London (1962).

Streeter. *Contrib. Embryol. Carneg. Instn.*, **32**, 135 (1948).

Taylor. *Trans. ophthal. Soc. U.K.*, **59**, 361 (1939).

Thompson. *Trans. ophthal. Soc. U.K.*, **20**, 97 (1900).

Todd, Beecher, Williams and Todd. *Human Biol.*, **12**, 1 (1940).

Törnquist. *Acta ophthal.* (Kbh.), Suppl. 39 (1953).

Weale. *Brit. J. Ophthal.*, **46**, 660 (1962).

Weiss. *Anat. Hefte*, **8**, 191 (1897).

Whitnall. *The Anatomy of the Human Orbit*, Oxon. (1921).

Wilmer and Scammon. *Arch. Ophthal.* (Chicago), **43**, 599 (1950).

Woinow. *Klin. Mbl. Augenheilk*, **12**, 407 (1874).

Worth. *Squint ; its Causes and Treatment*, London (1903).

INDEX